HORMONES
AND
CARCINOGENESIS

HORMONES
AND
CARCINOGENESIS

Aurel Lupulescu, M.D., M.S., Ph.D.

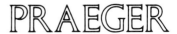

PRAEGER SPECIAL STUDIES • PRAEGER SCIENTIFIC

Library of Congress Cataloging in Publication Data

Lupulescu, Aurel.
   Hormones and carcinogenesis.

   Includes index.
   1. Carcinogenesis. 2. Hormones—Physiological
effect. 3. Hormone therapy. I. Title. [DNLM:
1. Hormones—Adverse effects. 2. Neoplasms—
Etiology. QZ 202 L966h]
RC268.5.L86   1983   616.99'4071   82-15110
ISBN 0-03-061697-2

Published in 1983 by Praeger Publishers
CBS Educational and Professional Publishing,
a Division of CBS Inc.
521 Fifth Avenue, New York, NY 10175 USA

3456789 052 987654321

Printed in the United States of America
on acid-free paper.

PREFACE

During the past five decades, since the discovery of most hormones, their role in carcinogenesis has been postulated and discussed in an expanding list of publications. Although there is no direct evidence that hormones are carcinogenic per se, there is ample evidence that hormones are crucial factors in controlling the development, propagation, and regression of several neoplasms.

Although hormones are widely used in the treatment and management of cancer, their effects are not yet fully understood and, in many cases, hormone therapy is still used on an empirical basis. With the use of modern methods, many achievements have been made regarding the mechanism of action of hormones at the cellular and macromolecular levels, namely, DNA, RNA, and protein synthesis. Despite this improved understanding of hormones and their role in carcinogenesis, the basic mechanism(s) of neoplastic transformation remain unsolved. As Goethe said, "What we need we do not know, and what we know we do not need."

Further investigation is required, namely, the study of initial cellular events by which normal cells are transformed into precancerous cells and then into cancer cells. It seems likely that the destiny of precancerous cells and premalignant lesions is largely dependent on the hormonal environment or "hormonal milieu."

In addition to the role of hormones in carcinogenesis, it was also found that many neoplastic cells can synthesize identic hormones (ectopic hormones) to authentic hormones secreted by the endocrine cells. This intriguing phenomenon provides a solid link between endocrinology, oncology, and molecular biology. Thus the new and fascinating field of hormonal oncology has recently emerged.

The primary purpose of this book is to emphasize the role of hormones in the etiology and pathogenesis of cancer, hormones as potential therapeutic agents, their intrinsic mechanism of action, as well as their role in tumor biology in general.

CONTENTS

Chapter 1

HORMONES AND CANCER: AN HISTORIC REVIEW

Despite the explosion of clinical and experimental observations of the past five decades regarding the relationship between hormones and carcinogenesis, few such observations were made before hormones were discovered and their role in carcinogenesis established.

For a more accurate description, it is better to describe these early observations as having occurred during the so-called *prehormonal era* (before hormones were discovered) and the period of research after hormones were isolated and their role in cancer development more widely investigated, the *hormonal era* (Table 1-1).

The role of hormones in carcinogenesis has been a subject of controversy during the past few decades. Most of these observations refer particularly to the role of gonads, sex steroids, and their synthetic analogues.

PREHORMONAL ERA

Sporadic observations during the past four centuries demonstrated some relationships between endocrine glands and cancer. In 1616, Sir William Harvey noted a shrinkage of testes and prostate gland of hedgehogs during hibernation, the first such association (8). Later, Ramazzini, in 1713, noted in his classic treatise on occupational health an apparent high incidence of breast cancer in nuns (16) and John Hunter, in 1786, observed that prostate gland failed to develop normally when the testes had been removed (9). By the end of the last century, in 1896, Beatson, a British surgeon, reported clinical improvement of breast cancer in women after surgical castration and the administration of thyroid extract (1).

In his intuitive studies, Beatson assumed that hormones play a major role in etiology of breast cancer and he wrote in his study concerning advanced mammary cancer, "that we are to look at an altered condition of the ovary and testicle as the real exciting cause of cancer, and if so, the sooner we direct our

1

energies into that channel the better. So there are grounds for the belief that the etiology of cancer lies in an ovarian or testicular stimulus" (1).

Later, in 1916, Lathrop and Loeb found that the hormonal milieu of multiple pregnancies predisposed to carcinoma formation and that an early ovariectomy prevented the occurrence of mammary gland neoplasms in large numbers of mice (11,14). Although this important experimental evidence suggests that estrogens can be significant carcinogens, it was overlooked or lightly dismissed by many because of a prevalent belief that the body should be able to metabolize these physiologic compounds without toxic effects. Also, the value of animal experimental models and their relevance to human carcinogenesis was highly questionable at that time.

A few years later, Engel reported that various glandular extracts (called optonen), such as hypophyseal (hypophysis opton), thymus (thymus opton), ovarian (ovarial opton), and thyroid (thyroid opton) exert an important role in development and transplantation of mouse carcinomas. Thus, hypophyseal extract was shown to have a slight stimulatory effect, whereas thyroid, and particularly thymus opton, exert a significant preventative or inhibitory influence on carcinoma formation (4).

This was the experimental basis for the wide use of glandular extracts (opotherapy) in different types of tumors during the 1920's through 1930's.

HORMONAL ERA

During the past five decades, a variety of naturally occurring hormones were isolated. Synthetic estrogens, progestins, androgens, and corticosteroids were manufactured and widely used for the treatment of cancer, prevention of abortion, contraception, and other therapeutic purposes without consideration of their carcinogenic potential.

In 1929, when Doisy extracted the first hormone, estrone, from the urine of pregnant women (3), the modern era of hormonal carcinogenesis began.

A few years later, in 1932, the role of estrogens in carcinogenesis was demonstrated for the first time. In his original experiment, Lacassagne induced mammary adenocarcinomas in mice after long-term administration of estrone benzoate. This was the first experimental evidence to indicate the significant carcinogenic potential of steroid hormones for mammalian tissue (10).

Since Lacassagne's experiment, the relationship between hormones and carcinogenesis was repeatedly demonstrated. In 1938, Dodds et al. synthesized the nonsteroid compound diethylstilbestrol (DES), which exhibits estrogenic activity and was the first chemotherapeutic drug used in cancer treatment. Thus, the era of cancer chemotherapy began (2). Also, because of its estrogenic activity, DES was recommended for estrogen replacement in surgically castrated women and was advocated as a treatment for so-called

Table 1-1 HISTORICAL EVENTS IN HORMONAL CARCINOGENESIS

1616	William Harvey noted a relationship between testes and prostrate of hedgehogs during hibernation (8).
1713	Ramazzini noted a high incidence of breast cancer in nuns (16).
1786	Hunter noted a shrinkage of the prostate gland after castration (9).
1895	White reported on the effects of castration in prostate hypertrophy (19).
1896	Beatson reported clinical improvement of advanced human breast cancer after castration and thyroid extract administration (1).
1916	Lathrop and Loeb reported that early castration prevents carcinoma formation in mice (11,14).
1922	Reports of several endocrine extracts on carcinoma formation appeared (4).
1929	Folliculin was extracted from urine of pregnant women (3).
1932	Lacassagne induced mammary carcinomas by injecting folliculin into male mice (10).
1938	Dodds et al. synthesized diethylstilbestrol (DES) (2).
1938– 1939	Reports concerning carcinogenicity of several estrogens, including DES, in laboratory animals appeared (5,13).
1941– 1944	Huggins et al. reported on the effects of hormones and castration on human prostate carcinoma (8).
1944	Heilman and Kendall reported dramatic effects of cortisone on malignant tumors in mice (6).
1962– 1969	Ectopic hormones were isolated from various neoplasms; ectopic hormone syndromes were reported (12).
1972– 1977	Reports appeared on the increased risk of hepatocellular neoplasms and adenocarcinoma in the endometrium of women exposed to androgens and oral contraceptives (7,15,18,20).

high-risk pregnancies (17). DES was also used extensively to caponize poultry and to increase cow's milk production, mainly in the United States.

However, during 1938 and 1939, the carcinogenicity of various estrogens, including DES, in the vagina and cervix of mice was reported (5,13). Meanwhile, Huggins and his associates, from 1941 to 1944, found hormones to be an important factor not only in cancer development, but in tumor regression and extinction as well. For example, hormones were demonstrated both to induce prostate cancer and to bring about a regression or extinction of prostate tumors (8). Huggins also advocated the use of DES as a form of anti-androgen therapy for carcinoma of the prostate.

Between 1944 and 1946, Heilman and Kendall induced a complete regression of transplanted lymphosarcomas in female mice after administering large doses of cortisone (6). This cornerstone observation quickly prompted the use of cortisone and adrenocorticotropic hormone (ACTH), producing dramatic results in various forms of human leukemias and lymphosarcomas.

By the early 1960s, the concept of hormone-dependent cancer was established. Several experimental and clinical observations employing such modern methods as electron microscopy, autoradiography, scanning electron microscopy, and hormone-receptor estimation, provide strong evidence that some neoplasms are totally dependent in development, propagation, and regression of specific hormones. These are called hormone-dependent cancers, as opposed to the hormone-independent tumors, which are more independent in evolution.

Also, by 1962, an intriguing phenomenon was recognized: the synthesis and secretion of several hormones by cancerous or nonendocrine tissues, which are very similar or identical to authentic hormones. These tumor-secreted hormones were called *ectopic hormones* (12). They produce clinical syndromes known as ectopic hormone syndromes. These hormones do not obey the normal regulatory mechanisms, a phenomenon that raises questions regarding the specificity of endocrine cells for hormone secretion. Thus, neoplastic cells as well as some embryonic or fetal tissues might acquire significant endocrine activity during differentiation by derepressing either inactive or repressed genes.

The important link between endocrinology, molecular biology, and oncology was thus established. Another interesting observation was made during the early 1970s, when hormones were being used extensively as contraceptives. Reports were published regarding the induction of various neoplasms after exposure to steroid hormones such as vaginal adenocarcinoma in women exposed to DES in utero, hepatocellular carcinoma in patients receiving anabolic steroids, hepatocellular neoplasms reported in women using oral contraceptives, and increased risk of adenocarcinoma of the endometrium in women using exogenous estrogens, including sequential oral contraceptives (7,15,18,20).

All these experimental and clinical observations deserve increased attention, since they suggest a strong association between hormones and carcinogenesis. Because hormones can function as potent carcinogens, their use for different therapeutic purposes (e.g., menopause, contraceptive "pills") should be more cautiously recommended.

REFERENCES

1. Beatson, G.: On the treatment of inoperable cases of carcinoma of the mamma: Suggestions for a new method of treatment with illustrative cases. *Lancet 2*: 104–162 (1896).
2. Dodds, E., Golber, L., Lawson, W., and Robinson, R.: Oestrogenic activity of certain synthetic compounds. *Nature 141*:247–248 (1938).
3. Doisy, E., Veler, C., and Thayer, S.: Folliculin from urine of pregnant women. *Am. J. Physiol. 90*:329–330 (1929).
4. Engel, D.: Experimentalle studien über die beeinflussung des tumor wachstum mit abbauprodukten (Abderhaldenschen optonen) von endokrinen drüsen bei maüsen. *Z. Krebsforsch. 19*:339–380 (1922).
5. Gardner, W., and Allen, E.: Malignant and non-malignant uterine and vaginal lesions in mice receiving estrogens and estrogens and androgens simultaneously. *Yale J. Biol. Med. 12*:213–234 (1939).

6. Heilman, F., and Kendall, E.: The influence of 11-dehydro-17-hydroxycortico-sterone (compound E) on the growth of a malignant tumor in the mouse. *Endocrinology 34*:416–420 (1944).

7. Hoover, R., Gray, L., and Fraumeni, J.: Stilbestrol (diethylstilbestrol) and the risk of ovarian cancer. *Lancet 2*:533–534 (1977).

8. Huggins, C., Stevens, R., and Hodges, C.: Studies on prostatic cancer. II. The effects of castration on advanced carcinoma of the prostate gland. *Arch. Surg. 43*:209–223 (1941).

9. Hunter, J.: *Observations on Certain Parts of the Animal Oeconomy*, London, Biblioteca Osteriana, 1786, p. 39.

10. Lacassagne, A.: Apparition de cancers de la mammelle chez la souris mâle soumise à des injections de folliculine. *Compt. Rendu. Acad. Sci (Paris) 195*: 630–632 (1932).

11. Lathrop, A., and Loeb, L.: Further investigations on the origin of tumors in mice. III On the part played by internal secretion in the spontaneous development of tumors. *J. Cancer Res. 1*:1–19 (1916).

12. Liddle, G., Nicholson, W., Island, D., Orth, D., Abe, K., and Lowder, S: Clinical and laboratory studies of ectopic humoral syndromes. *Rec. Prog. Horm. Res. 25*:283–305 (1969).

13. Lipschütz, A.: *Steroid Hormones and Tumors*. (Baltimore, Williams & Wilkins, 1950).

14. Loeb, L.: Further observations of the endemic occurrence of carcinoma, innoculability of tumors. *Univ. Penn. Med. Bull. 20*:2 (1907).

15. Lyon, F.: Development of adenocarcinoma of endometrium in young women receiving long term sequential oral contraceptives. *Am. J. Obstet. Gynecol. 123*:299–301 (1975).

16. Ramazzini, B.: *De Morbis Artificum, Diatriba [Diseases of Workers]*. The latin text of 1713, translated by W. C. Wright. (New York, Hafner, 1964), p. 191.

17. Smith, O., Smith, G., and Hurwitz, D.: Increased excretion of pregnanediol in pregnancy from diethylstilbestrol with special reference to the prevention of late pregnancy accidents. *Am. J. Obstet. Gynecol. 51*:411–415 (1946).

18. Sweeney, E., and Evans, D.: Hepatic lesions in patients treated with synthetic anabolic steroids. *J. Clin. Pathol. 29*:626–633 (1976).

19. White, J.: The results of double castration in hypertrophy of the prostate. *Ann. Surg. 22*:1–80 (1895).

20. Ziel, J., and Finkle, W.: Increased risk of endometrial carcinoma among users of conjugated estrogens. *N Engl. J. Med. 293*:1167–1170 (1975).

Chapter 2

TUMOR CELL CYCLE AND HORMONES

GENERAL CONSIDERATIONS

Although hormones are not essential components of the mitotic cycle (i.e., cells can enter mitosis and divide in their absence), the overall regulation of cell division and proliferation and mitotic homeostasis in general appear to fall under their control. Since its formulation about 30 years ago (31), the concept of the cell cycle has had a great impact on cell biology, tumor cell homeostasis, and cancer chemotherapy.

Our knowledge regarding the cell cycle and its sequences (phases or gaps) emerged from the use of light microscopic autoradiography and ^{3}H-thymidine. DNA synthesis was shown to take place only during a discrete period of the cell cycle, called the S phase. Using more sensitive methods, such as high-resolution autoradiography, it was demonstrated that only a limited amount of nuclear chromatin incorporates ^{3}H-thymidine, the aminonucleo-tide essential to DNA synthesis and chromosome formation known as heterochromatin (or genetic chromatin), whereas large areas are only metabolically active (euchromatin). Later, two additional fundamental pro-cesses in molecular biology—transcription and translation—were described. It was also shown that hormones can influence the genetic regulatory mech-anism(s) by modulating gene expression (78).

Research on the animal cell cycle has thus entered a new era during recent years, providing important data for an improved understanding of tumor cell biology and DNA replication as well as for a rationale basis of cancer therapy. This chapter briefly describes the cell cycle with an emphasis on the role of hormones in controlling the cell cycle, especially the tumor cell cycle.

The cell cycle can be defined as the interval between the midpoint of one mitosis and the midpoint of the subsequent mitosis in one or both daughter cells, as well as the cyclic biochemical and cellular events associated with this period. Thus, the original or stricto senso definition of the cell cycle as the interval between two consequent mitoses is broadened to include all structural and biochemical events that take place during this period.

The cell cycle is the road map for each individual cell. Any normal or abnormal cell in order to divide and proliferate should enter the cell cycle and undergo its phases, or gaps. The movement of cells during the cycle is a highly ordered phenomenon that occurs in specific temporal sequences. However, the time for completion of these sequences in the cell cycle is highly variable in normal and abnormal cells. An understanding of the cell cycle, its phases, and the factors governing its mechanism is of crucial importance for selection and use of chemotherapeutic drugs. During the past 20 years, the use of such new methods as high-resolution autoradiography, biochemical and scanning electron microscopy for the study of DNA, RNA, protein synthesis, and dynamics of cell membranes in the study of cell replication and cell cycle has improved our understanding of molecular biology of cell division.

Although the outlines of the cell cycle have been established, the factors that initiate and stimulate the reentry of the cells into the cycle, as well as the factors governing the transition from one phase, or gap, to another, remain largely unknown. Cell kinetic studies show that not all cells enter cell cycle. It is well demonstrated that at any given time, a normal or abnormal tissue is composed of three different and interchangeable compartments: a compart-ment of actively dividing cells that continuously follow the cell–cycle pattern; a compartment of nondividing cells or cells that undergo cytolysis and die or differentiate to specialized cells; and a compartment containing a large cell population of quiescent, silent, or dormant cells, that is, cells that are temporarily in a nondividing or dormant stage, but that can easily be stimulated to reenter the cell cycle and follow a similar pattern, as they previously do. The equilibrium among these three cellular compartments is critical in the selection of chemotherapeutic drugs that will kill the cancer cells.

The cell cycle of mammalian cells was described in detail nearly 30 years ago (31,62). At that time, the cell cycle (i.e., the interval between mitosis) was believed to be of shorter duration in neoplastic cells than in normal cells, hence cancer cells would proliferate faster than do normal cells. This contention was disproved a few years later, when autoradiography with ^{3}H-thymidine was used to show that the cell cycle of epithelial cells from jejunal mucosa of mice is of shorter duration than is that of tumor cells, suggesting that neoplastic cells do not proliferate faster than do normal cells (4,62). Thus, the proliferation rate of neoplastic cells depends not only on the cell cycle, but on two other functions or characteristics, as well: growth fraction and cell loss (or cell death). Growth fraction is the ratio or number of cycling cells or dividing cells; the higher the growth fraction, the faster the increase in cell number and proliferation rate. Cell loss is the ratio of dying cells per unit of time. Hence the growth of neoplastic cells depends on these three parameters. In growing normal and neoplastic tissues alike, cell cycle length and growth fraction are predominant over cell loss; hence, in these rapidly dividing tissues, more cells are born than die and ultimately the number of cells is increased per unit of time. (This is also valid for normal tissues, such as bone marrow and certain mucosal epithelium.) When the number of cycling cells is equal to the number of dying cells, growth of adult tissue ceases, bringing these normal or abnormal tissues or organs into a steady state. Hence, the growth of neoplastic and normal cells is largely dependent on cell-cycle time, growth fraction, and cell death (3).

Thus, the length of the cell cycle is variable in different tissues; the cell cycle is very important for cellular homeostasis and regulation of cell proliferation. In order to maintain this equilibrium during the course of the cell cycle, each cell must double its mass before mitosis. Thus all cellular components increase twice their number. Any cycling cells that do not double their mass progressively decrease in size and eventually disappear.

There are no specific biochemical or cellular events for neoplastic cells as compared with normal cells, so that no specific "markers" of cancerous cells were demonstrated. Not all normal or neoplastic cells are entering the cycle continuously. After mitosis, each cell makes its own decision as to reentry of the cell cycle. Thus, in a cellular compartment, there are at any given time both cycling and noncycling cells. The predominance of cycling cells is indicative of an increased proliferative rate, which frequently occurs in neoplastic tissues.

Once a cell enters the cycle, it follows a highly ordered pattern that occurs in specific temporal sequences, the cell-cycle phases or gaps. Each cell rigidly undergoes each phase of the cycle. This ordered sequential pattern constitutes an important facet for selecting the multidrug regimens or combined therapeutic methods for cancer treatment. Most of these drugs are cell-cycle specific (CCS), acting primarily during one phase of the cycle (29,79).

The determination of these sequential events and the progression through the cell cycle appear to be based on a program regulated by a set of cell-cycle genes and consisting of sequential transcriptions and translations (61). However, the intrinsic mechanism of the events in the cell cycle and the progress through it have not been satisfactorily explained and remain to be elucidated (58).

In recent years, a random transition model (RTM) for the cell cycle has been proposed in order to explain the variations in cell cycle times. An alternative to the classic concept of the cell cycle has been also proposed and this involves a *chromosome cycle (CC)*, which includes DNA replication and mitosis (chromosomes) and is determined mainly by genetic factors and the *growth cycle (GC)*, which is related to cytoplasmic growth and protein synthesis. The length of the GC is determined primarily by growth conditions (51).

Possible humoral factors, mainly hormones and hormonelike substances, interfere with the cell cycle and can modulate the length of cell cycle phases. The following discussion describes the phases of the cell cycle, the basic mechanism(s) of cycling cells, the role of hormones and hormonelike substances on the cell cycle, the role of the cell cycle in carcinogenesis, and the action of CCS drugs.

CELL CYCLE PHASES

All cycling cells progress through various phases, periods, or gaps. Basically, these phases are described as G_1, S, G_2, and M, a nomenclature introduced by Howard and Pelc (31). Recently a great deal of attention was paid to a new state termed the G_0 *state or* G_0 phase. Both normal and neoplastic cells can move out of the cycle or become arrested for extended periods of time in a silent, or quiescent G_0 state. These so-called silent or dormant cells are neither in the state of cycling nor of dying and can be reactivated at any time by appropriate stimulus to reenter the cycle. The cells enter the G_0 stage after leaving the G_1 phase (Fig. 1). Non-dividing cells (noncycling cells) that have left the cycle forever are destined to die. The cell cycle phases exhibit a great variability in length and are accompanied by several biochemical and molecular events that occur only in dividing cells and are cell cycle specific.

Phase G_1

The *phase G_1 (gap 1)* is the most variable phase of the cell cycle; its length largely influences the duration of the cell cycle and the rate of cell

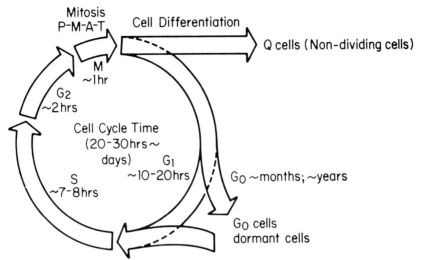

Figure 2-1 The cell cycle and its phases, illustrated in plant, animal, and tumor cells.

proliferation. This is a pre-DNA synthesis period, in which preparation for DNA synthesis takes place, especially enzyme DNA polymerases are required for synthesis of DNA precursors. RNA and protein synthesis are also necessary for cells to move from G_1 to the S phase. However, RNA and protein synthesis are almost the same during the cell cycle, except during mitosis (M phase) when they reach the peak (maximum). The length of the G_1 phase is highly variable (10–20 hr to 2–5 days); it is very short (2–3 hr) or practically absent in rapidly proliferating erythropoietic stem cells or in ascites tumor cells. Thus, G_1 (presynthetic period) represents a vital control period in the cell life cycle. During this stage, a cell still has the option to enter the cycle and to progress to S, G_2, and M periods or to leave the cycle and remain for a long period of time in the G_0 stage. The control of cell cycle can thus be achieved by extension of the G_1 phase. G_1 (Gap 1) is the period between mitosis and the onset of DNA synthesis. Thus normal cells in G_1 can make a choice between division and proliferation or quiescence (dormancy). However, most neoplastic cells, upon entering G_1 phase, move rapidly toward the S, G_2, and M phases. G_1 cell population generally refers to cycling or dividing cells. The number of chromosomes remains the same (46 chromosomes), as in normal cells. Cells with a longer G_1 phase are slowly growing population cells; conversely, cells with a shorter G_1 phase are rapidly growing population cells. During the G_1 period, the cell is awaiting a triggering mechanism whereby it can enter the S period. These triggering factors are not yet fully understood. The possibility of switching between G_1 phase and G_0 stage is of paramount importance in growth regulation and cell proliferation. Drugs that kill rapidly proliferating cells will also kill certain normal cells.

It was recently found that cells can be arrested during the G_1 period, interrupting the entire cell cycle. Some cells can be arrested at the starting point. This starting point is located in the early to midpart of G_1 period in yeast cells (61).

G_0 Phase

G_0 state (dormant, silent, or quiescent state) represents "G_0" population of cells, or cells which are going in this "out-of-cycle" state and remain quiescent for extended period of time. There is a special point in G_1 called the restriction point (57) where the cells make the commitment to enter G_0 state or to continue to proliferate by entering the cell cycle. It is possible that some tumor cells are defective in their restriction point control. Several factors, including high cell density, some amino acids, growth factors, presence of certain drugs, and especially hormones, can help a cell "quit" the cycle, go into G_0 state, and remain dormant. For instance, drugs such as streptovitacin A and caffeine or glucocorticoids have been shown to arrest fibroblasts from chick embryo. There is still some controversy as to whether the cells arrested in G_0 by different mechanisms are actually in identical physiologic states. There is no DNA synthesis or S phase in this cell population, and no labeled cells can be seen. G_0 cells can be stimulated by different factors, including hormones, to reenter the cell cycle. However, G_0 cells take longer to reach the S period than do G_1 cells progressing to S (Fig. 1).

Not all cells can leave the cycle and enter G_0 stage. When the cellular environment is impaired by restrictions of certain nutrients or growth factors, normal cells can enter the G_0 stage and survive. However, virally transformed cells, which are incapable of entering G_0 stage, rapidly die. Chemically transformed cells (by using carcinogens) are also incapable of entering G_0 stage. They are mostly stopped or arrested in G_1 phase (50,68). Clearly, normal cells require growth factors (hormones and polypeptides) to reenter the cycle, whereas neoplastic cells are in need of nutrients (amino acids and carbohydrates). Normal cells can be manipulated by hormones and polypeptides, whereas in neoplastic cells this can be done by nutrients. Hence, the factors that control the cell cycle of normal cells and of neoplastic cells are different.

The shift of G_1 and G_0 populations is of crucial importance in controlling the proliferation rate of neoplastic cells and the therapeutic use of antineoplastic drugs. Thus, some cancerous cells are defective in their restriction point control, whereas other transformed cell lines retain the ability to enter G_0 (resting state) and can later be reactivated under some conditions (50).

S Phase: DNA Synthesis

The S phase is the period during which DNA replication takes place and proteins are manufactured and released for the newly synthesized DNA. The number of chromosomes and chromosomal proteins is doubled. A number of enzymes related to DNA synthesis (thymidine kinase, DNA polymerase, dihydrofolate reductase, and ribonucleotide reductase) are greatly increased. These enzymes are formed in the cytoplasm, arranged in a multienzyme complex, and moved into the nuclear chromatin. The transit of a cell from G_1 to S period is not accompanied by specific molecular events. Protein synthesis is needed for the cell to transit G_1 period. It is not known whether one or more proteins are needed to initiate S phase. Thus protein and RNA synthesis are necessary for a cell to enter S phase. Also a unique copy gene transcription is required for the initiation of S phase. A temperature sensitive enzyme RNA polymerase II is necessary for the active form; if this enzyme is inactive, the cells are unable to enter S phase (63).

The length of S phase is remarkably constant (approximately 7–8 hr) in plant and animal cells. However, tumor cells often have a longer S period than that of normal cells. Normal and tumor cells in S phase can be easily recognized by the use of autoradiography with ^{3}H-thymidine. Cells incorporate thymidine in the S period required for DNA synthesis. The factors that trigger DNA synthesis remain unknown. It is generally accepted that a cell enters the S phase, automatically moves through G_2, and is committed to mitosis. Although S phase is remarkably constant in most cells at approximately 7 hr, there are a few exceptions, such as mouse ear epidermal cells, in which the S phase is exceptionally long (approximately 18 hr). Cells can be either stimulated in S phase by different mitogenic stimulants, such as hormones, growth factors, nutrients, or arrested by chemotherapeutic drugs.

G_2 Phase: Gap$_2$ or Post-DNA Synthesis

G_2 phase is a short period (approx. 1.5–4 hr). During this phase, cells synthesize RNA and proteins, but not DNA. Using puromycin and amino acid analogs, it was shown that all protein synthesis essential for normal mitosis takes place in G_2 period. Arrest in S period with amethopterin for as long as 8 hr does not affect G_2 period. Thus, the length of G_2 period does not depend on S period, although the completion of DNA synthesis triggers the initiation of events in G_2. Studies (58,61) showed that RNA synthesis is required as well, but that this synthesis takes place before protein synthesis. Actinomycin-D, which selectively inhibits the synthesis of ribosomal RNA does not affect entry in mitosis. All these data demonstrate that transcription of RNA (mRNA) is required until mid to late G_2 and that protein synthesis is required until very late G_2. Electrophoretic analysis showed that proteins synthesized in G_2 are of varying mobility. It is possible that some of these proteins are required for operation of mitotic apparatus, while others are needed for chromosome condensation. The length of G_2 period is short, varying between 1.5 and 4 hr. The transition between G_2 and M, that is, mitosis, is poorly understood. The transition is not marked by any characteristic changes in cell metabolism, and RNA and protein synthesis continue into prophase.

Arrest of the cycle in G_2 in normal condition was discovered by Gelfant and Candelas (23) in the mouse ear epidermis. Normally, only few cells (2 to 6 percent) are arrested in G_2; they are the first to enter mitosis when epithelium is stimulated by wounding. The cells can remain in G_2 indefinitely. The molecular basis for G_2 arrest or block is unknown, although it is possible that some genes are responsible for the transit of G_2 and are repressed by factor(s) present in early phases (G_1 and S).

In G_2 phase the cells contain twice their normal complement of chromosomes. Although most mammalian cells spend less than 6 hr in G_2, some cells stop in G_2 and differentiate: hepatocytes, some lymphocytes, and neurons. Whereas most cells arrested in G_1 period (epithelial cells of duodenum) are diploid cells, almost all cells arrested in G_2 period (rabbit osteocytes, enamel cells, and a few mouse ear epidermal cells) contain at least twice the amount of DNA of interphase diploid cells; these are polyploid cells. Most tumor ascites cells, some rodent liver cells, and almost all human myocardial cells can be stopped, remaining in G_2 period; from this period, they can be stimulated to enter mitosis.

Inasmuch as most cells are arrested in G_1 or G_0 phase (diploid cells), some cells (tetraploid cells) can be also arrested in G_2 period. Despite the fact that length of the cell cycle is regulated mostly by G_1 period, G_2 is a short period and lasts mainly 1 to 4 hours, with few exceptions (e.g., mouse ear epidermis, rabbit enamel cells, mouse ascites tumors, and spermatogonia) in which G_2 ranges from 6 to 9 hours.

M Phase: Mitosis

After completing G_2 phase, the cells progress sequentially through the classic phases of mitosis: prophase, metaphase, anaphase, and telophase. During mitosis, protein synthesis reaches a minimum and RNA synthesis declines rapidly in late prophase; all RNA synthesis stops before metaphase, with the exception of continued synthesis of some RNA precursors (4S and 5S) during mitosis. RNA synthesis resumes in late telophase and rapidly rises to a steady rate a few minutes after the completion of telophase. The mechanism by which RNA synthesis is blocked during mitosis is unknown. The end result of mitosis is the reduction in the ratio of DNA per cell to the diploid value characteristic of the species (e.g., 46 chromosomes for humans), with the formation of two daughter cells.

The duration of M phase varies in different tissues from 30 minutes to 2.5 hours, averaging 1 hour for most mammalian cells (3,4,61).

Some investigators suggest two cell cycles: one regulating cytoplasmic and cell growth and another controlling DNA replication. Both cycles converge to produce mitosis using two distinct pathways. Thus, the cell cycle that controls DNA replication is dependent on a functional enzyme called RNA polymerase II, whereas the cell cycle that regulates cell growth does not depend on RNA polymerase II. It is therefore possible to use drugs that can kill individual cells by inhibiting their growth or by inhibiting DNA replication alone (3).

The length of the cell cycle varies both in normal as well as in neoplastic tissues, primarily in the G_1 phase. The major portion of the life-span of most cells is usually spent in G_1. Some neurons of the central nervous system remain stationary in G_1 throughout their entire life, whereas muscle cells leave G_1 period only if replication occurred because of the death of adjacent cells.

Thus, the duration of the cell cycle is as short as 18 hr in bone marrow stem cells, of average length in crypt cells from colon epithelium, at 39 hr and from rectum (48 hr), and quite long in mouse ear epidermis (3 to 5 days) and human bronchus epithelial cells (about 10 days) (3). Also, it is variable in human cancers; for instance, it is approximately 72 hr in carcinoma of the stomach, between 80 and 120 hr in acute and chronic myeloid leukemia, nearly 220 hr in carcinoma of bronchus, and also varies between 60 and 90 hr in some squamous cell carcinomas of human skin (7). Since the average length of cell cycle in most plant, animal, and tumor cells ranges between 20 and 30 hours or several days, it appears that the length of the cell cycle of neoplastic cells is no longer than that of normal cells. The rapid proliferation of tumor cells depends, in addition to cell cycle length, on growth fraction (the fraction of cycling cells) and the rate of cell loss, while the proliferation of normal cells is mostly dependent on the duration of the cell cycle. Generally, the cell cycle includes two phases, that is, A phase (interphase; G_1, S, and G_2) and B phase (mitosis). In addition to these classic phases, two other important compartments can play a substantial role in the normal and abnormal growth of cell populations: one is the dormant (quiescent compartment of cells in G_0 period and are only temporarily "out of cycle" and can reenter the cycle at any time after appropriate stimulation) and the other is a compartment of cells irreversibly leaving the cycle (called Q cells), and are going to differentiate. These differentiated Q cells are distinct from G_0 cells, as demonstrated by autoradiography, scanning electron microscopy, and flow cytometric studies.

Dormant cells (G_0 phase) can be brought into the cycle at any time by an appropriate stimulus, such as growth factors, hormones, and nutrients. Whereas they represent only a small fraction of normal cells, dormant cells can reach a significant proportion in several neoplasms. The tumor dormant state represents a large proportion of neoplastic cells restrained in their growth for prolonged periods (about 10 years); they are temporarily noncycling cells (G_0 cells). Dormant tumor cells are indistinguishable from normal cells and cycling tumor cells. For example, thyroid cells (normal, hyperplastic, or neoplastic) are capable of surviving even in other tissues, particularly in lung, for long intervals. An appropriate stimulus, however, such as thyroxine deficiency (induced by administration of methylthiouracil), can stimulate these cells to reenter the cycle and form typical follicles.

The mechanisms by which a cell leaves the cycle for a variable period of time are more complex; several different mechanisms might be involved in the establishment and maintenance of the dormancy of different tumors (84).

The cell cycle of both normal and neoplastic cells is represented diagrammatically in Figure 2-1.

Cell Surface Changes During the Cell Cycle

Recently a relationship between the cell surface changes and cell cycle phases was demonstrated, showing differences in glycolipid synthesis and organization in the cell cycle. It has been proposed that surface modulating assemblies consisting of glycoprotein receptors, microtubules, microfilaments, and associated membrane contractile proteins regulate the growth signals from the cell surface to the interior. Thus, colchicine, which disrupts the microtubules, blocks the transition from G_0 to S in chick embryo fibroblasts and neuroblastoma cells (58). Also, concanavalin A (Con A), which inhibits surface receptor mobility, inhibits entry into S phase; cytochalasin, which inhibits microfilaments, is involved in lymphocyte activation. Scanning electron microscopic examination has exhibited significant cell surface changes in synchronized populations of Chinese hamster ovary (CHO) cells during the cycle. Cells in G_1 exhibit large numbers of microvilli, blebs, and ruffles. During S phase, the surfaces are more flat and free of blebs; they show only microvilli and ruffles and become relatively smooth, forming a thin layer. During G_2 phase, the number of microvilli increases and the cells thicken and round up for mitosis (M phase) (60). Clearly, there is a relationship between the cell surface and its internal structure, especially the cytoskeleton apparatus (microtubules and microfilaments), which plays an important role in chromosomal arrangement and movement. This phenomenon is better visualized by high-voltage electron microscopy (HVEM) and SEM.

From a general biologic aspect, cell and tissue aging can occur as a result of the transition of cycling to noncycling cells (G_1 and G_2 blocked cells) (24). Hormonal and immune mechanisms could be responsible for cellular aging; these mechanisms are discussed later in this chapter.

MECHANISM(S) OF CYCLING CELLS: THE OPERON MODEL

The intrinsic mechanism(s) that influence cells regarding reentry into the cycle or leaving it to remain out of cycle either for a period of time in a dormant state or forever by differentiation are not fully understood. In recent years various models elaborated by computer studies regarding the controlling mechanisms of cell cycle in prokaryote cells and some lower eukaryote cells strongly suggest that initiation of the cell cycle and functional homeostasis in living cells are achieved by different operon groups (e.g., functional operon, mitotic operon).

The operon model proposed by Jacob and Monod (32) results from their original studies of enzyme synthesis in *Escherichia coli*. According to the operon model, each operator gene acts as a switch that turns the synthetic activity of the structural genes on or off, synthesizing mRNA which goes to the ribosomes and act as a template for protein synthesis. A single operator gene can control several structural genes arranged in a linear sequence in the chromosomes. This assembly of operator genes and its cluster of structural genes is called an operon. According to Jacob and Monod, there are two different operons: induced operon and repressor operon (operons prevented from functioning). However, the original operon model cannot be fully applied to eukaryotes, wherein chromosomes are a complex of DNA and proteins (histones). It is more likely that induction and repression of enzyme or protein synthesis in eukaryote cells are primarily attributable to histones. In turn, the repressor and corepressor proteins control DNA synthesis. The initiation of DNA synthesis and subsequently of cell entry into mitosis is brought about by a specific protein called initiator protein (P). The synthesis of initiator protein is controlled in turn by mRNA. The synthesis of mRNA is ordinarily repressed by a repressor–corepressor protein complex. Repressor and corepressor proteins are continuously synthesized and are highly specific for each cell line. Repressor proteins tend to remain intracellular, while corepressor proteins are labile, equilibrating with the extracellular environment. The production of repressor proteins is regulated for the most part by factors coming from the cytoplasm. Thus, the initiation of DNA synthesis and the commitment of cells of mitosis depend on a repressor–corepressor protein complex. Hormones, heat, wounding, and probably mutations in the precancerous cells of the repressor genes might be responsible for controlling the inhibitory mechanism of DNA synthesis (Fig. 2–1).

It has also been postulated that two different operons control the cell cycle. Operon F controls the synthesis of functional proteins (P_f) and operon M the synthesis of specific mitotic proteins (P_m). Operons M and F are connected by the repressor protein (R_m and R_f). Operon M is responsible for the synthesis of all cellular proteins required for the mitotic cycle. It also produces a repressor protein that inhibits the action of the functional operon (operon F). Thus, operons M and F are in reversible equilibrium, which in turn is controlled by various factors, namely hormones and hormonelike substances, such as growth factors and chalones. Hormones appear to affect the production of repressor or derepressor proteins and thus may activate in turn, the cell cycle (Fig. 2-1) (19,23). However, the factors that influence the cells to leave the cycle temporarily (dormant cells, G_0 cells, cells arrested in G_1 or G_2 period) or permanently leave the cycle (differentiated cells, Q cells) remain still unknown.

Elucidation of the molecular control of initiation of DNA synthesis and the cell cycle will provide further details of the regulatory mechanisms of normal and abnormal cell division and proliferation. There is only a short period (about 4 hr) between the commitment of cells to DNA synthesis and the initiation of DNA synthesis.

Although it has been demonstrated that hormones can act as mitogenic stimulants, there is no convincing evidence that hormones act directly on operon M or F. According to the original operon model described 20 years ago by Jacob and Monod, DNA synthesis and the commitment of cells to enter cell cycle and mitosis is regulated primarily by cytoplasmic factors called repressors. Repressors can be either inactivated through induction or activated through repression.

The two types of genes—structural genes and genetic (functional genes)—have two operons—a functional operon (F operon), which controls the functional proteins, and a mitotic operon (M operon), which directly controls the DNA synthesis and mitotic cycle. However, the F operon can indirectly influence the M operon, as a result of its reversible equilibrium, which is in turn regulated by functional repressor (R_f) and mitotic repressor (R_m). Hence, the M operon controls by a specific mitotic mRNA ($mRNA_M$), which acts on mitotic ribosomal RNA ($rRNA_M$), which regulates the synthesis of mitotic proteins (P_m) (Fig. 2-2). All operon controlling mechanisms are negative, thus they operate by inhibition rather than activation. Derepression is the process by which an inducer combines with an active repressor, resulting in activation of a previously repressed operator gene, followed by enzyme synthesis. It is possible that derepression phenomena play an important role in controlling the mitotic homeostasis of neoplastic (precancerous and cancerous) cells. These two operon models (F and M operons) could also explain the existence of two cell cycles: one functional cell cycle regulating the cell growth and another controlling cellular DNA replication.

Recent advances were made using recombinant DNA techniques. Thus, certain small, oncogenic DNA viruses, such as SV 40 (simian virus 40) and polyomavirus can induce mitosis in mammalian cells. In this way we can obtain mutant genes, deriving from the entire gene or fragments of gene; these mutant genes will be predominantly mitotic genes, and when microinjected into human cells are inducing mitosis (74).

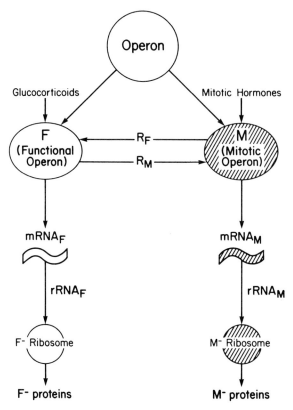

Figure 2-2 The operon model, showing functional (F) and mitotic (M) operons.

Although the operon model works beautifully in prokaryotes, the mechanism(s) which controls the cell cycle and mitotic homeostasis in eukaryote cells are more complex and not yet fully understood. It has been also proposed that the cell membrane can regulate the cell cycle, by sending signals from the exterior to the interior (nuclear chromatin) through its cell surface glycoprotein receptors, cytoskeleton (microtubules, microfilaments) and associated contractile proteins. Disorganization of microtubules by colchicine administration can block the transition from G_0 to S in chick embryo fibroblasts (15).

Recent studies demonstrate that microtubule depolymerization is sufficient to initiate both DNA synthesis and events leading to cell cycle and cell division and suggest that microtubule depolymerization may be a required step in initiating cell proliferation. Administration of colchicine or other microtubule disrupting drugs significantly increase the ^{3}H-thymidine incorporation. There is a correlation between DNA synthesis and the synthesis of tubulin (principal protein in microtubules) visualized by immunofluorescence. It seems that some hormones and growth factors exert their mitogenic effects through the cytoskeleton, which acts as a modulator of cell-surface events and initiates DNA synthesis (13). There is an apparent loss of microtubule integrity in many transformed fibroblasts and neoplastic cells and it is possible that microtubule depolymerization is causally involved in neoplastic transformation. Thus, administration of Taxol (antitumor drug), which stabilizes cytoplasmic microtubules, prevents the initiation of DNA synthesis. By using tritium-labeled Taxol (^{3}H-taxol) it has been shown that Taxol binds directly to cytoplasmic microtubules. It enhances microtubule formation. Conditions which depolymerize microtubules inhibit the binding of ^{3}H-taxol.

It is also possible that hormones and growth factors bind to cell surface receptors and through a phenomenon called receptor-mediated endocytosis are going into cells and act on DNA synthesis (25). However, there is no direct evidence that initiation of DNA synthesis and the start of cell cycle requires a cellular internalization of hormones or hormonelike substances.

HORMONAL REGULATION OF THE CANCER CELL CYCLE

In addition to the above discussion suggesting that hormones can regulate the initiation of DNA synthesis and commitment of cells to mitosis by inducing cell surface changes, there is no direct evidence that hormones act through the operon model. According to this model (32), the hormones are presumed to act as inducers by antagonizing specific gene repressors (histones or other chromosomal proteins) and consequently increasing the synthesis of mRNA. Thus, steroid hormones increased RNA synthesis, which is blocked by actinomycin-D.

RNA synthesis occurs rapidly (about 2 minutes) after hormone administration. Estrogen administration increases ^{3}H-uridine incorporation and RNA synthesis as early as 2 minutes in ovariectomized rats. New species of mRNA and also an increase of preexisting species occurs in hormone-treated tissues. By using autoradiography and ^{3}H-labeled hormones a nuclear localization and binding of radioactive hormones to chromatin was frequently reported. Chromosomal puffing always occurs in polytene chromosomes from ecdysone-treated insect larvae. All these findings strongly suggest that hormones primarily act at transcriptional level by facilitating gene transcription (19,78).

In addition to the above findings which indicate that steroid hormones control DNA transcription directly, there is also the possibility that hormones may act at the post-transcriptional level in gene expression. Thus, tyrosine amino-transferase synthesis in cultured hepatoma cells was shown to be induced by corticosteroids only in late G_1 and S phases of the cell cycle, while inducer-independent enzyme synthesis occurs during the rest of the cycle. Hence, the enzyme synthesis is controlled by both a steroid-insensitive transcriptional process and a steroid-sensitive, posttranscriptional process (78). Hormones may act by derepression of either F operon (glucocorticoids) or M operon (mitogenic hormones). In some instances, such as in estrogens in vaginal epithelium, they can activate both F and M operons.

Bullough suggested that homeostatic mechanisms of mitosis and the cell cycle are controlled by a combination between hormones and chalones (tissue-specific mitotic inhibitors). He suggested that mitogenic hormones exert their main effects on target tissues by neutralizing the effect of tissue chalones (chalones are basic glycoproteins) (8).

Recently it was shown that epidermal chalones inhibit the cell cycle at the G_1–S, S–G_2, and G_2–M transitions in mouse epidermis (17). In addition to these intracellular mechanisms by which steroid hormones intervene in the cell cycle, thereby regulating the mitotic homeostasis, polypeptidic hormones (insulin, prolactin, thyroid hormones, pituitary hormones) may act on the cell membrane by combining with specific receptors and forming hormone–receptor complexes.

Hence, the above studies imply that hormones act in different ways on the cell cycle and in more than one site in a cell (Fig. 2–3).

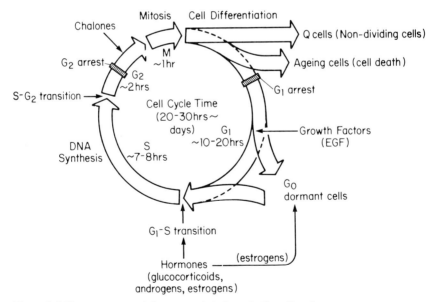

Figure 2-3 Hormones, growth factors, and chalones in the cell cycle.

Since most of the cells that have entered S phase are commited to mitosis, the control of S phase (DNA synthesis) is a key event in controlling the cell cycle of normal and abnormal cells. Thus, most studies regarding the effects of hormones on the cell cycle are focused on their effects on S phase. Our studies regarding the effects of hormones on DNA synthesis (S phase) in neoplastic epidermal cells using ^{3}H-thymidine light and electron microscopic autoradiography and DNA labeling indicated marked changes of DNA synthesis of the nuclei of both squamous cell carcinoma and basal cell carcinomas induced by 3-methylcholanthrene (3-MCA) in rodents. Thus, thyroxine, estradiol, calcitonin, and prostaglandin $F_{2\alpha}$ ($PGF_2\alpha$) markedly enhance DNA synthesis in the nuclei of neoplastic cells, whereas a notable inhibition occurs after administration of cortisol or after hypophysectomy or gonadectomy. There are also interesting changes regarding the distribution of labeled cells in the proliferative and nonproliferative compartments. Thus, the labeled nuclei are located mostly at the periphery of epithelial pearls in squamous cell carcinoma, whereas no labeled nuclei can be seen in horn pearls (Figs. 2–4 and 2–5). In basal cell carcinoma, only the nuclei of dark cells are heavily labeled, whereas only few nuclei of light cells are labeled (Fig. 2–6). Electron

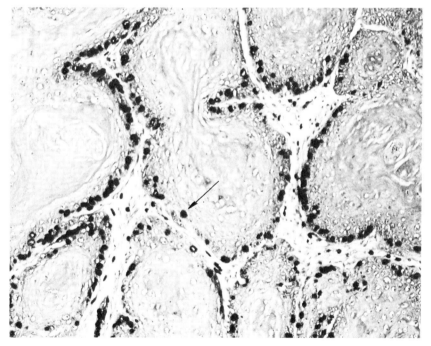

Figure 2-4 Light microscopic autoradiogram of a mouse squamous cell carcinoma, induced by 3-methylcholanthrene and PGF_2. ^{3}H-thymidine-labeled nuclei are located primarily at the periphery of tumor masses (arrow). Paraffin section, NTB_2 nuclear emulsion, H & E stain, $\times 400$.

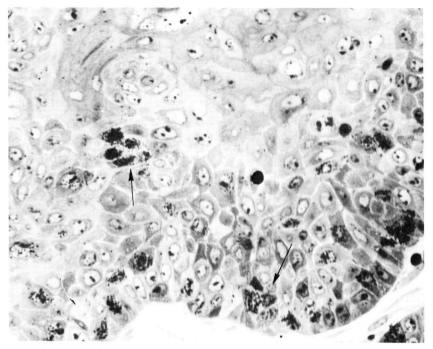

Figure 2-5 Light microscopic autoradiogram showing the characteristic distribution of ^{3}H-thymidine-labeled nuclei. Several labeled nuclei (arrows) are located only at the periphery of tumor. No labeled nuclei are seen in the horn pearls (middle) of the squamous cell carcinoma. Plastic thick section ($\sim$ 1 μm), NTB$_2$ emulsion, toluidine blue stain, $\times$400.

microscopic autoradiography shows most developed grains (filaments) to be distributed over dense chromatin (heterochromatin, genetic chromatin) and no grains to occur over loose chromatin (euchromatin, or metabolic chromatin) (Fig. 2-7). Estradiol induced a peculiar, peripheral distribution, namely over the peripheral chromatin and nuclear envelope (Fig. 2-8). These findings suggest that hormones mainly affect the S phase of the cell cycle of cancerous cells; thus hormones and hormonelike factors can change the cellular evolution and modulate carcinogenic process by interfering with DNA synthesis (43).

Steroid Hormones and the Cell Cycle

Early investigations using ^{3}H-thymidine autoradiography regarding the effects of steroid hormones on target endocrine and nontarget cells led many investigators to consider the nucleus as the primary site of hormone action (5,21). Later investigations were undertaken to clarify what period of the cell cycle of each tissue was affected by steroid hormones (4,5,19,21,43,54).

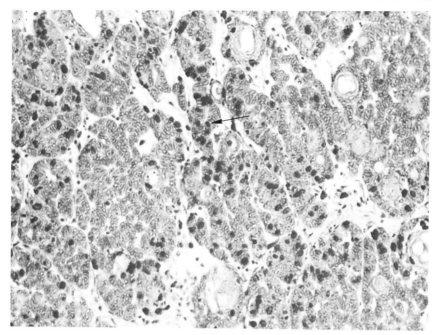

Figure 2-6 Light microscopic autoradiogram showing a different distribution of ^{3}H-thymidine in basal cell carcinoma induced in a rat by 3-MCA. Most heavily labeled nuclei are in the dark cells (arrow). Paraffin section, NTB$_2$ nuclear emulsion, H & E stain, $\times 400$.

Previous investigations regarding the role of estrogens on the cell cycle revealed in both target (uterine epithelium) and nontarget (corneal epithelium) tissue that estrogens mainly act on early phases (transition G$_1$–S), suggesting common estrogen-sensitive system (stage of DNA precursor synthesis) (16,18). Recently it has also been shown that in chick oviduct, estrogens dramatically increase DNA synthesis in oviduct and cell proliferation (54). To ascertain the precise phase of the cycle, chicks were given simultaneous injections of estrogens and inhibitors of DNA synthesis, that is, fluorodeoxyuridine (FdU) and hydroxyurea (HU); estrogens were shown to act before completing DNA synthesis (G$_1$–S transition). Thus, estrogens stimulate G$_1$ cells to enter S phase (54). However, different effects of estrogens on the cell cycle were reported in the uterine and cervical epithelium of neonatal mice. Thus, in the uterine epithelium, estradiol reduces the length of the total cell cycle (T$_c$) from 18 to 16 hr and the duration of S phase from 6.7 to 5.1 hr, whereas it lengthened the cell cycle from 21 to 47 hr and later to 61.2 hr in the cervical epithelium of neonatal mice (16). The effect is most pronounced in G$_1$. In addition to the estrogen effect on DNA synthesis, in target and nontarget tissues, estrogens as well as progesterone markedly stimulated the mRNA synthesis in target tissues and stimulated the synthesis of new species of mRNA and proteins (avidins) in chick oviducts. Recent data suggest that

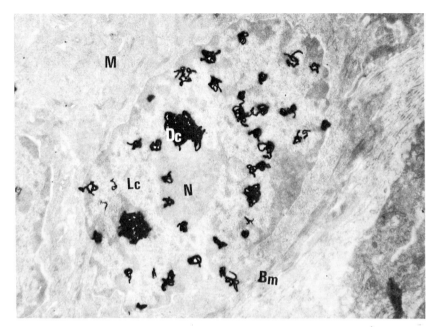

Figure 2-7 Electron microscopic autoradiogram showing a specific distribution of ^{3}H-thymidine as heavily developed grains over the dense (heterochromatin) chromatin of neoplastic nuclei (DC); no developed grains (filaments) are seen over the light chromatin (LC) or other cell organelles. Mitochondrion (m), nucleolus (N), and basement membrane (Bm). Chemically induced mouse squamous cell carcinoma (3-MCA). Epon section, Ilford L$_4$ nuclear emulsion (3 to 4 months' exposure), lightly stained with uranyl acetate and lead citrate, ×11,000.

both estrogens and progesterone act on the nucleus of target cells to promote mRNA synthesis. Estrogens also stimulate the reentry of dormant cells into the cell cycle in several estrogen-dependent tumor cells. However, the direct mitogenic role of estrogens versus indirect mechanism on cell cycle and cell proliferation has not yet been solved. Thus, in vitro experiments using different tumor cell lines (mammary, pituitary, and kidney) showed that estrogens exert their action by increasing the synthesis of specific growth factors. Hence, the estrogens or other steroid hormones alone are not sufficient to promote the growth of tumor cells but require specific growth factors (71).

Estrogens, however, inhibit DNA synthesis in rat mammary tumors in vitro. These conflicting results could be attributable to the estrogen doses used in experiments. Recently small doses of estradiol were shown to increase the DNA synthesis in a human mammary tumor cell line (MCF-7) two- to fourfold, whereas high doses of estradiol inhibit DNA synthesis in the same cell line (41).

Progesterone also stimulates a small fraction of cells to undergo mitosis

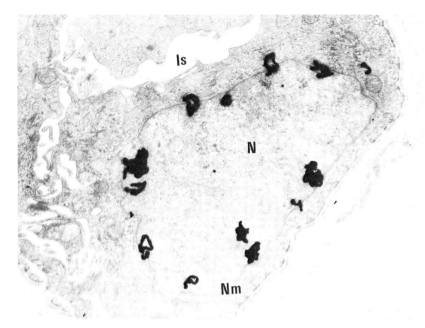

Figure 2-8 A peculiar peripheral distribution of developed grains only over nuclear membrane (N_m) of cancerous cells in a mouse squamous cell carcinoma treated with estradiol propionate. N (nucleus) and Is (intercellular spaces). Epon section, Ilford L_4 nuclear emulsion (3 to 4 months' exposure), lightly stained with uranyl acetate and lead citrate, $\times 11,000$.

in the epithelium of immature chick oviduct. Although most of the data show that progesterone combined with estrogens acts synergistically on the cell cycle by increasing DNA synthesis and S phase, progesterone alone can exhibit a dual action. First, it stimulates the mitotic cycle in a small fraction of cells (stromal cells), and second, it blocks the normal progress of proliferating epithelial cells through the cycle by triggering these cells to pass into the G_0 period, or dormant state. Progesterone also increases the synthesis of mRNA (transcriptional stage) and possibly acts on the cytoplasmic repressors (translational stage) (19,53).

Androgens

It is well known that continuous administration of androgens or estrogens induces a decrease in mitotic activity in target tissues, whereas when this treatment is discontinued, a sharp rise in mitosis can be observed (18,19). Previous observations suggest that testosterone increased cell production in castrated animals by increasing the growth fraction of crypt cells. This increase occurred only in the crypt cells of small bowel of castrated rats, but not in intact adult male rats given physiologic quantities of testosterone. Thus,

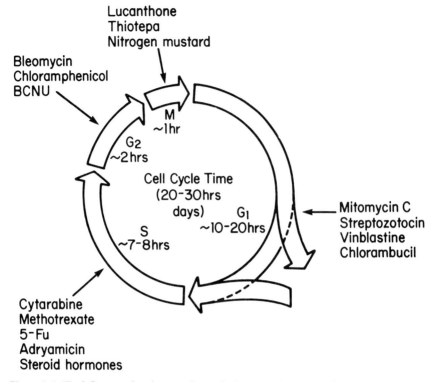

Figure 2-9 The influence of various carcinostatic drugs on the phases of the cell cycle.

testosterone increases DNA synthesis in the crypt cells of castrated rats. It has been suggested that effects of testosterone might have resulted from conversion of some of administered testosterone to estrogens. However, this conversion of testosterone to estrogen was not confirmed by using radio-immunoassay of serum samples from adult rats treated with testosterone (48).

Studies using synchronized cell populations showed that testosterone and 4-androstene-3β, 17β-diol reduced the cell cycle of synchronized popula-tions of the androgen sensitive human cell line NHIK 3025 cultured in MEM-type medium. Dexamethasone prolonged the cell cycle, while estradiol had no effect.

These results might be attributable to a shortening of G₂ period, but were not exclusively located in one particular phase of the cell cycle. They are in accordance with previously described data in asynchronous cell populations (56). Previous studies using electron microscopy indicated a loss of endo-plasmic reticulum and shrinkage of the cytoplasm, as well as a decrease in mitochondrial respiratory enzyme concentrations, observed in castrated postpuberal male rats. These data are consistent with the fact that testosterone should have specific and early stimulatory effects on the synthesis of nucleolar RNA, DNA polymerase, and DNA in the target tissues (53,54). ^{3}H-testosterone has been used to study the autoradiographic distribution in the nuclei of several cells. Changes in DNA synthesis occur approximately 10 hr after testosterone administration, whereas changes in cell morphology occur later (1 day). This finding suggests that androgens, and possibly glucocorticoids, affect cell proliferation both directly and indirectly (through the cell membrane), acting on the cytoskeleton, and consequently on DNA and RNA metabolism (38).

Effects of *corticosteroid hormones* on the cell cycle were previously reported (5,21); it was shown nearly 15 years ago that glucocorticoids play an important role in the initiation of DNA synthesis and in the commitment of cells to enter mitosis and cell division. Thus, injection of hydrocortisone 9 hr before the transition of cells to S phase inhibits the initiation of DNA synthesis in the squamous epithelial cells of the mouse forestomach, whereas hydrocortisone has no effect on DNA synthesis when it is injected 3 to 6 hr before its transition to the S phase. Epinephrine and actinomycin D exert similar effects. Thus, the effects of these hormones occur in G_1 (presynthetic period) and are connected with synthesis of DNA polymerases and RNA necessary for DNA synthesis (RNA–DNA-dependent synthesis) (21). It is possible that weakening of mitotic homeostatic mechanisms with aging is caused by weakening of the adrenal cortex function, favorable for carcinogenesis (8). Autoradiography using labeled cortisol (^{3}H-cortisol) demonstrates a rapid incorporation (about 20 min) of ^{3}H-cortisol by isolated rat liver nuclei. The incorporation of hormone is temperature dependent and is blocked by actinomycin D (5). Studies regarding the effects of prednisolone on mouse lymphoma-cultured cells showed that the depression in growth rate was caused by an increase in cell cycle length. Also, in synchronous cell populations obtained by successive treatment with thymidine and colcemid, prednisolone should be in contact longer than a complete cell cycle in order to inhibit cell multiplication. No particular phase of the cycle was found more sensitive than any other (76). Also, glucocorticoids do not appear necessary for the maintenance of DNA synthesis in normal mammary tissue or rat tumor explants in organ culture. High concentrations have been shown to be deleterious. Maximum effect appears when glucocorticoids inhibit the DNA synthesis in both target and nontarget tissues; their effect on the cell cycle should be considered still inconclusive. However, the lymphatic system (lymph nodes, spleen, and thymus) should be considered a target tissue for corticosteroids. Hydrocortisone significantly decreases the DNA synthesis in mouse and rat thymus and lymph nodes within 2 to 3 hr after hormone administration. It is possible that hydrocortisone inhibits the DNA synthesis by preventing cells from entering S phase (inhibiting especially the transition G_1–S period), while G_0, G_2, and M remain unaffected.

The effects of corticosteroids on the cell cycle of nontarget tissues have been studied by several investigators. Thus, hydrocortisone inhibits the transition G_1–S period and the initition of DNA synthesis in the squamous epithelial cell of the mouse forestomach. It is interesting to note that normal cells are more sensitive than are hyperplastic cells (21). Also, cortisol inhibits the DNA synthesis in rat liver nuclei, and especially in epidermal neoplastic cells of both squamous cell carcinoma and basal cell carcinoma. The latter experiments have shown, by estimating DNA content and ^{3}H-thymidine incorporation with light and electron microscopic autoradiography, that administration of cortisol (hydrocortisone) markedly reduces the DNA synthesis of neoplastic cells in vivo (43,45).

Although the antimitotic effects of glucocorticoids are mainly attributable to their interference in DNA synthesis (S phase), it is likely that corticosteroids act as well during the transcription stage, thereby increasing mRNA synthesis. These are required to induce the synthesis of new protein species, for phenotypic expression of hormone effects, and can also act on the cell membranes. However the effects of corticosteroids on the cell membrane are not yet fully investigated.

Thus, administration of hydroxyurea, an inhibitor of DNA synthesis, does not prevent cortisol action. According to our knowledge there are not significant differences regarding the corticosteroid action between normal and tumor cells. Inhibitory effects of glucocorticoids failed to appear when these hormones are administered concomitantly with antibiotics on tumor cells (75). Thus, corticosteroid hormones (cortisone, cortisol, dexamethasone, fluocinomide, and fluocinolone acetamide) were all found to be potent inhibitors of epidermal DNA synthesis and liver DNA synthesis, and also act in tumor cells (solid Ehrlich tumor and hepatomas). Most of these steroids act during S phase or late G_1 (especially transition G_1–S). There is a good correlation between the inhibition of DNA synthesis induced by these steroids and their ability to inhibit epidermal carcinogenesis (35,43,69).

Liver DNA synthesis has also been reported to be inhibited by glucocorticoids (28). However, if the liver or epidermis is given a stimulus in order to regenerate, as in partial hepatectomy or inflicted wounds, then glucocorticoids induce only a partial inhibition of DNA synthesis and cell proliferation (28). What causes the epidermis and liver to lose their sensitivity to glucocorticoids when they are regenerating is unknown. Inhibition of DNA synthesis by corticosteroids have been also reported in fibroblasts, solid Ehrlich tumor, and hepatoma cells in culture (42), hence the strong correlation between the inhibitory effects of glucocorticoids on DNA synthesis and their inhibition of carcinogenesis.

Polypeptide Hormones and the Cell Cycle

Adrenocorticotropic hormone (ACTH) exerts opposite effects on DNA synthesis, stimulating DNA synthesis in vivo (67) and inhibiting DNA synthesis of normal and tumor adrenal cells (30). These divergent effects on DNA synthesis can be attributable to the concentration of cyclic AMP in the medium (increased in vitro, decreased in vivo). Thus, cyclic AMP is necessary for ACTH to express its effects on DNA synthesis.

Prolactin, when added to cell cultures of some mammary tumors, stimulates DNA synthesis (two- to fourfold). Also, the numbers of ^{3}H-thymidine-labeled nuclei are increased approximately 30-fold when prolactin is added to a medium containing insulin or cortisol (66). Thus, prolactin alone can stimulate DNA synthesis in primary cultures of DMBA-induced mammary tumors. Insulin and glucocorticoids are necessary for prolactin to exert its stimulatory effects in monolayers of normal rat mammary tissue and also to maximize this effect on tumor cells.

Somatomedin C belongs to growth hormone-dependent peptides; it is related to insulin and is capable of inducing DNA synthesis and mitosis in cell cultures. In vivo somatomedin C restores DNA synthesis and mitosis, which are eliminated by hypophysectomy in frog lens epithelium. It is possible that somatomedin C acts on G_0 cells blocked by hypophysectomy, stimulating them to reenter and traverse G_1 phase and the entire cell cycle. Thus, somatomedin C restores in vivo the capacity of G_0/G_1 blocked cells of hypophysectomized frogs to reenter and traverse the cell cycle and achieve mitosis (64). Growth hormone, prolactin, thyrotropin, and triiodothyronine also restore and promote lens cell proliferation in vivo, but not in vitro. Insulin and epidermal growth factor stimulate cell growth in rabbit lens epithelium in vitro. Growth hormone (GH) as well as insulin, is involved in DNA synthesis but does not affect the rate of DNA replication (80).

Insulin increases the DNA synthesis in tissue cultures of some rodents and human mammary tumors (83) and in a continuous cell line derived from a human breast cancer (55). The degree is maximal in cultures of virgin mammary gland; it appears to be maximal at 24 to 48 hr after the addition of prolactin to the stimulating action of insulin, suggesting that the insulin is the mitogenic hormone (52). Studies regarding the cell cycle analysis and binding of ^{125}I-labeled insulin on mouse melanoma cells (CCL 531) showed the highest binding activity during S phase. Thus, insulin acts mainly during the S phase of the cell cycle (especially late G_1 and transition to S phase) (70). However, findings derived from our investigations regarding the effects of insulin on DNA synthesis in epidermal neoplastic cells are inconclusive (see Chapter 4).

Glucagon, the hyperglycemient pancreatic hormone, was also investigated during the cell cycle and DNA synthesis. Glucagon was shown to stimulate DNA synthesis of the intestinal epithelial cells after resection. The effect was maximal at the physiologic dose (20). Our investigations also demonstrated that exogenous glucagon markedly increases DNA synthesis in epidermal cancerous cells, especially during S phase in rodents (44).

Recent evidence suggests a direct mitogenic role of *thyroid hormones* in vitro. Thus, the growth of a rat pituitary tumor cell line (GH 3/C14) was stimulated 3.5-fold by the addition of thyroxine (T_4) or triiodothyronine (T_3).

The physiologic concentrations of thyroid hormones are directly mitogenic for these tumor cells in vitro (36). The effect of T_3 on the cell cycle was also studied in cultured GC cells, a thyroid hormone-sensitive rat pituitary cell line that produces GH. Thus, in hypothyroid calf serum, an increase in the cell cycle stages of GC cells was observed, that is, a 7.9-fold increase in the duration of G_1, a 2.2-fold increase in G_2, and a 1.35-fold increase during the mitotic (M) stage. No changes in the duration of S period were apparent. Addition of T_3 to this medium effected a 3.9-fold increase in growth rate owing to a decrease in G_1, G_2, and M phases of the cell cycle (14). Thyroid hormones increase the mitotic rate also in frog lens, rat liver, and rat intestinal mucosa in vivo. Addition of T_4 increased the growth rate of cultured human kidney epithelial cells; it was suggested that this effect resulted from a decrease in the pre-DNA-synthetic period (G_1) of the cell cycle (9). Some rat pituitary cell lines can grow in a defined serum-free medium supplemented with hormones. Hormones are required for the cell growth. Thus, rat pituitary cell line GH_3 can grow in a serum-free medium supplemented with T_3, thyrotropin-releasing hormone (TRH), parathyroid hormone, and a partially purified somatomedin. BHK and HeLa cells can grow in serum-free medium supplemented with a mixture of 25 hormones (GH, TSH, prolactin, glucoagon, insulin, calcitonin, prostaglandin E_1, somatomedin A, and transferrin) (27). Some polypeptide hormones and glucocorticoids interact with plasma membrane receptors, subsequently affecting DNA synthesis. Thus, insulin receptors in G_0 Balb/3 T_3 cells were 2–9-fold higher than in growing cells and the number of glucocorticoid receptors per HeLa cell doubled between late G_1 and S (10).

Hormonelike Substances (Prostaglandins, Epidermal Growth Factor, Chalones) and the Cell Cycle

Prostaglandins E_2, $F_{2\alpha}$ and A_2 (PGE$_2$, PGF$_{2\alpha}$, PGA$_2$) can modify the cell cycle by interfering with S phase. Recent investigations from our laborabory, using ^{3}H-thymidine autoradiography and DNA content, demonstrated that PGE and PGF$_{2\alpha}$ markedly enhanced the ^{3}H-thymidine incorporation and DNA synthesis of tumor cells from chemically induced epidermal neoplasms (both squamous cell and basal cell carcinomas) in rodents. Thus, labeling and mitotic index of epidermal neoplastic cells are markedly increased after administration of PGE$_2$, but primarily after PGF$_{2\alpha}$.

These findings suggest that prostaglandins, which are ubiquitous tissue hormones, affect the cell cycle of neoplastic and normal epidermal cells by interfering with DNA synthesis, especially S phase (45). The initiation of cell proliferation by PGF$_{2\alpha}$ was markedly potentiated by insulin and inhibited by hydrocortisone (34).

The role of *growth factors*, for example, epidermal growth factor (EGF), fibroblast growth factor, the cartilage-derived factor, and the nerve growth factor in the cell cycle regulation of normal and transformed cells was recently reviewed (59). Some data suggest that the primary event of action of EGF on transformed cells (HeLa, KB) is a stimulation of RNA synthesis followed by an increase in protein synthesis. Effects of epidermal growth factor (EGF) are mainly due to the presence of EGF receptors on the cell surface. Studies regarding the effects of EGF on transformed and normal cells (SV_3T_3, 3T3) indicate that the entry in S phase is not affected by the cellular RNA level and consequently none of the events induced during the G_1 phase studied in 3T3 cells is essential for DNA synthesis initiation under normal conditions (50). Also, studies regarding the effects of EGF on tumor cells showed that EGF stimulated DNA synthesis and the mitotic index in the cells of mammary adenocarcinoma of mice. EGF also increases DNA synthesis and RNA and protein synthesis in HeLa cells and KB cells derived from a human tumor of the rhinopharynx (12).

Unlike fibroblast growth factor, which requires glucocorticoids to exert its maximal effect, the cartilage-derived factor can alone stimulate DNA synthesis in 3T3 cells.

Effects of chalones (from the Greek *chalao,* meaning "inhibit") were extensively studied in the cell cycle of normal and neoplastic cells, from which some speculative conclusions were drawn (8). It is suggested that each tissue is controlled by its own specific chalone. Chalones are basic glycoproteins and the effects of epidermal chalone were mostly investigated. Bullough (8) suggested that chalones play an important role in the mitotic cycle and that mitogenic hormones exert their effects by combining and neutralizing tissue chalones. It is possible that the epidermal chalone–epinephrine complex does not affect DNA synthesis and exerts its action later in the cell cycle. Thus, epinephrine inhibits mitosis by acting and increasing the chalone activity. Hormones and chalones complexes intervene and act in the mitotic homeostasis of normal and transformed cells as a negative feedback mechanism in which the antimitotic chalone molecule acts as the messenger. It has been shown that the epidermal chalone–epinephrine complex does not directly interfere with DNA synthesis and exerts its action later in the cell cycle. Thus, chalones are mitotic inhibitors which can control the cell cycle, not only in epidermal cells, but in other rapidly dividing cells (granulocytes, tumor cells). Hence, chalones exert this inhibitory or antimitotic effects by preventing the cells from entering mitosis and also by lengthening the cell cycle phases.

Recently it was shown that epidermal chalones inhibit the cell cycle at the G_1–S, S–G_2, and G_2–M transitions in the hairless mouse epidermis. The inhibition at the G_1–S transit was stronger than that at S–G_2 and G_2–M transitions (17). There are two types of chalones: chalone I and chalone II. In conclusion, chalones inhibit mitosis both in vitro and in vivo; their action is reversible and they are not cytotoxic; and they are circulating substances, which are tissue specific, but not species specific.

Originally, an important role of chalones was assumed in the control of mitotic homeostasis of neoplastic cells; this role has not yet been fully demonstrated, however.

Therefore, from a therapeutic standpoint, it is important to know that cell homeostasis depends on the number of mitotic, or permanently dividing cells, cells that are continuously "in the cycle" and those cells that are nondividing or permanently "out of cycle" (differentiated cells or aging cells) or temporarily "out of cycle" (dormant, quiescent or G_0 cells). Some cells are reversible out of cycle (dormant or G_0 cells), while others are irreversible (differentiated cells, aging cells) (79). After mitosis is completed, the daughter cells make their own decision to enter the cycle and divide again, or get "out of cycle," either temporarily or permanently. Although this decision is mainly gene dominated (genetically determined), it can be strongly influenced by cellular environmental factors, such as hormones, growth factors, and nutrients. According to the operon concept, the controlling mechanism(s) of mitosis, function, and aging in a tissue cell are operating by different operons: mitosis operon (M operon), function operon (F operon) and aging operon (A operon) (8). These operon groups are activated or inactivated by both repressor and derepressor factors (19,32).

A normal tissue has a constant equilibrium or balance between the mitotic or dividing cells and the rate of cell loss caused by death; however, in an abnormal or neoplastic tissue, this equilibrium is shifted in favor of dividing cells and is always a cell gain; the growth fraction is always larger than the cell loss. This appears to be the essential difference between the tumor and its tissue of origin.

THE CELL CYCLE AND CARCINOGENESIS

It is well demonstrated that carcinogens (chemical, radiation-induced, or viral), in order to exert their action, require cell proliferation (1). Carcinogens cannot induce neoplasms in the absence of a proliferative state. There is also sufficient evidence to suggest that cycling, or dividing, cells are more vulnerable to carcinogenic agents than are normal cells and that the sensitivity to carcinogens can vary at different stages of the cell cycle. Thus, the liver of newborn mice or the regenerating liver (partial hepatectomy) of adult mice is more sensitive to chemical carcinogens or to radiation, as compared with controls. A single dose of urethane administered to adult mice at various intervals after parial hepatectomy (4, 18, 32, and 46 hr) corresponding to cell cycle stages (G_1, S, G_2, and M) produced a variable incidence of hepatomas. Thus, at 13 months after urethane administration, the percentages of hepatoma induction was 10, 68, 42, and 77 percent of treated animals, compared with only 3 percent in untreated mice, or with 6 percent in those treated with urethane only. These findings indicate a clear-cut relationship between the induction of hepatoma and the intervals after hepatectomy, which roughly correspond to the cell cycle phases of hepatocytes (82). The high tumor yield in S, G_2, and M phases can be explained by the variation in the DNA binding to carcinogen, which can be quantitatively high at this time. In addition, susceptibility to carcinogens is a function of sex. For example, female newborn mice developed only few hepatomas as compared with males, possibly attributable to hormonal influences on tumor development. These experiments clearly indicate that neonatal tissues and regenerating liver are highly susceptible to chemical carcinogens as compared with resting adult liver, strongly suggesting that cycling cells, especially S-phase cells, are the most sensitive to the initiating action of chemical carcinogen. Also, carcinogens (chemical, viral, and radiation induced) cannot transform cells in which DNA synthesis was inhibited (46).

Experiments in vitro using a cloned line (M_2) of mouse fibroblasts, which is susceptible to chemical carcinogens, showed that malignant transformation in tissue culture is also cell-cycle dependent. Thus, administration of two chemical carcinogens—7-12-dimethylbenz(a)anthracene-5-6-oxide (DMBA-5, 6-oxide) and N-methyl-N-nitro-N-nitrosoquanidine (MNNG)—at various times in the synchronized mouse fibroblasts (M_2) demonstrated malignant transformation only when cells were treated during the G_1 or S phase of the cell cycle. The induction of malignant transformation was significantly greater in the S phase as compared with that observed in the G_1 phase, whereas no malignant transformation was observed in the cells treated during G_2 or M phase of the cell cycle (46). It is interesting that only carcinogenic action was cell cycle dependent, while the toxicity caused by both agents was not cell cycle dependent. However, when abnormal cells from ataxia telangiectasia (AT) are exposed to various carcinogens, they exhibit primarily a diminished inhibition of DNA replication and increased lethality (33).

The interactions of hormones and chemical carcinogens are also cell cycle related. Thus, the hormone combination of cortisol with insulin + prolactin + aldosterone enhances the incidence of nodulelike alveolar lesions (NLAL) of mouse mammary cells by DMBA, whereas hormone combination insulin + prolactin + cortisol was unfavorable and the combination of aldosterone + insulin + prolactin was only moderately effective. The highest incidence of NLAL occurred when mammary glands were treated with DMBA for 24 hr between days 3 and 4 of culture, the period corresponding to the second wave of DNA synthesis in the gland. These data strongly suggest that DMBA induction of NLAL in mammary glands in organ culture involves a complex carcinogen–hormone–cell cycle interaction (40). It is possible that hormones activate DNA synthesis and consequently cell proliferation, creating a favorable environment for the induction of preneoplastic and neoplastic lesions.

Recent data also indicate that metastatic lung colony formation is cell cycle dependent. Thus, exponentially growing FSA 1233 (isolated from a mouse fibrosarcoma) cells in vitro were separated into subpopulations corresponding to specific phases of the cell cycle (G_1, S, G_2, M) by centrifugal elutriation and were injected intravenously to determine the efficiency of lung colony formation (LCF). The LCF showed a marked cell cycle and cell size dependency, being the lowest at G_1, highest at S phase, and declining slightly at G_2. Thus, the metastatic colony formation in lungs depends on stage in cell cycle, being the highest in the S phase cells. Always, the large cells (S, G_2, M) appear to be more efficient in forming lung colonies than are small cells (G_1) (77).

Hence, these findings strongly suggest that neoplastic transformation and metastatic colony formation are cell cycle dependent.

CELL CYCLE SPECIFIC DRUGS

Experimental and clinical observations indicate that most cytostatic drugs are acting mainly on dividing or cycling cells and thus are cell cycle specific (CCS) drugs. During the last decade, as a result of kinetic studies of tumor growth and neoplastic cell populations, significant achievements in cancer chemotherapy were made, enabling us to select better drugs for adjuvant chemotherapy. The cell cycle specificity of cytostatic drugs was demonstrated approximately 20 years ago (8).

When in cycle, the cells are more sensitive to cytostatic agents; consequently, the most successful application of cytostatic chemotherapy is more evident in those tumors showing rapid proliferation (leukemias, lymphomas, chorio-epithelioma, and testicular tumors). CCS agents exhibit a specific toxicity and kill mainly the dividing or proliferating cells. They are primarily effective in rapidly growing tumors or in tumors exhibiting a high "growth fraction" (the percentage of tumor cells proliferating at any given time). CCS drugs can act during any phase of the cell cycle, although most act selectively during S phase. Cytarabine is an excellent example of a drug exhibiting selective toxicity only during the S phase of the cell cycle. In addition to cytarabine, CCS agents include mercaptopurine, fluorouracil (5-FU), methotrexate (MTX), vincristine, bleomycin, and certain steroid hormones. During G_1 phase, these agents are mitomycin C, streptozotocin, vinblastine, and chlorambucil; during S phase, they are cytarabine, daunomycin, adriamycin, MTX, 5-FU, vincristine, and some steroid hormones; during G_2 phase, they are bleomycin, BCNU, and chloramphenicol; and during M phase, they are mitomycin C, nitrogen mustard, thiotepa, and lucanthone (Fig. 2–9).

A second major group of drugs are defined as *cell cycle nonspecific (CCNS) agents*, which act by complexing with DNA and are capable of doing this regardless of whether the cells are proliferating. Examples are the alkylating agents: cyclophosphamide, melphalan, and antibiotics. Both CCS and CCNS are discussed in detail in Chapter 10.

There are many difficulties to overcome, since the cell cycle time of neoplastic cells is similar to that of their surrounding normal cells; thus, the same drugs can kill both neoplastic and normal cells. The study of cell cycle phases and drug dependence provides significant advantages in the design of optimal chemotherapeutic schedules (29,81).

COMMENTS AND CONCLUSIONS

Studies of the cell cycle and its phases began nearly 30 years ago, with the use of ^{3}H-thymidine. Light microscopic autoradiography, and especially high-resolution autoradiography, demonstrated that this nucleotide is specifically incorporated during the synthesis of DNA (called DNA synthesis or S phase). The use of ^{3}H-uridine makes more data available; it was found that this nucleotide is specifically incorporated in mRNA. ^{3}H-Leucine, another radionucleotide, produced accurate data regarding the protein synthesis at its ribosomal stage.

In the early studies, two phases of the cell cycle were defined: a long interphase (A phase) and mitosis (B phase) (31,49). All phases from interphase were preparative stages required for mitosis (mitotic cycle). In most of these phases, euchromatin or metabolic chromatin was synthesized, with the exception of S phase, wherein heterochromatin or the genetic chromatin was synthesized. The purpose of current investigations is twofold: (1) to learn more about the dividing or cycling cells in tumors, and (2) to determine the predominant phase or cell cycle stage in which hormones act on neoplastic cells.

It has been well demonstrated that tumors are composed of heterogeneous cell populations. Some compartments are composed of dividing cells, other nondividing cells (silent or dormant cells), and finally, dead cells. It is well known that dividing or cycling cells are more sensitive to carcinogens and are also more vulnerable to cytostatic drugs. It is also known that some phases of the cell cycle are more susceptible to carcinogens and are also more vulnerable to cytostatic or chemotherapeutic agents. Hormones, growth factors, and nutrients play an important role in controlling the cell cycle and its phases. Through the use of hormones, we can manipulate a cell to get "into the cycle" or get "out of the cycle" and stay in a dormant or quiescent stage for several months or years. Thus, we can modulate the proliferative state or *"growth" fraction*, which is extremely important in making therapeutic decisions. By using synchronized cell populations, with a double ^{3}H-thymidine block, it was shown that some cell cycle phases are specifically more aggressive in proliferating, invading, and metastasizing, whereas other cell cycle phases are more vulnerable to chemotherapeutic agents.

Modern methods provide interesting data that have shown that the cell cycle and its phases can be modulated by changing the environmental (milieu interieur) factors. Thus, the commitment or decision of a cell to stay "in the cycle" or to "leave the cycle," either permanently or temporarily, is not rigidly and genetically determined, as was generally believed, but it can be markedly influenced by the action on the cell by environmental factors, such as hormones. Some phases of the cell cycle are more hormone dependent, while others are more influenced by growth factors, hormonelike substances, or nutrients. Also, the use of modern methods has shown that the length of cell cycle or its duration are not significantly greater or longer in cancerous cells as compared to their original cells. In fact, some dividing normal cells have a shorter cell cycle than that of many tumor cells. What makes the difference is the predominance of cycling cells, dividing cells, or cell proliferation, which is always higher in tumors as compared with their original, normal, tissue. The growth fraction is much higher in tumors, as compared with that found in normal tissue, in which there is a balance among dividing cells, dying cells, and noncycling cells.

The dormant cells represent an important cell compartment in tumor cell homeostasis. These cells are reversible cells; they can be influenced at any time to reenter the cell cycle and to start to divide again. We also can remove dividing cells temporarily from the cycle and keep them for months or years in this dormant stage. It was also a general belief that by influencing only the G_1 period (shortening or lengthening), we can markedly change the cell cycle. All phases of cell cycle (including S phase) can be influenced by environmental factors or hormones. Of special significance is the last stage of G_1 period, or G_1–S transition, in which the cells, after being committed to mitosis, enter S phase. It is a short period of time between the commitment of a cell and its final decision to enter S phase, and thus undergo mitosis. After a cell enters S phase, it cannot change its "mind" and leave the cycle; the cell will definitely undergo mitosis. Thus by changing and modulating the cell cycle and its phases, we can markedly influence and shift tumor cell homeostasis and make it more favorable and cooperative to our therapeutic decision. Although the intrinsic mechanism by which hormones intervene in the cell cycle is not yet fully understood, it seems likely that hormones can control the cell cycle in more than one way. Thus, they can interfere with DNA synthesis (S phase or more likely the transition G_1–S), or through operon groups, influencing the equilibrium between the repressor and corepressor factors, which can result in derepression (19,23). The derepression phenomenon was thought responsible for the unlimited proliferative capacity of neoplastic cells.

In addition to a direct means (DNA synthesis or operon models), hormones can intervene in the cell cycle in an indirect way, affecting the cell membrane and consequently cytoskeleton. The cytoskeleton is an important apparatus, composed of motile structures, such as microtubules and micro-filaments, recently demonstrated to play an important role in mobility and transport of chromosomes. This phenomenon was better visualized with the aid of high-voltage electron microscopy (HVEM). Depolymerization of these motile structures is sufficient to initiate DNA synthesis. It has been suggested that androgens, and possibly glucocorticoids, are capable of acting in both ways. Thus, the mechanism by which hormones control the cell cycle and mitosis is more complex.

Although the hormones are not critical factors in mitosis—the mitosis can go on without hormones—they can markedly change the duration of cell cycle, and thus the proliferative rate. Since the rapid mitosis remains the hallmark of cancerous cells, the elucidation of mechanisms by which hormones enhance mitosis (mitogenic hormones) or inhibit it are of crucial importance.

Extrapolation of data obtained in in vitro systems, using synchronized cells for the study of the effects of hormones, growth factors, or cytostatic drugs, is not always appropriate, because in vivo cell systems are in different phases of the cell cycle. Although most investigations strongly suggest that the passage or transition of a cell through the cycle goes into four phases, or gaps, other investigations, using statistical methods, suggest a random transition through the cell cycle (51,72). Studies regarding the cell cycle should not be limited only to the four phases or to the passage of a cell from one mitosis to another, which is stricto senso the cell cycle, but should include all biochemical and morphologic phenomena which accompany this passage. Although there are no significant differences between the duration of the cell cycle of normal and cancerous cells, cancerous cells often have a shorter G_1 period and longer G_2 and S periods than those of normal cells (3).

Recently some cell cycle mutants were obtained. Cell lines blocked mostly in G_1 have been isolated. Thus, using a recombinant-DNA form by gene transfer from a methotrexate-resistant cell line into mouse bone marrow cells, it was possible to alter the genotype and make mouse bone marrow cells resistant to methotrexate (11). The implications of these experiments are of great significance. In the future, it will be possible to make normal cells more resistant to the toxic effects of cytostatic agents.

Although the outlines of the cell cycle and its phases have been established, establishing a clearer definition of cell growth and reproduction, still to be determined are the transition from one stage to another and the arrest of the cycle in G_1 or G_2, in order to provide regulation of cell reproduction. It seems likely that the basic mechanism in neoplasia is the abnormal cell growth and reproduction caused by a genetic lesion or defect in the initiation of DNA synthesis (transition G_1–S) and chromosome replication. Since all events of cell reproduction are encompassed in the cell cycle, it was logical to assume that by controlling the phases of the cell cycle, namely the G_1 period, we might regulate cell reproduction. Thus, the major task is to study and determine the genetic and environmental factors that initiate and coordinate the sequences of the cell cycle, as well as the molecular events that accompany its phases, that is, the decision of a cell to enter the cycle and divide again into two daughter cells or to leave the cycle and differentiate, or to enter it only temporarily (in a dormant state for prolonged periods). Early investigations have provided hope that by controlling the G_1 period, or more precisely the transition from G_1 to S, it will be possible to control the cell reproduction in cancer.

Unfortunately not all data obtained from animal models and in vitro studies can be extrapolated to in vivo models. Hence, the cell cycle phases and its controlling factors are not yet understood and well documented in vivo, that is, in human neoplasms, which exhibit a great variability from one to another (4,29,58,79). Most of the data available from the cell cycle analysis in a number of regenerating tissues, as well as in neoplasms, indicate that in addition to genetic factors regulating and modulating the events of the cell cycle, there are environmental factors, especially hormones, growth factors, and nutrients, which can dramatically affect cell reproduction by influencing the cell cycle.

We have to keep in mind that we can control the mitotic cell homeostasis in neoplasia at least in two different ways: (1) by controlling the cycling or dividing cells, and (2) by controlling the temporarily noncycling, dormant, or restrained cells (G_0 period) (3,24,58,61,79). The dormant state represents an important cell reservoir in controlling the homeostasis of tumor cells. The dormant cells can remain in this silent, or quiescent, state for long periods and resume their proliferative capacity by entering the mitotic cycle whenever a stimulus is added (e.g., environmental, hormones, growth factors). Although the dormant state is well documented in tumor animal models, it is only presumed in human cancers, since breast tumors and melanomas can recur and metastasize after a long period of apparent curative treatment of primary tumors. During this quiescent phase, G_0 cells restrain their growth. In addition to hormones and hormonelike substances, other factors (e.g., vascularization, mechanical, and tissue enzymes) can induce the dormancy of cells. It is possible that cells in this state exhibit a reduced transcriptional activity. The deeper the cells are involved in this state (e.g., for several years), the more difficult their rescue. Although the G_0 cells can at any time reenter the cycle and reach S phase, the time it takes to reach S phase is longer than it is for cells in a normal G_1 period. Thus, up to 96 percent of G_0 chick embryo cells become labeled only after a long period (120 hr) of continuous exposure to ^{3}H-thymidine (65). A restriction point between G_0 and S phase was found in some cells; for example, BHK cells can be restricted at this point with caffeine, 5-fluoromacil, and puromycin (57). Also, the sulfated polysaccharides were shown to block the transition from G_0 to S in BHK cells and interferon was shown to suppress the transition from G_0 to S in 3T3 cells (73). Thus, the kinetic and biochemical studies using thymidine and uridine transport suggest only slight qualitative differences between G_0 and G_1 phases; these two quiescent populations are not identical (37). These cells take more time to reach S phase from G_0 period than from their G_1 period; they make different proteins, lack polysomes, have reduced RNA content, and display reduced transport activities (57).

The transition from G_0 state to S phase can be also influenced by cytoskeleton (microfilaments and microtubules), and disrupting agents (colchicine) can block the transition from G_0 to S in chick embryo fibroblasts. Hence, the temporary withdrawal of cells in G_0 stage can be deterministic (genetic and cell environmental factors) or probabilistic. According to the probabilistic cell cycle model, the cell cycle has two states: an A state, which includes G_0 cells and a portion of G_1 phase, and a B phase, which includes S, G_2, and M, and which may include a portion of G_1 phase as well. The transition of a cell from A to B phase is probabilistic and is strongly influenced by the cell type and environmental factors, including hormones. Hence, we still do not know with certainty if the animal cell cycle is a linear sequence of dependent events or whether it consists of relatively independent biochemical events (51,72). Thus, the cell proliferation can be regulated primarily by interruption in G_1 period (G_1 arrest) several hours before the initiation of DNA synthesis or by a reversible shift into G_0 phase. Studies of the factors controlling these phases will be of great significance in understanding the proliferation rate of neoplastic cells. Recruitment of dormant neoplastic cells which are biochemically and antigenically different from normal cells, as well as more drug resistant to the growth fraction of the cell cycle, makes them more vulnerable to both immune and chemotherapeutic agents that act in the S phase (84). There are also drugs, called "protective" drugs, that can shift reversibly and selectively the rapidly proliferating cells of normal tissues (bone marrow, lymph nodes, and intestinal epithelium) into a dormant state and thus protect them from the adverse effects of cytostatic drugs.

Hence, the primary objectives of cancer chemotherapy will be (1) to bring the dormant cells back into the cell cycle and eradicate them with chemotherapeutic drugs, and (2) to reverse the rapidly proliferating normal cells into a dormant state, where they will be protected (by means of protective drugs) from the toxic effects of cytostatic drugs (57,84). Thus, data from animal models suggest that our therapeutic approaches should be designed to either prolong the tumor dormant state or to recruit all dormant cells into the cycle and destroy them. However, the mechanism(s) that regulate and maintain the human neoplastic dormant cells are more complex and are not yet fully understood. The study of factors that can modulate or shift the dormant cells (modulator factors), including hormones, hormonelike substances, and immune factors, will be of crucial significance in attempting a rational approach to cancer chemotherapy.

Recent kinetic studies on tumor cells and drug sensitivity demonstrated that there are cell cycle specific (CCS) drugs and phase-specific drugs in different systems. In large and slow-growing tumors associated with necrosis and a large compartment of dying cells, the use of chemotherapeutic CCS drugs or phase-specific drugs does makes no significant difference; however, in small tumors with a high proliferation rate, cell sensitivity is significantly increased with the use of both CCS or phase-specific drugs, although a prolonged drug level is more effective for phase-specific drugs. Thus, cytostatic chemotherapy is evidently successful in rapidly dividing tumor, where most of the cells are in cycle. Since most of the cytostatic drugs act in the same way on normal rapidly dividing cells (bone marrow, lymph nodes, or intestinal epithelium), and the suppression of bone marrow hematopoiesis is one of the main limitations of intensive treatment with antineoplastic drugs, it is important to enhance their drug resistance. This will be possible using recombinant DNA procedures and gene transfer from drug-resistant cell lines into intact animals. For instance, MTX-resistant cell lines exhibit elevated levels of dihydrofolate reductase (DHFR). MTX exerts its antineoplastic effects by inhibiting this enzyme. It was recently shown that mice receiving bone marrow inoculated with MTX-resistant DNA tolerate high doses of MTX for long periods without toxic effects on bone marrow (11). Recent findings also indicate that S phase is not as rigidly constant (about 7 to 8 hr) as was previously assumed (49), but that it can be influenced by cell environmental factors, such as hormones and hormonelike substances.

In addition to hormones, temperature and nutrients can also affect the S phase. Most light and electron microscopic autoradiographic studies using ^{3}H-thymidine strongly suggest that hormones are potential factors in controlling the cell cycle of normal and neoplastic cells by interfering with DNA synthesis (S phase), and especially the transition G_1–S. The role of hormones on the cell cycle is more complex, however; hormones can also act on operon groups, cell membranes, and presumably on the cytoskeleton. The cell cycle and its linear sequences are primarily determined genetically; nevertheless, environmental cell factors, especially hormones, can markedly influence the cell cycle and its phases.

Kinetic studies have shown that the cell cycle is variable in normal tissues as well as in different tumors. There are no marked differences, however, between the cell cycle of normal cells as compared with that of abnormal cells, as was originally believed. Cells undergo profound ultrastructural, enzymatic, and surface changes during the cycle. Scanning electron microscopy demonstrated that synchronized cells in different phases of the cycle exhibit characteristic features (i.e., microvillous, blebs), making it possible to distinguish among cell cycle phases (60). Although the decision of a cell to enter the cycle is largely determined by genetic factors, it is important to know that such factors as hormones and hormonelike substances (growth factors, prostaglandins, chalones) can markedly influence this decision, as well as the cell's commitment to mitosis. Once a cell enters the cycle, it can still be arrested in G_1 (G_1 arrest) or later in G_2 (G_2 arrest); also, the cell can temporarily withdraw from the cycle and remain in a dormant, silent, or quiescent state for long periods of time. At any time, dormant cells can be stimulated by various factors, including hormones, to reenter the cycle and divide again.

Since cycling cells are more sensitive to anticancer drugs than are noncycling cells, it is important to recruit these cells into a cycle and thus make them more vulnerable to the actions of various drugs. Hence, we can manipulate the mitotic homeostasis of neoplastic cells and significantly improve our therapeutic decisions.

Unfortunately, not all data obtained either in vitro or in animal models can be extrapolated to human cell cycle. The in vitro systems are inadequate tools for the study of in vivo systems because most human neoplasms are composed of a mosaic of cell populations, having different growth fractions. Some cell lines are more rapidly dividing than others. Also, the cell cycle and its phases are slightly different in these cell populations, and the effect of cytostatic drugs will be different in these nonsynchronized cells from in vitro studies.

Perhaps these difficulties will be overcome, and more effective and safe drugs will be available in the future. Recent kinetic cellular studies have also shown that most normal and seemingly malignant cells have only a limited capacity to go into a cycle and proliferate; after dividing a restricted number of times they die. Only a small fraction (10 percent of tumor cells) have an unlimited capacity to enter the cycle and divide; because they are capable of an indefinite number of divisions, these cells are called stem cells, or tumor stem cells. Stem cells are responsible for the renewal and propagation of neoplastic cells (22,26,47).

In summary, the role of hormones and hormonelike substances in controlling the cell cycle and its phases, as well as in modulating tumor cell homeostasis and cancer therapy, is emphasized.

REFERENCES

1. Adamson, R., Banerjee, M., and Medina, D.: Susceptibility of mammary tumor virus free BALB/c mouse mammary nodule outgrowth cells in DNA synthesis to 3-methylcholanthrene tumorigenesis. *J. Natl. Cancer Inst. 46*:899–907 (1971).
2. Baserga, R.: The relationship of the cell cycle to tumor growth and control of cell division: A review. *Cancer Res. 25*:581–591 (1965).
3. Baserga, R.: The cell cycle. *N. Engl. J. Med. 304*:453–459 (1981).
4. Baserga, R., and Kisieleski, E.: Comparative study of the kinetics of cellular proliferation of normal and tumorous tissue with the use of tritiated thymidine I. Dilution of the label and migration of labeled cells. *J. Natl. Cancer Inst. 28*:331–339 (1962).
5. Beato, M., Homoki, J., and Sekeris, C.: On the mechanism of hormone action. *Exp. Cell Res. 55*:107–117 (1969).
6. Bresciani, F., Paoluzi, R., Benassi, M., Nervi, C., Casake, C., and Ziparo, E.: Cell kinetics and growth of squamous cell carcinoma in man. *Cancer Res. 34*: 2405–2415 (1974).

7. Berry, R.: Comparison of effects of some chemotherapeutic agents and those of x-rays on the reproductive capacity of mammalian cells. *Nature 203*:1150–1153 (1964).

8. Bullough, W.: Mitotic and functional homeostasis: A speculating review. *Cancer Res. 25*:1683–1727 (1965).

9. Burki, H., and Tobias, C.: Effect of thyroxine on the cell generation cycle parameters of cultured human cells. *Exp. Cell Res. 60*:445–448 (1970).

10. Cidlowski, J., and Michaels, G.: Alteration in glucocorticoid binding site number during the cell cycle in HeLa cells. *Nature 266*:643–645 (1977).

11. Cline, M., Stang, H., Mercola, K., Morse, L., Rubrecht, R., Browne, G., and Salser, W.: Gene transfer in intact animals. *Nature 284*:422–425 (1980).

12. Covelli, I., Mozzi, R., Rossi, R., and Frati, L.: The mechanism of action of the epidermal growth factor. *Hormones 3*:183–191 (1972).

13. Crossin, K., and Carney, D.: Evidence that microtubule depolymerization early in the cell cycle is sufficient to initiate DNA synthesis. *Cell 23*:61–71 (1981).

14. DeFesi, C., and Surks, M.: 3,5,3′-Triiodothyronine on the growth rate and cell cycle of cultured GC cells. *Endocrinology 108*:259–267 (1981).

15. Edelman, G.: Surface modulation in cell recognition and cell growth. *Science 192*:218–226 (1976).

16. Eide, A.: The effect of estradiol on the cell kinetics in the uterine and cervical epithelium of neonatal mice. *Cell Tissue Kinet. 8*:249–257 (1975).

17. Elgjo, K., Clansen, O., and Thorud, E.: Epidermis extracts (chalone) inhibit cell flux at the G_1–S, S–G_2 and G_2–M transitions in mouse epidermis. *Cell Tissue Kinet. 14*:21–29 (1981).

18. Epifanova, O.: Mitotic cycles in estrogen treated mice: A radioautographic study. *Exp. Cell Res. 42*:562–577 (1966).

19. Epifanova, O.: Effects of hormones on the cell cycle. In Baserga, R. (ed.): *The Cell Cycle and Cancer.* (New York, Dekker, 1971), pp. 143–190.

20. Fatemi, S., Cullan, G., Crouse, D., and Sharp, J.: Relative roles of gastrin and glucagon in the control of intestinal cell proliferation. *In Vitro 13*:685–686 (1980).

21. Frankfurt, O.: Effect of hydrocortisone, adrenalin and actinomycin D on transition of cells to the DNA synthesis phase. *Exp. Cell Res. 52*:222–232 (1968).

22. Gavosto, F., and Pilieri, A.: Cell cycle of cancer cells in man. In Baserga, R. (ed.): *The Cell Cycle and Cancer.* (New York, Dekker, 1971), pp. 99–128.

23. Gelfant, S., and Candelas, C.: Regulation of epidermal mitosis. *J. Invest. Dermatol. 59*:7–12 (1972).

24. Gelfant, S., and Smith, J.: Aging: noncycling cells an explanation. *Science 178*:357–361 (1972).

25. Goldstein, J., Anderson, R., and Brown, M.: Coated pits, coated vesicles and receptor mediated endocytosis. *Nature 279*:679–684 (1979).

26. Hamburger, A., and Salmon, S.: Primary bioassay of human tumor stem cells. *Science 197*:461–463 (1977).

27. Hayashi, I., and Sato, G.: Replacement of serum by hormones permits growth of cells in a defined medium. *Nature 259*:132–134 (1976).

28. Henderson, J., and Loeb, J.: Hormone induced changes in liver DNA synthesis: Effects of glucocorticoids and growth hormone on liver growth and DNA polymerase activity. *Endocrinology 94*:1637–1643 (1974).

29. Hill, B.: Cancer chemotherapy: The relevance of certain concepts of cell cycle kinetics. *Biochem. Biophys. Acta 516*:389–417 (1978).

30. Hornsby, P., and Gill, G.: Hormonal control of adrenocortical cell proliferation: Desensitization to ACTH and interaction between ACTH and fibroblast

growth factor in bovine adrenocortical cell cultures. *J. Clin. Invest. 60*:342–352 (1977).

31. Howard, A., and Pelc, S.: Synthesis of deoxyribonucleic acid in normal and irradiated cells and its relation to chromosome breakage. *Heredity 6*(suppl.): 261–273 (1953).
32. Jacob, F., and Monod, J.: Genetic regulatory mechanisms in the synthesis of proteins. *J. Mol. Biol. 3*:318–356 (1961).
33. Jaspers, N., DeWitt, J., Regulski, M., and Bootsma, D.: Abnormal regulation of DNA replication and increased lethality in ataxia telangiectasia cells exposed to carcinogenic agents. *Cancer Res. 42*:335–341 (1982).
34. Jimenez de Asua, L., Carr, B., Clingan, D., and Rudland, P.: Specific glucocorticoid inhibition of growth promoting effects of prostaglandin $F_{2\alpha}$ on 3T3 cells. *Nature 265*:450–452 (1977).
35. Kalkoff, K., and Born, W.: Zur Wirkung von Fluocinolon acetomid auf die DNA synthese in der Epidermis. *Klin. Wochenschr. 43*:1335–1337 (1965).
36. Kirkland, W., Sorrentino, G., and Sirbasku, D.: Control of cell growth III. Direct mitogenic effect of thyroid hormones on an estrogen dependent rat pituitary tumor cell line. *J. Natl. Cancer Inst. 56*:1159–1164 (1976).
37. Kohn, A.: Differential effects of isoleucine deprivation on cell motility, membrane transport and DNA synthesis in NIL8 hamster cells. *Exp. Cell Res. 94*: 15–22 (1975).
38. Lenk, R., and Pemman, S.: The cytoskeletal framework and polio virus metabolism. *Cell 16*:289–301 (1979).
39. Lewis, D., and Hallowes, R.: Correlation between the effects of hormones on the synthesis of DNA in explants from induced rat mammary tumors and the growth of the tumors. *J. Endocrinol. 62*:225–240 (1974).
40. Lin, F., Banerjee, M., and Crump, L.: Cell cycle related hormone carcinogen interaction during chemical carcinogen induction of nodule like mammary lesions in organ culture. *Cancer Res. 36*:1607–1614 (1976).
41. Lippman, M., and Bolan, G.: Oestrogen responsive human breast cancer in long-term tissue culture. *Nature 256*:592–593 (1975).
42. Loeb, J., Corek, C., and Young, L.: Suppression of DNA synthesis in hepatoma cells exposed to glucocorticoid hormones in vitro. *Proc. Natl. Acad. Sci. (USA) 70*:3852–3856 (1973).
43. Lupulescu, A.: Hormonal regulation of DNA synthesis in cancerous epidermal cells. *J. Cell Biol. 87*:103a (1980).
44. Lupulescu, A.: Enhancement of carcinoma formation by glucagon. *J. Cell Biol. 91*:207a (1981).
45. Lupulescu, A.: Hormonal regulation of epidermal tumor development. *J. Invest. Dermatol. 77*:186–195 (1981).
46. Marquardt, H.: Cell cycle dependence of chemically induced malignant transformation in vitro. *Cancer Res. 34*:1612–1615 (1974).
47. McCullough, E., Siminovitch, L., and Till, J.: Spleen colony formation in anemic mice of genotype WW. *Science 144*:844–846 (1964).
48. McLaughlin, D., Breitkreuz, J., Lipscomb, G., and Sharp, J.: Effect of testosterone and estrogen on DNA synthesis in rat small bowel. *In Vitro 13*:669a (1980).
49. Mitchison, J.: *The Biology of the Cell Cycle.* (New York, Cambridge University Press, 1971), pp. 244–250.
50. Moses, H., Proper, J., Volkenant, M., Wells, D., and Getz, M.: Mechanism of growth arrest of chemically transformed cells in culture. *Cancer Res. 38*: 2807–2812 (1978).

51. Nelson, S., and Green, P.: The random transition model of the cell cycle: A critical review. *Cancer Chemother. Pharmacol.* 6:11–18 (1981).

52. Oka, T., and Topper, Y.: Is prolactin mitogenic for mammary epithelium? *Proc. Natl. Acad. Sci. (USA)* 69:1693–1696 (1972).

53. O'Malley, B.: Hormonal regulation of nucleic acid and protein synthesis. *Trans. NY Acad. Sci.* 31:478–503 (1969).

54. O'Malley, B., and Means, A.: Female steroid hormones and target cell nuclei. *Science* 183:610–620 (1974).

55. Osborne, C., Bolan, G., Monaco, M., and Lippman, M.: Hormone responsive human breast cancer in long term tissue culture. Effect of insulin. *Proc. Natl. Acad. Sci. (USA)* 73:4536–4540 (1976).

56. Ostgaard, K., Wibe, E., Lindmo, T., and Eik-Nes, K.: Effects of steroids and different culture media on cell cycle of the androgen sensitive human cell line NHIK 3025. *J. Cell Sci.* 48:281–290 (1981).

57. Pardee, A., and Dubrow, R.: Control of cell proliferation. *Cancer* 39:2747–2754 (1977).

58. Pardee, A., Dubrow, R., Hamlin, J., and Kletzien, R.: Animal cell cycle. *Annu. Rev. Biochem.* 47:715–750 (1979).

59. Paul, D., Brown, K., Rupmiac, H., and Ristow, J.: Cell cycle regulation by growth factors and nutrients in normal and transformed cells. *In Vitro 14*: 76–84 (1978).

60. Porter, K., Prescott, D., and Frye, J.: Changes in surface morphology of Chinese hamster ovary cells during the cell cycle. *J. Cell Biol.* 57:815–836 (1973).

61. Prescott, D.: The cell cycle and the control of cellular reproduction. *Adv. Genet.* 18:99–177 (1976).

62. Quastler, H., and Sherman, F.: Cell population kinetics in the intestinal epithelium of the mouse. *Exp. Cell Res.* 17:420–438 (1959).

63. Rossini, M., Baserga, S., Huang, C., Ingles, J., and Baserga, R.: Changes in RNA polymerase II in a cell cycle specific temperature sensitive mutant of hamster cells. *J. Cell Physiol.* 103:97–103 (1980).

64. Rothstein, H. VanWyk, J., Hayden, J., Gordon, S., and Weinsieder, A.: Somatomedin C: Restoration in vivo of cycle traverse in G_0/G_1 blocked cells of hypophysectomized animals. *Science 208*:410–412 (1980).

65. Rubin, H., and Steiner, R.: Reversible alterations in the mitotic cycle of chick embryo cells in various states of growth regulation. *J. Cell. Physiol.* 85:261–270 (1975).

66. Rudland, P., Hallowes, R., Durbin, H., and Lewis, D.: Mitogenic activity of pituitary hormones on cell cultures of normal and carginogen-induced tumor epithelium from rat mammary glands. *J. Cell Biol.* 73:561–577 (1977).

67. Saez, J., Morera, M., and Gallet, D.: In vivo opposite effects of ACTH and glucocorticoids on adrenal DNA synthesis. *Endocrinology 100*:1268–1275 (1977).

68. Schiaffonati, L., and Baserga, R.: Different survival of normal and transformed cells exposed to nutritional conditions nonpermissive for growth. *Cancer Res.* 37:541–545 (1977).

69. Schwartz, J., Viaje, A., Slaga, T., Yuspa, S., Hennings, H., and Lichti, U.: Fluocinolone acetonide: A potent inhibitor of mouse skin tumor promotion and epidermal DNA synthesis. *Chem. Biol. Interact.* 17:331–347 (1977).

70. Shimizu, N., Shimizu, Y., and Fuller, B.: Cell cycle analysis of insulin binding and internalization on mouse melanoma cells. *J. Cell Biol.* 88:241–244 (1981).

71. Sirbasku, D.: Estrogen induction of growth factors specific for hormone-respon-

sive mammary, pituitary and kidney tumor cells. *Proc. Natl. Acad. Sci. (USA)* 75:3786–3790 (1978).

72. Smith, J., and Martin, L.: Do cells cycle? *Proc. Natl. Acad. Sci. (USA)* 70:1263–1267 (1973).

73. Sokowa, Y., Watanabe, Y., Watanabe, Y., and Kawade, Y.: Interferon suppresses the transition of quiescent 3T3 cells to a growing state. *Nature* 268:236–238 (1977).

74. Soprano, K., Rossini, M., Croce, C., and Baserga, R.: The role of large T antigen in simian virus 40 induced reactivation of silent RNA genes in human-mouse hybrid cells. *Virology* 102:317–326 (1980).

75. Stevens, J., and Stevens, Y.: Cortisol (F) induced loss of tumor lymphocyte cell membrane integrity. *Proc. Am. Assoc. Cancer Res.* 18:710a (1977).

76. Story, M., and Melynkovych, G: Growth inhibition of mouse lymphoma cells, L5178Y, in vitro, by glucocorticoids. *Exp. Cell Res.* 77:437–449 (1973).

77. Suzuki, N., Frapart, M., Gardina, D., Meistrich, M., and Withers, H.: Cell cycle dependency of metastatic lung colony formation. *Cancer Res.* 37:3690–3693 (1977).

78. Tomkins, G., and Martin, D.: Hormones and gene expression. *Annu. Rev. Genet.* 4:91–106 (1970).

79. Tormey, D.: The cell cycle. In Bergevin, P., Blom, J., and Tormey, D. (eds.): *Guide to Therapeutic Oncology.* (Baltimore, Williams & Wilkins, 1979), pp. 80–82.

80. Turkington, R.: Induction of milk protein synthesis by placental lactogen and prolactin in vitro. *Endocrinology* 82:575–583 (1968).

81. VanPutten, L.: Cell cycle specificity of anticancer agents. *Antibiot. Chemother.* 23:128–134 (1978).

82. Warwick, G.: Effect of the cell cycle on carcinogenesis. *Fed. Proc.* 30:1760–1765 (1971).

83. Welsch, C., DeIturri, G., and Brennan, M.: DNA synthesis of human, mouse and rat mammary carcinoma in vitro. *Cancer* 38:1272–1281 (1976).

84. Wheelock, E., Weinhold, K., and Livich, J.: The tumor dormant state. In Klein, G., and Weinhouse, S. (eds.): *Advances in Cancer Research*, vol. 34. (New York, Academic Press, 1981), pp. 107–140.

Chapter 3

HORMONAL REGULATION OF PRECANCEROUS AND CANCEROUS CELL POPULATIONS

Evidence in recent years has mounted offering strong support to the concept of tumor progression (26). According to this concept, a neoplastic, or cancerous cell always starts out as a normal cell that, under the influence of various oncogenic or carcinogenic agents—chemical, viral, physical, or hormonal—undergoes a series of progressive changes. This transformation is depicted in Figure 3–1.

The cellular changes that occur during carcinogenesis are called neoplastic transformation and illustrate several changes in cellular differentiation. A cancer cell is an altered phenotype that expresses certain properties from those of the normal cell from which it evolved. Cancer appears to be a disease of cellular differentiation. In a tissue exposed to a carcinogen, whether chemical, viral, or physical, initiating changes can take place at the genome level by altering DNA synthesis and DNA repair mechanisms; later, tumor progression primarily results from the effect of cocarcinogens and tumor promoters. Most of these agents are hormones or hormone mimetic agents that enhance random gene expression and the production of multiple cell phenotypes, among them the phenotype associated with the development of cancer.

A precancerous cell is thus an intermediate, obligatory stage between the normal cell and cancerous, or malignant, cell (Fig. 3–2).

Hence, an initiating carcinogen induces different cellular alterations in a

46

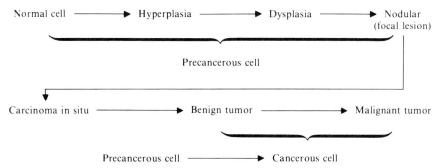

Figure 3-1 Cellular evolution and tumor progression from normal cell, to precancerous cell, to cancer cell.

normal cell population. Some of these cells exhibit distinct structural, autoradiographic, antigenic, and cell surface changes as compared with those of the normal cells from which they derive; consequently, these cells have a putative carcinogenic potential for progressing toward transformation into cancerous, or malignant, cells. These cells are precancerous, premalignant, or preneoplastic, depending on the final stage—neoplasm, malignant tumor, or cancer. However, the morphological variations in cellular differentiation from normal cells represent only minor variations at the level of transcription of the genome. Although after initiation, cellular changes take place at the DNA level, mostly in nonreplicating DNA material, the cell carries miscoded information, yet remains an unexpressed phenotype for several years. In order for the cell to express an altered phenotype, a promoter has to act on it, inducing morphological alterations, mainly at the post-transcriptional translation stage. By increasing the opportunity to express any previously altered information induced by initiating carcinogen, and also by increasing the rate of mitosis, promoters increase the opportunity for abnormal phenotypic expression. Thus, hormones can have an important role in the early stage of expression of an altered phenotype, explaining the occurrence of preneoplastic cells (32). These intially altered cells have the ability to form a focal area of proliferation, subsequently acquiring a certain degree of autonomy in their growth.

After induction, preneoplastic cells can be selected by an appropriate environment in which to proliferate. It has been also suggested that preneoplastic cells are already present in the target tissue and that the carcinogens are not induced altered cells, but rather encourage the selection of already altered cells (73). However, this argument does not seem likely, since a promoter cannot induce neoplastic transformation in the absence of initiation

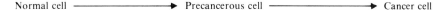

Figure 3-2 Transformation of normal cell into cancerous cell.

by a carcinogen. Thus, preneoplastic cells are primarily initiated cells and phenotypically altered cells, not selected abnormal cells. Most information regarding the characteristics and behavior of precancerous cells derives from studies on skin carcinogenesis and liver carcinogenesis. Mammary carcinogenesis and thyroid carcinogenesis have provided interesting data regarding precancerous lesions or carcinoma in situ.

Numerous studies from this and other laboratories have provided data indicating an ultrastructural, autoradiographical, and antigenic relationship of precancerous cells from epidermis, liver, thyroid, and mammary gland to cancerous or malignant cells in these target tissues (23,45,58,76). Thus, the development of cancer in skin, liver, thyroid, and mammary gland is a stepwise process involving recognizable precancerous lesions, as in carcinoma in situ, Bowen's disease, nodular hyperplastic lesions in liver and thyroid, and precancerous mastopathy (13). The progression of precancerous mastopathy toward an invasive mammary carcinoma—or transformation of precancerous cells into cancer cells—is largely determined by hormonal, immunological, and genetic factors (13).

Early detection of precancerous or premalignant lesions is of great importance for cancer prophylaxis and therapy. Studies of precancerous cells are only beginning to be undertaken; results thus far are mainly from animal cancers, which are easier to investigate during the early stages, whereas later stages (i.e., cancerous cells) are chiefly investigated in human cancers.

Although hormones and hormonelike substances (hormonoids) are known to have a profound effect on cell growth and differentiation, we lack convincing evidence that hormones are able to induce normal cells into becoming neoplastic cells directly through neoplastic transformation (51,57). Although hormones can sometimes be considered carcinogenic or oncogenic per se, prolonged exposure to hormones markedly increases the progression of precancerous cells toward becoming cancerous or malignant cells. It is still uncertain as to whether precancerous cells move obligatorily toward the state of cancer cells or whether they can remain for years as an independent cell population whose neoplastic transformation can later be triggered by various oncogenic or environmental factors, including hormones. Thus, a hormonal environment, or hormonal milieu, is required for the development of both precancerous and cancerous cells. Behavior and cell biology can be significantly influenced and their ratio changed by various hormonal treatments.

Several studies, including ours, using electron microscopic high-resolution autoradiography and SEM, have shown, however, that precancerous and cancerous cells are heterogeneous cell populations displaying different behavior and hormone responsiveness. Not all precancerous cells exhibit the same putative carcinogenic potential and presumably undergo neoplastic transformation. Some can remain precancerous cells for several years. Even after a long time, hormones can stimulate this pool of precancerous cells and convert it into cancerous cells.

The factors that have the ability to accelerate or restrain the progression of precancerous cells toward cancerous or malignant cells are still poorly understood. However, electron microscopic observation of nodular, or focal, lesions in thyroid, epidermis, and liver has shown that they contain a mixed cell population of both precancerous and cancerous cells. It is known that liver or epidermal tumors can occur from one cell or from just a few cells; our task is to detect these few precancerous cells from the surrounding noninvolved or normal-appearing cells. A cancerous cell is a new and different cell as compared with the normal cell from which it is derived; it displays a great lack of control (76).

Neoplastic transformation is a complex phenomenon accompanied by changes in almost all cell organelles. Ultimately in a normal cell the basic functions are coordinated and controlled according to the sequence depicted in Figure 3–3.

Cancerous and precancerous cells manifest several specific defects in control mechanisms reflected in their structure and ultrastructure; antigenic capacity; enzymatic activity; hormone responsiveness; and autoradiographic patterns, including those of DNA, RNA, and protein synthesis, as well as cell surface and membrane biogenesis.

Although it is known that cancerous cells develop from precancerous cells, the progression is an unpredictable process that cannot be determined on the basis of morphological appearance alone. The period required for the progression of precancerous toward cancerous cells is variable, from a few months to many years. Virtually nothing is known about the biological behavior, the molecular mechanisms, and factors governing the capricious behavior of precancerous cells.

Further research is needed in order to identify and classify precancerous cells, their cell biology, morphological characteristics, and the controlling factors of their progression toward the cancerous state (32,45). Experimental and clinical investigations demonstrate that a large proportion of precancerous lesions (e.g., carcinoma in situ) never develop into overt neoplasia. This evidence strongly suggests that neoplastic transformation can be restrained and maintained in a precancerous state for a long period of time, thereby holding new hope for the prevention and treatment of cancer. Identification of precancerous cells and elucidation of those factors that might control and restrain the progression of precancerous cell toward neoplastic cells are of crucial importance in understanding carcinogenesis, hence its prevention and treatment.

Research from this laboratory as well as from others suggests that hormones and hormonomimetic agents (hormonelike substances) are impor-

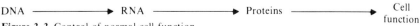

DNA ⟶ RNA ⟶ Proteins ⟶ Cell function

Figure 3-3 Control of normal cell function.

tant homeostatic factors in controlling cell growth and proliferation. This study deals with the role of hormones as factors (57,61) that can accelerate or restrain the induction of precancerous cells and their transformation into cancerous cells.

WHAT IS A PRECANCEROUS CELL?

As a generalization, a precancerous cell is a new cell—an altered or transformed cell—as compared with the normal cell from which it was derived. A precancerous cell can be more appropriately defined as a transitional or intermediary stage between a normal and cancerous cell. It is also an obligatory stage in neoplastic transformation. There is no convincing evidence that cancerous cells directly emerge from normal cells. Furthermore, there is enough evidence from this laboratory and others, using ultrastructural, autoradiographic, and cell surface studies, to suggest that a normal cell population, when exposed to an initiating carcinogen (mostly chemical carcinogens) undergoes a progressive transformation exhibiting alterations in almost all its cell organelles, enzymes, antigens, membrane biogenesis, and ability to incorporate amino acids in synthesizing new DNA, RNA, and proteins. However, the cellular alterations occur to a much lesser degree as compared with those seen in cancer cells, making it difficult to identify these cells in a mixed cell population.

It is likely that when a carcinogen acts on a normal cell population, only few precancerous cells are produced; earlier cellular changes are detected only with great difficulty. It would appear that all precancerous cells originate from normal cells (Fig. 3-4).

Precancerous cells are therefore induced or transformed by an initiating chemical or hormonal carcinogen. Personally, I am not convinced that precancerous cells are already present in a normal cell population or that carcinogens (or oncogens) act mainly by selecting the precancerous cells, instead of initiating them as Prehn suggested (73).

If precancerous cells are only selected cells, and the selection hypothesis is correct, the promoters that specifically act on precancerous cells, transforming them into cancerous cells, would have to induce neoplasms in the absence of initiating carcinogens—which of course is not the case. Although precancerous cells do originate in the surrounding normal cells, their transformation into cancerous cells is not obligatory, as they can remain precancerous cells for months or even years (32,45). Electron microscopic, autoradiographic, and SEM observations of the early stages of hepatocarcinogenesis, epidermal carcinogenesis, and thyroid carcinogenesis show

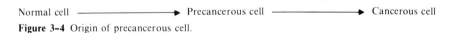

Normal cell ⟶ Precancerous cell ⟶ Cancerous cell

Figure 3-4 Origin of precancerous cell.

precancerous cells to be heterogeneous cell populations, exhibiting different degrees of hormone responsiveness, antigenicity, and a variable putative carcinogenic potential. Recent studies of precancerous hepatocytes obtained from hepatic nodules induced in rats by the carcinogen 2-acetylaminofluorene (AAF) demonstrated significant and progressive DNA damages. DNA damages of precancerous hepatocytes from focal lesions progressed in the absence of any carcinogen, suggesting that DNA damages initiated by a carcinogen are irreversible (78). Histological observations of focal or nodular hepatic lesions showed at least four different cell populations, that is, hypoplastic or enzyme-deficient areas; early hyperplastic nodules; late hyperplastic nodules (neoplastic nodules), and hyperbasophilic foci (23). Similar focal lesions (papillomas) were observed in skin carcinogenesis. Most nodular lesions from liver and mouse epidermis mature and regress, with only a few persisting and becoming neoplasms. Histochemical analysis of these liver hyperplastic nodules shows various enzymic and metabolic alterations of the precancerous hepatocytes, such as increased γ-glutamyltranspeptidase activity (γGT), a decrease of glucose 6-phosphatase (G6P), nucleotide polyphosphatase, β-glucoronidase, glycogen phosphorylase, and ATPase activities.

Other alterations include secretion of α-fetoprotein, altered nucleic acid metabolism, decreased iron uptake or metabolism, decreased breakdown of glycogen, and disturbances in cell mitosis. Thus, the metabolic control mechanisms are defective in precancerous liver cell (19,76). These enzymic alterations also indicate that liver nodules are composed of mixed or heterogeneous precancerous cell populations, so that only a few nodules present one enzyme alteration and a single nodule can have a mixed cellular population. The histochemical procedures are accurate enough to permit distinction of precancerous cells from the surrounding normal hepatocytes.

Precancerous cells grow more easily in tissue culture than in vivo. Carcinogenesis is a multisequential or multistage process and precancerous cells are an intermediate stage.

Experimental observations show that many papillomas, hyperplastic liver nodules, or hyperplastic alveolar mammary nodules, composed predominantly of precancerous or preneoplastic cells, can regress and return to a normal morphology. Preneoplastic cells have at least three choices, that is, to progress toward cancerous cells; to regress to normal cells; or to remain for several months or years in this stage as latent tumor cells (see Fig. 3–5).

These choices are largely dependent on genetic, immunological, and mainly environmental factors, especially hormones, hormonomimetic agents, growth factors, chalones, and nutrients. The most detailed studies regarding structural morphology, membrane biogenesis, and DNA metabolism of preneoplastic cell populations were carried out on the liver, mammary gland, tracheobronchial epithelium, and skin. Considerable experimental evidence shows that neoplastic transformation from a normal cell to a precancerous

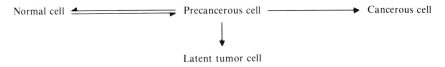

Figure 3-5 Transformation of normal cell into precancerous and cancerous cell.

cell, and later to a neoplastic or cancerous cell, is accompanied by a sequential series of cellular changes involving nearly every cell organelle. Most of these early changes are similar in different experimental models as well as in clinical observations.

The earliest changes observed in preneoplastic liver cells are called focal alterations. Light microscopy shows these foci to be clear, eosinophilic, or basophilic. Their cytoplasm, nuclei, cell membranes, enzymatic activity, and DNA metabolism are different from those of the surrounding hepatocytes. Nevertheless, these changes are only minimal, exhibiting minimal deviation. Later, they evolve into such hyperplastic nodules as carcinoma in situ and invasive anaplastic neoplasms composed entirely of cancerous or malignant cells.

Ultrastructural studies demonstrate that preneoplastic hepatocytes occurring during DAB (diazoaminobenzen) hepatocarcinogenesis in hyperbasophilic foci are heterogeneous cells. At least two different types, dark and clear cells, can be seen. The dark cells exhibit an ultrastructural pattern similar to that of normal hepatocytes, while the clear cells exhibit a different ultrastructural pattern, close to that of benign liver tumors or hepatomas. They are poorly differentiated cells, with increased smooth endoplasmic reticulum (SER) and increased polysomal populations. Other specific organelles, such as microbodies, biliary canaliculi, and glycogen granules, are greatly decreased or even absent. Mitochondrial alterations are also observed with blurred mitochondrial cristae and intramitochondrial granules. In addition, nuclear alterations are frequent, accompanied by nuclear hypertrophy, an irregular nuclear envelope, clumping of nuclear chromatin, increased mitotic figures, a high nuclear/cytoplasmic ratio, and prominent nucleoli. Cells are usually separated by widened intercellular spaces, with few microvilli and the appearance of bundles of pericanalicular microfilaments (38). Scanning electron microscopic observations also exhibit interesting cell surface changes in preneoplastic cells different from those of normal cells and cancerous cells. In early or focal alterations, membrane changes are minimal and close to those of normal hepatocytes. Some dilatation of microvilli and a few blebs are also observed (81).

Alterations of the intracellular membrane system and cell surface membrane are frequently observed in preneoplastic cells, but display great variability. This variability can be explained by the fact that most early nodules or foci regress toward a normal cell morphology, while only a few evolve toward neoplasms. It will be interesting to study preneoplastic cells, namely those arising from these resistant nodules that will undergo neoplastic transformation. Ultrastructural and SEM characteristics of preneoplastic cells vary greatly from those of minimally altered to those close to neoplastic cells or poorly differentiated cells, thereby reflecting the heterogeneity of the precancerous cell population.

Through the use of transmission electron microscopy (TEM) and SEM, we can detect and identify not only different cell types, but different subtypes of precancerous and cancerous cells and the initial lesions at the epidermal-dermal junction as well, especially those of basal lamina. Early cell surface changes were observed by TEM and SEM on the preneoplastic cells from premalignant nodular epidermal hyperplasia induced by chemical carcinogens, such as 3-methylcholanthrene (MCA), 7, 12-dimethylbenzanthracene (DMBA),or hormones. Characteristic features, such as the occurrence of numerous microvilli, elongated or club shaped, and blebs, as well as cell extension, can be seen in mouse epidermal preneoplastic cells (Fig. 3–6). Similar SEM observations regarding skin carcinogenesis and cocarcinogenesis were also recently made in mice treated with tetradecanoylphorbol acetate (TPA). Chemical carcinogens (DMBA) and a tumor promoter (TPA) show distinctive and progressive cell surface changes more distinctly at basal membrane

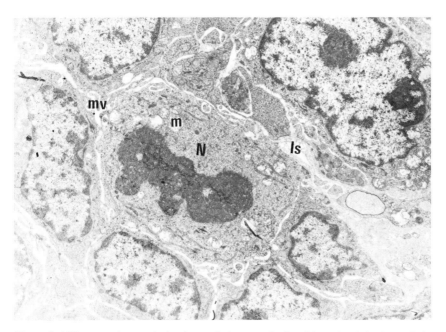

Figure 3-6 Electron micrograph showing typical preneoplastic epidermal nodular hyperplasia. Nuclear (N) changes include mitosis, microvilli (mv), and swollen mitochondria (m). Is, enlarged intercellular spaces. Epon section, uranyl acetate and lead citrate stain. (× 11,000.)

(basal lamina). A marked disintegration of basal lamina is frequently observed, in mice treated with both DMBA and TPA, whereas these changes are reversible in TPA-treated mice only (43).

Autoradiographic studies using ^{3}H-thymidine show that only poorly differentiated hepatocytes or clear cells exhibit a higher ^{3}H-thymidine incorporation, appear as labeled cells, and are rapidly proliferating cells; the others (i.e., dark cells) do not incorporate ^{3}H-thymidine and are not labeled.

Most recent studies indicate that development of hepatocarcinoma (hepatocarcinogenesis) is a multistep process (23,38,76) in which ultrastructural and enzymatic deficiencies occur. Hyperplastic hepatocytes display abundant SER and enzymatic alterations, suggesting a specific irreversible change responsible for malignant transformation. Sequential steps are described as occurring after partial hepatectomy and exposure to a single dose of diethylnitrosamine (DENA). After 2 months, islands or altered foci are detected. These islands grow, forming hyperplastic nodules by 9 months; after 12 to 15 months, these nodules evolve into hepatocarcinomas in rats. Hepatocytes from these hyperplastic nodules from normal surrounding area and from hepatocarcinomas were tested in vitro for their invasiveness, providing a good marker for malignancy.

Hepatocytes from hyperplastic nodules show progressive invasion in the same manner shown by hepatocarcinoma cells in vitro. Control (normal) hepatocytes show no invasion. Therefore, only the cells from these nodules are precancerous cells and must be considered malignant altered hepatocytes (86). These cells display the characteristics of preneoplastic cells, as shown by ultrastructural, cell surface, and autoradiographic studies, distinguishing them from normal cells and neoplastic cells. Preneoplastic hepatocytes are also different from embryonic liver or regenerating liver cells (postpartial hepatectomy).

Similar ultrastructural changes have been seen in tracheobronchial epithelium, mammary gland, and epidermis after exposure to carcinogens. In tracheobronchial epithelium of both humans and experimental animals, the lesions progress from goblet cell hyperplasia to epidermoid metaplasia, carcinoma in situ, and invasive neoplasm. Some of these early metaplastic or dysplastic changes are reversible. As the preneoplastic cell population evolves, a defective activity on the occurrence of carcinoembryonic antigen (CEA) accompanies this event.

No convincing evidence has been accumulated regarding either the role of the cytoskeleton or the number of microtubules in preneoplastic versus neoplastic cells. Thus, some workers (66) have concluded that the number of microtubules is reduced in preneoplastic and neoplastic cells, whereas others (82) have found no significant differences between the population and organization of microtubules of normal and preneoplastic and neoplastic cells. However, alterations in one (tubulin) or more components of the cytoskeleton can adversely affect cell shape, membrane mobility, and cell–cell adhesion and play an important role in preneoplastic and neoplastic cell behavior.

Important observations regarding the cell biology and behavior of preneoplastic cells have been made from the study of preneoplastic cells in mammary tumorigenesis. For example, a sequential expression of preneoplastic and neoplastic mouse mammary epithelial cells was observed in organ culture. Two characteristic preneoplastic lesions were mainly described in DMBA-induced mouse tumorigenesis: hyperplastic alveolar nodules (HAN), and nodulelike alveolar lesion(s) (NLAL). HAN, a type of mammary epithelial cell dysplasia, is composed primarily of preneoplastic cells that exhibit a variety of altered physiological and biochemical characteristics, such as deviation from normal hormone-mediated growth regulation and potential for indefinite cell proliferation. Also, transplantation studies have established that mammary tumors appear more frequently in HAN than in outgrowth from normal mammary tissue (63). Thus, both NLAL induced by DMBA in the mammary gland in vitro and HAN in the mammary gland in vivo are analogous, containing preneoplastic cells of high neoplastic potential. The hyperplastic outgrowth produced by the explants of dissociated cells are derived from nonapparent preneoplastic cells (37). Expression of nonapparent preneoplastic cells has also been observed after transplantation of dissociated cells from virus-induced mammary tumors in BALB/CH₃H mice.

Hormones enhance expression of preneoplastic cells and their progression toward neoplastic cells by mitogenic stimulation.

Observations in dogs and humans on mammary tumorigenesis as well as in other organs, such as liver and skin indicate that neoplastic transformation is the consequence of a multistep sequential transformation of epithelial cells into neoplasms. It is possible that preneoplastic cells from these hyperplastic nodules evolve by some unknown mechanism(s) into neoplastic cells or that both preneoplastic and neoplastic cells coexist in the initial lesion, with the neoplastic cells eliciting a delayed expression (Fig. 3–7).

Interesting findings regarding the DNA polymerase activity and DNA synthesis in preneoplastic cells from nodular lesions (nodular outgrowths) of BALB/c and C₃H mouse mammary gland have also been reported. Unlike normal mouse mammary cells, both DNA polymerase activity and DNA synthesis in the preneoplastic cells are independent of ovarian hormones. The HAN outgrowth lines of both BALB/c and C₃H mice exhibit altered

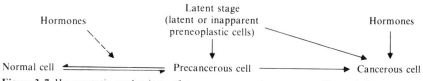

Figure 3-7 Homeostatic mechanisms of precancerous and cancerous cell populations.

responsiveness to normal regulation of DNA polymerase and DNA synthetic activities (9). Thus, mouse mammary carcinogenesis is characterized by a defined precancer precursor, HAN. The characteristic lobuloalveolar structures and the histology of HAN are virtually indistinguishable from normal mammary tissue of pregnancy. After serial transplantations into virgin hosts, HAN produces the same hyperactive lobuloalveolar pattern, indicating an irreversible altered responsiveness of preneoplastic HAN cells to hormonal regulation (8).

Generally, the term preneoplastic applies to cells that are more likely to give rise to neoplasms. The tumorigenic potential of preneoplastic cells from HAN induced by DMBA is more expressed, becoming evident after several transplantation generations. However, transplantation of a mixture of normal mammary epithelial cells and preneoplastic cells obtained from HAN delays the progression of preneoplastic cells and thereby the occurrence of neoplastic cells.

Preneoplastic mammary cells transplanted into virgin hosts exhibit a very low tumorigenic potential, whereas hormonally stimulated virgin hosts display a very high tumorigenic potential.

Thus, hormonal stimulation during the first generation enhances the expression of latent precancerous cells (Fig. 3–7). The role of hormones in the homeostatic mechanism(s) of preneoplastic and neoplastic cells is discussed in greater detail later in this chapter under endocrine regulation.

Another important procedure in distinguishing between the precancerous and cancerous mammary cell population is that of in vitro cytochalasin B-induced multinucleation.

In spite of recent studes concerning the cell surface and surface-related properties, which demonstrated no difference in lectin agglutinability (5), drug-induced modulation of lectin agglutinability (6), and cytoskeletal patterns of microtubules and actin-containing filaments, administration of cytochalasin-B in mammary epithelial cells in vitro is an accurate assay. Cytochalasin B was shown to induce multinucleation in epithelial cells in vitro. Cytochalasin B administration, 1 μg/ml for 48 hours showed the percentage of multinucleated cells to be 5 percent in normal mammary cells, 4 percent in precancerous mammary cells, 36 percent in primary mammary tumor cells, 70 percent in transplanted mammary tumor cells, 80 percent in carcinogenic established cell lines, and 5 percent in nontumorigenic established cell lines. The frequency of multinucleated neoplastic cells increased with serial transplantations in vivo and with several passages in vitro.

These results suggest that only cancerous or neoplastic cells within a primary tumor exhibit an uncontrolled nuclear division, whereas precancerous cells do not (64). This test is more accurate in distinguishing between precancerous and cancerous cell populations, is quick, easy, inexpensive, and reproducible, and can be correlated with in vivo carcinogenicity. Precancerous cells clearly behave differently than cancerous cells. Considerable data regarding the cell biology and behavior of precancerous cells were also obtained during the past 10 to 15 years from the studies of epidermal carcinogenesis in rodents or humans (59–61,74,90). Precancerous cells in animal and human epidermis have been studies mainly by light microscopic and biochemical procedures.

Few ultrastructural studies have been performed on mouse epidermis (74), rat epidermis (60), hamster cheek pouch (88), human cornea (80), and human epidermis (59). These studies reveal incipient cellular changes undetectable with the light microscope. Ultrastructural changes in preneo-plastic cells of mouse epidermis treated with a promoter agent (TPA) rather than a carcinogen show an increased number of polysomes, enlarged intercellular spaces, and occurrence of atypical dark cells accompanied by DNA, RNA, and protein synthesis (74).

Epithelial pseudopodia and enlarged intercellular spaces have also been described in chemically induced premalignant lesions in the hamster cheek pouch, but they disappear during the final phase of cancer development (88). Inasmuch as rat epidermis exposed to chemical carcinogens develops a great variety of neoplasms closely resembling those of human skin, we have studied the ultrastructural changes of epidermal cells both before (preneoplastic cells) and after the development of visible tumors (neoplastic cells) in order to elucidate the key question: Does cancer originate abruptly in a normal cellular surroundings, or by a progressive, stepwise process?

Our studies on rat epidermis exposed for several months to the chemical carcinogen 3-MCA showed some ultrastructural changes similar to those found in fully developed tumors, such as an increased number of free ribosomes (or polysomes), dilated and tubular rough endoplasmic reticulum (RER), several swollen mitochondria with disrupted cristae, irregular distri-bution and condensation (clumping) of tonofilaments, and hypertrophic nuclei with prominent nucleoli (Fig. 3–8). The finding of atypical electron-dense dark cells similar to those found in mouse epidermis after exposure to a tumor promoter (74) or in spontaneous human corneal precancer (80) indicates that these cells are only phenotypically different from their neighbors, the (light cells). Dark cells contain a granular material, increased polysome populations, condensed RER, and more mitochondria and tono-filaments as compared with the light cells. Although their origin is unknown, they have been found in a variety of premalignant lesions (precancerous rat liver) (38) and thyroid nodules (58), but they have not been found in normal epidermis.

Another striking ultrastructural feature, that of markedly dilated intercellular spaces with increased number of microvilli and disrupted desmosomes (Fig. 3–9), indicates an increased cellular mobility caused by a loss of cohesion, described earlier (18). The basal lamina is intact in most instances, also indicating a preneoplastic stage (60). Ultrastructural observa-tions of initiated epidermal cells (induced by application of a single dose of

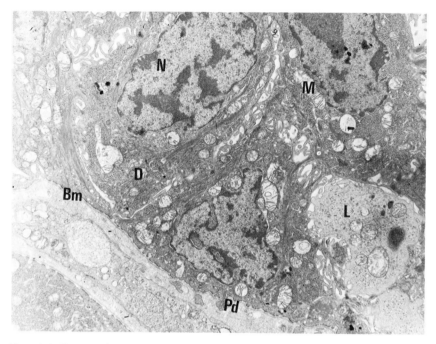

Figure 3–8 Electron micrograph showing precancerous dark (D) and light (L) cells in mouse skin exposed to chemical carcinogen (MCA). Nuclear (N) changes, several mitochondria (M), and pseudopodia (Pd) through basement membrane (Bm). Epon section, uranyl acetate and lead citrate stain, × 11,000.

3-MCA on mouse dorsal skin) also show the presence of dark cells, cellular hypertrophy, enlarged nuclei with prominent nucleoli, and widened intercellular spaces. The ultrastructural changes of these precancerous epidermal cells are accompanied by a moderate increase in DNA, RNA, and protein synthesis (61).

Ultrastructural studies of human precancerous cells in various premalignant conditions show interesting findings similar to those described in animal models. Ultrastructural studies in Bowen's disease (a precancer or carcinoma in situ) show advanced dyskeratosis, acantholysis attributable to dissolution of desmosomal tonofilament complexes, hypertrophied nuclei and nucleoli, increased polysome populations, mitochondrial alterations, and few nuclear inclusions (Fig. 3–10). The basement membrane remains intact. Occasionally atypical cells are seen undergoing cytolysis and are engulfed and phagocytized by neighboring cells, a process called apoptosis (40). Ultrastructural alterations of these human preneoplastic cells are accompanied by changes in DNA and protein synthesis (59).

The ultrastructural, autoradiographic, SEM, and biochemical findings strongly suggest several possibilities. First, early changes of preneoplastic cells

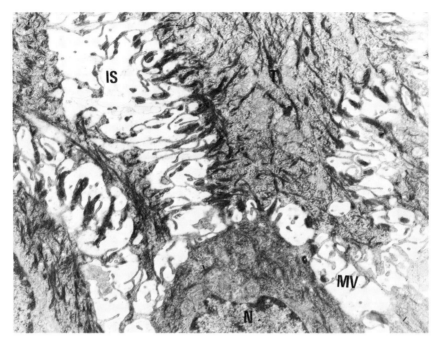

Figure 3-9 Preneoplastic cells from rat skin exposed to chemical carcinogen (MCA) separated by markedly enlarged intercellular spaces (IS) with microvilli (Mv). T, clumped tonofilaments; N, hypertrophied nuclei. Epon, uranyl acetate, and lead citrate, × 11,000.

occurring in animal precancers are similar to those occurring in human precancers or carcinoma in situ; they are also similar in several organs (liver, thyroid, epidermis). Second, the ultrastructural changes are rather variable in preneoplastic cells, ranging from minimal or close-to-normal cells to marked or closed to that of cancerous cells, strongly suggesting that precancerous cells are heterogeneous cell populations of different biology and behavior. Third, ultrastructural changes are always accompanied by changes in DNA, RNA, and protein synthesis. Fourth, these findings support the concept that neoplastic transformation results from progressive changes from normal to hyperplastic, carcinoma in situ (precancer), and fully malignant neoplasm (cancer). Thus carcinogenesis is accomplished by progressive cellular changes or cellular evolution; it is not a rapid process.

Hence, much of our present knowledge regarding the precancerous cell and cancerous cell populations comes from studies on epidermal carcinogenesis, the prototypical model of chemical carcinogenesis in human subjects and experimental animals during the past two to three decades.

The DNA distribution pattern is variable in preneoplastic cells of various organs, (such as the stomach and cervix uteri). In both stomach and cervix uterus normal cells, the DNA distribution is the same as would be expected for

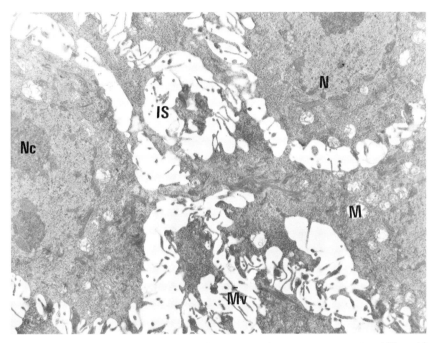

Figure 3–10 Precancer cells from human skin (Bowen's disease). Advanced cell mobility, with enlarged intercellular spaces (IS), microvilli (Mv), and many mitochondria (M). N, hypertrophied nuclei; Nc, nucleoli. Epon section, uranyl acetate and lead citrate, × 11,000.

a normal cell population. In chronic atrophic gastritis (a precancerous condition), however, the DNA distribution pattern is distinct and smaller, indicating a lower risk of chronic atrophic gastritis as compared with higher-risk or preneoplastic lesions of the cervix uteri for malignancy. Only in few cases is there a risk of preneoplastic cells of gastric mucosa converting into malignant or cancerous cells, as compared with the preneoplastic cells of carcinoma in situ of cervix uteri (87). Similar studies regarding nuclear DNA and the number of Barr bodies (sex chromatin positive cells) in premalignant and malignant lesions of the uterine cervix were also conducted. Recent research in cytogenetics and DNA synthesis demonstrates that the transition from mild to severe dysplasia is accompanied by increased DNA synthesis. The incidence of double Barr bodies was increased in cases of dysplasia, carcinoma in situ, and invasive carcinoma. Correlated with this, the DNA histograms show a decrease in the diploid mode and an increase in the tetraploid mode in those cells. Most cases showing an excessive increase in nonspecific chromatin were early invasive carcinoma of the cervix.

Thus, the content of nuclear DNA and the number of Barr bodies can be used as an accurate procedure for detecting and identifying preneoplastic cells from neoplastic cells in cervix uteri (69).

As was previously stated, neoplastic transformation is related to cell cycle phases (Chapter 2) and expresses a cell cycle dependency. Thus, studies using the chemical oncogen N-methyl-N'-nitro-N-nitrosoguanidine (MNNG), demonstrated that the progression of preneoplastic cells toward malignant cells (i.e., malignant transformation) attained maximum at the end of G_1 phase and at 4 hours before S phase (or at G_1-S boundary); hence neoplastic transformation is markedly cell cycle dependent (11). However, the molecular events that occur at this G_1-S boundary immediately before the onset of DNA synthesis, and the factors that trigger DNA synthesis are still poorly understood. It is possible that specific proteins are required for the start of DNA synthesis (27); surface membrane changes or hormones are also responsible for triggering the S phase, hence commitment of cells to DNA synthesis (3).

It is interesting that this G_1-S boundary is a so-called restriction (R) point (71). At this critical switching point, cells shift back and forth from cycling–noncycling states. Thus, malignant cells have lost their R-point control. An unscheduled DNA synthesis (UDS) was recently reported in some tumor cell lines from human melanoma with metastases (49).

Recent studies also suggest that the transition from precancerous cells into malignant or cancerous cells is accompanied by chromosomal abnormalities, such as congenital chromosomal anomaly syndromes, preleukemia with abnormal clones, chromosomal instability syndromes, and other situations. Occurrence of abnormal chromosomes enhances the transformation of a premalignant lesions into a malignant lesion, or neoplasm. It has also been suggested that a specific carcinogen might induce malignancy with a specific chromosomal aberration. Although appearance of an abnormal chromosomal clone enhances the risk of leukemia, a number of acute leukemias show normal diploid karyotypes. Sufficient data have been accumulated to show a definite association between specific chromosomal aberrations and specific types of malignancy (15).

According to the mutation somatic theory of cancer, neoplastic transformation is the result of two consecutive mutations. First, mutation occurs during germinal stage, after which a second somatic mutation triggers the neoplastic transformation (42). Sporadic cases have shown both mutations to occur in the somatic cell (42).

We do not know whether chromosomal aberration is the primary triggering event in malignant transformation or whether it is only the result of toxic action of a carcinogen. Although chromosome studies represent a relatively crude attempt at investigating genetic changes in cell populations, they have led to a hypothesis regarding tumor progression termed clonal evolution (70). According to this hypothesis, most tumors are clones derived from a single cell of origin. Tumor progression results from genetic instability in the neoplastic population, with increasingly mutated subpopulations within the original clone. This genetic instability of preneoplastic and neoplastic cells can be an inherited defect in all cells of the body in rare instances, as in the chromosome breakage syndromes (15); more usually, it appears to be an acquired defect caused by activation of a mutation gene in the neoplastic cells (70). At this time, new mutants continue to appear within the neoplastic clone, along with an increasingly abnormal subpopulation, often with visible chromosomal changes.

As a result, some preneoplastic cells will exhibit chromosomal aberrations; continuing selection will result in increasing numbers of neoplastic cells displaying malignant behavior, predominating with increasing malignancy and associated loss of differentiation by cancerous cells.

Hence, chromosomal studies suggest that preneoplastic and neoplastic cells are clones of unicellular origin and that tumor progression and neoplastic transformation are attributable to an acquired genetic instability in the neoplastic cell populations, leading by a sequential selection to increasingly mutant subpopulations (48,70).

Further investigations are needed to identify the specific chromosomal sites at which genes important in neoplastic development are apparently healed (48).

It is postulated that after exposure to carcinogens, a single cell initially undergoes mutational changes; later, the progeny of that cell will form new mutated subpopulations from which the neoplastic cells will predominate and grow as a neoplasm via sequential selection (Fig. 3–11).

Recent studies show that microtubules and microfilaments, which are the primary components of the cytoskeleton in eukaryotic cells, are both connected to macromolecules in the plasma membrane and participate in regulating a number of membrane-associated cellular events, such as cell motility, cell spreading and adhesive properties, maintaining contact inhibition, mobility of cell surface receptors for immunoglobulins and lectins, and binding of hormones to cell surface receptors (6).

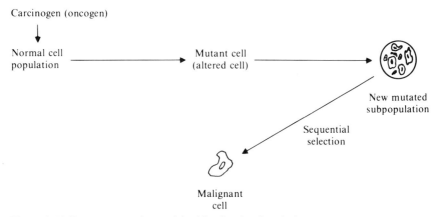

Figure 3–11 Tumor progression explained by the clonal evolution.

However, examination of microtubules and actin-containing filaments of normal, preneoplastic, and neoplastic mouse mammary epithelial cells in primary cultures using indirect immunofluorescence with antibodies to tubulin and actin or electron microscopy shows no consistent differences in these cytoskeleton components. These results suggest that the lesion(s) in growth control and neoplastic progression of mammary cells might not involve any growth alterations in the morphology of microtubules and microfilaments (4). Hence, the precancerous or preneoplastic cells are distinct cell populations that exhibit ultrastructural, autoradiographic, cell surface, and antigenic characteristics. Also, they exhibit an altered hormone responsiveness, as compared with the normal cell population from which they arose.

However, precancerous cells are a heterogeneous cell population. Some of these cells exhibit only minimal structural and cell surface changes and closely resemble normal cells; they are detected with difficulty, whereas other cells exhibit a more advanced degree of ultrastructural, cell surface, autoradiographic, antigenic capacity, and hormone responsiveness, as well as a loss of cell differentiation and contact inhibition. These precanerous cells behave more aggressively and exhibit a carcinogenic potential and greater autonomy.

WHAT IS A CANCEROUS CELL?

This section deals with one of the most intriguing problems of carcinogenesis: Is the cancer cell a new cell or is it a transformed cell?

Recent studies using electron microscopy, high-resolution autoradiography, cell surface and immunologic procedures, and hormone receptors demonstrate that cancerous cells are a heterogeneous cell population. Cancerous (neoplastic) cells are not homogeneous cell lines, but exhibit great variability as regards ultrastructural organization, autoradiographic distribution, surface changes, antigenic capacity, and hormone responsiveness.

Their fine structure, mobility, adhesiveness, and ability to synthesize DNA, RNA, and proteins varies in different types of neoplasms, although ultrastructural, autoradiographic, and cell surface studies indicate that cancerous cells are not markedly different from the normal or preneoplastic cells from which they were derived. Cancerous cells exhibit no new organelles or peculiar characteristics that might characterize them as a new cell species.

Conversely, their ultrastructural and cell membrane organization as well as their capacity to incorporate the required isotopes for DNA, RNA, and protein synthesis are similar to that of normal and preneoplastic cells, but differ only quantitatively. For instance, an increased number of polysomes, mitochondria, lysosomes, tonofilaments, increased amount of nuclear chromatin, increased number of microvilli, pseudopod(s), and blebs or protuberances on their cell surfaces, with a loss in the intercellular connections (such as desmosomes or tight junctional complexes) are often seen in cancerous cells in

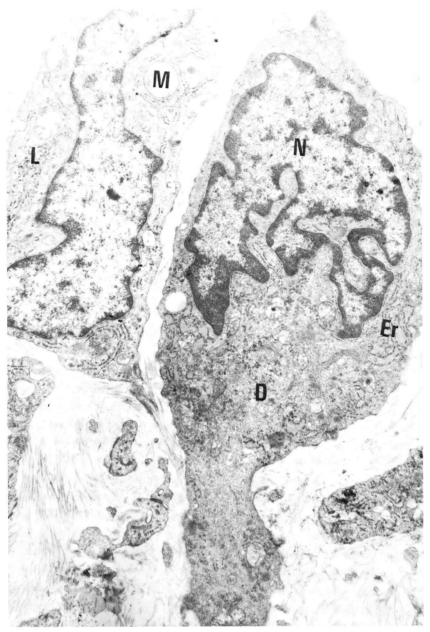

Figure 3-12 Electron micrograph showing cancer cells from mouse squamous cell carcinoma. Heterogeneous cells, dark (D) and light (L) cells with marked nuclear (N) atypicality. Poorly differentiated endoplasmic reticulum (Er); swollen mitochondria (M). Epon section, uranyl acetate and lead citrate, × 11,000.

various neoplasms. (Fig. 3–12) However, no new organelles specific to cancerous cells have been demonstrated.

These findings strongly suggest that cancerous cells are transformed cells that are only quantitatively, but not qualitatively, different from their original normal cells. However, the cancerous cells exhibit some ultrastructural, autoradiographic, and membrane changes which distinguish these cells from the normal cells from which they were derived.

1. All cancerous cells are abnormal cells that have lost their differentiation to differing degrees, as well as their capacity to synthesize hormones (54), enzymes, fetal antigens, or other antigens. Furthermore, this loss of differentiation is often accompanied by synthesis of abnormal proteins, antigens, or ectopic hormones.

2. Cancerous cells are rapidly dividing cells, exhibiting an increased mitotic index as well as a labeled index. (Fig. 3–13) Most cancerous cells are cycling cells (growth fraction), and only a small proportion are resting cells; in normal tissues the cycling and noncycling cells are almost equal.

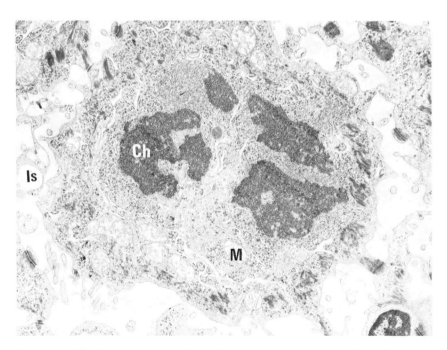

Figure 3–13 Mitotic cancer cells (metaphase) from a mouse squamous cell carcinoma induced by chemical carcinogen (MCA) and treated with thryoxine. Several chromosomes (Ch), enlarged intercellular spaces (Is), with microvilli (Mv), and mitochondrion (M). Epon, uranyl acetate, and lead citrate, × 15,000.

3. Cancerous cells exhibit a great lack of control, having lost their homeostatic mechanisms (systemic, regional, and intrinsic). They proliferate continuously, a capacity that is not more controllable (or at least in a lesser degree) by genetic, hormonal, or immunologic factors.

4. Cancerous cells are often, but not invariably, associated with chromosomal abnormalities in both number and structure. Their degree of malignancy can be related to the chromosomal abnormalities; conversion of neoplastic to nonneoplastic cells or the reverse is very much a function of the balance between different numbers or pattern of chromosomes. Also, existing evidence suggests that human diseases with chromosomal instability have a strong predisposition for different types of cancer.

5. Cancerous cells exhibit an advanced degree of mobility, loss of contact inhibition, and tendency to metastasize. The metastatic potential is a key property of cancerous cells and can be used to identify many neoplastic cell lines.

6. The use of genetic markers such as glucose-6 phosphate dehydrogenase isoenzymes and antigens has suggested a monoclonal origin for cancerous cells (25).

7. Electron microscopic, cell surface, autoradiographic, and hormone receptor studies of cancerous cell populations in different types of neoplasms strongly suggest that cancerous cells are heterogeneous cell populations with different degrees of differentiation, metastatic capacity, antigenic properties, and hormone responsiveness. According to their loss of hormone receptors, some still maintain their hormone responsiveness, whereas other are hormone irresponsive. These observations are of greatest importance, from the standpoint of therapy, and can be correlated with clinical response. Also, the capacity to incorporate isotopes and the number of labeled cells can be used as a good criterion for the effectiveness of chemotherapy and hormonotherapy. Patients in whom a significant increase in labeling index was seen after hormonotherapy or chemotherapy had a favorable clinical response, with tumor cell regression. By contrast, in patients in whom no increase in labeling index and no alteration in growth fraction could be induced by hormono- or chemotherapy, no clinical response and tumor regression was observed (87).

8. Cancerous cells exhibit characteristic surface membrane changes that can distinguish them from normal and preneoplastic cells. (Fig. 3-14) Generally, the plasma membrane of cancerous cells is less morphologically specialized than is that of the normal cell (81). A derangement in membrane biogenesis and structure is critical for carcinogenesis, as cancer is postulated to be a membrane disease (85). According to this theory, the most likely target membrane is

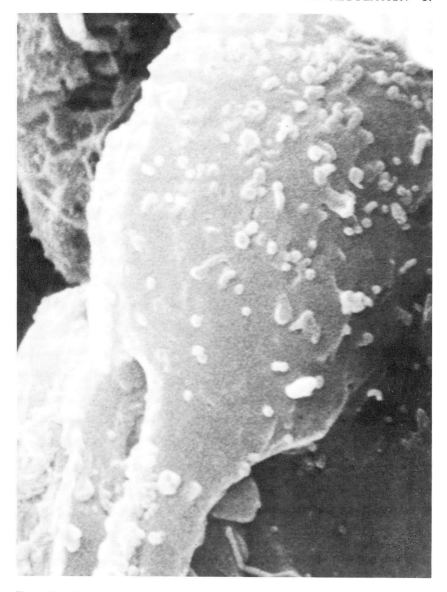

Figure 3-14 Scanning electron micrograph showing cancer cells from mouse squamous cell carcinoma induced by carcinogen MCA and treated with thyroxine. Cancer cells exhibit marked surface changes with numerous microvilli, blebs, and ruffles. CO_2 critical point method and gold-coated cells, $\times$ 10,000.

the plasma membrane, but other membranes (mitochondrial, nuclear, microsomal) might play an important regulatory role.

9. No new DNA or altered DNA is convincingly demonstrated in cancerous cells and only very little "new" mRNA is demonstrated in the nucleic acid hybridization experiments.

10. In some instances, cancerous cells are associated with the presence of developmental antigens (α-fetoprotein, oncodevelopmental, and carcinoplacental antigens) (25). Some early work suggested that these antigens might be useful markers for precancerous cells, since they appeared in the precancerous hepatocytes long before cancers appeared.

Thus, studies employing modern methods in detecting the progressive changes from normal cell to precancerous and cancerous cells generally indicate that cancerous cells are phenotypically altered and transformed cells similar to the normal cells that had lost control over differentiation. The abnormal differentiation of these cancerous cells is expressed only phenotypically; they still preserve or maintain some of the characteristics of the original, or so-called normal, cells from which they were derived. They are not new mutant cells, that are genetically different from the original cells—they differ only phenotypically from their normal counterparts. Therefore, the neoplastic transformation is a stepwise, progressive process evolving from normal cells transformed first into preneoplastic cells and later into malignant or cancerous cells.

Since it is difficult to detect these subtle changes, especially the borderline stages, some researchers believe that cancerous cells are new mutants and genetically different cells.

In the absence of a good model for the study of preneoplastic or premalignant lesions, the problem remains open for debate. Most of our knowledge regarding the cell biology and behavior of precancerous cells comes from work on experimental tumors in animal models. Furthermore, data regarding the behavior of precancerous cells are primarily from in vitro studies, since these cells are deprived of their natural microenvironment, data cannot always be extrapolated to human preneoplastic cells.

ENDOCRINE REGULATION OF PRECANCEROUS AND CANCEROUS CELLS

Since precancerous cells and some well-differentiated cancerous cells still preserve their morphological, antigenic, and hormone responsiveness because of the presence of hormone receptors on their cell surface, it seems likely that hormones and hormonelike substances (or hormonomimetic) agents might influence precancerous and cancerous cell populations.

Hormones might regulate or modulate the homeostasis of precancerous and cancerous cells in different ways, such as

1. Influencing the rate of transformation or progression of precancerous cells to cancerous cells.
2. Influencing the induction of precancerous cells by stimulating cell proliferation and hyperplasia, resulting in premalignant or precancerous lesions.

3. Preferentially stimulating proliferation of these abnormal cell populations, inasmuch as both precancerous and cancerous cell populations are heterogeneous cell populations, involving cells with minimal morphological alterations to abnormal cells.
4. Stimulating the DNA, RNA, and protein synthesis essential to fixation of transformed cells.
5. Reactivating the latent or dormant precancerous and cancerous cells, thereby increasing the growth fraction and ultimately tumor invasiveness and malignancy.

Clearly, the mechanisms whereby hormones and hormonelike (or hormonomimetic) substances regulate the homeostasis of these two cell populations are more complex and not yet fully understood (Fig. 3–15).

Although there is no conclusive evidence that hormones can induce the occurrence of preneoplastic and neoplastic cells per se (with few exceptions), since hormones exert important roles in cell growth, mitosis, and cell proliferation, it is possible that hormones and hormonomimetic agents have an important role in controlling the homeostasis (or equilibrium) of precancerous and cancerous cells. Thus, hormones are important cellular homeostatic factors, and hormonal environment or hormonal milieu is a critical factor in maintaining this cell homeostasis.

More recently, it was demonstrated that long-term administration of estrones, especially DES or 17β-estradiol, in the diet of virgin female C_3H/He mice induced neoplastic and preneoplastic lesions. These animals have a high titer of the mammary tumor virus factor (MMTV). In estrogen-treated mice, an increased incidence of cervical adenosis and of mammary HANs was observed and the time to development of mammary adenocarcinomas was shortened. These changes increase with dose and time and appear earlier in the C_3H/He mice. Other multiple tumors included cervical and endometrial adenocarcinomas, cervical granular cell myoblastomas, vaginal squamous cell carcinomas, ovarian teratomas, osteosarcomas, pheochromocytomas, and thyroid carcinomas occurred. Very few spontaneous tumors occurred in the same mouse strain. Thus, estrogens can induce various preneoplastic and neoplastic lesions in the female C_3H mouse and can serve as an animal model for uterine adenocarcinomas and adenosis in women exposed to estrogens (33). Likewise, preneoplastic and neoplastic lesions in livers of rats and mice treated with some component steroids of oral contraceptives should be more

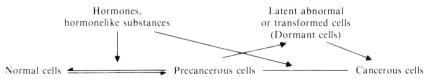

Figure 3–15 Survey of possible hormone influences in homeostasis of precancerous and cancerous cells.

prophetic for the development of hepatocellular carcinoma in women using oral contraceptives or in patients receiving androgens for anemia (51).

Another intriguing and as yet unexplained phenomenon is that most human cancers of nongenital organs occur more frequently in males at all ages (34). It is possible that females are better equipped to resist carcinogenesis because of immune factors located on X chromosomes. Because the female has two X chromosomes, she has a better chance than the male, with only one X chromosome, to recognize and inactivate the preneoplastic genes coding for hormone synthesis and hormone receptors, genes controlling production of enzymes that activate or inactivate chemical carcinogens also located on sex chromosomes. Since mouse mammary carcinogenesis is characterized by a definite preneoplastic stage (i.e., HAN), the role of hormones in controlling the precancerous cells, as well as their progression to cancerous cells, were studied mostly in this model. Thus, HAN formation in mice is stimulated by daily injections of prostaglandin E_2 (PGE$_2$) and of progesterone but not of prolactin. Hence, HAN formation in mice is mainly dependent on progesterone, and not on prolactin (68).

Also, induction of premalignant mammary lesions as well as mammary adenoacanthoma and carcinomas by a tumor virus in BALB/c female mice is hormonally dependent. The same hormones that generated tumors in normal glands greatly accelerated tumor development in precancerous hyperplasia but did not amplify viral RNA or antigens either in hyperplasia or in tumors derived from them, suggesting a defective replication of murine mammary tumor virus in hormone-induced neoplasms (30).

The induction and progression of another preneoplastic lesion (NLAL) under hormone influences has also been studied in organ culture. NLAL induced by DMBA (or methylcholanthrene) in female BALB/c mice was greatly modified by hormone supplementation. Thus, a marked increase in NLAL formation was detected in the presence of insulin + prolactin + aldosterone + cortisol in the medium. The hormone combination of insulin + prolactin + cortisol was unfavorable for NLAL induction by DMBA and the combination of aldosterone + insulin + prolactin was only moderately active.

Thus, the presence of cortisol with insulin + prolactin + aldosterone enhances the NLAL incidence of precancerous cells by DMBA. The highest incidence in a period corresponding to maximum DNA synthesis, which suggests that DMBA induction of precancerous NLAL in mammary glands in organ culture involves a complex carcinogen–hormone–cell cycle interaction (50). Thus, a favorable hormone environment is required for increased frequency of NLAL in organ culture. Also, hormonal regulation of preneoplastic NLAL cells in organ culture is similar to that of HAN in vivo.

Both in vitro (organ culture) and in vivo studies regarding the endocrine physiology of mouse mammary gland show that growth and development of mammary tissue is under hormonal control. Lobuloalveolar growth of the mouse mammary gland requires prolactin and growth hormone plus estrogen and progesterone. Insulin, and possibly aldosterone, also have a role, as was indicated by organ culture studies (8). Exogenous estradiol and progesterone given to virgin mice leads to lobuloalveolar development similar to that observed in pregnancy (10).

As in rat uterus and chick oviduct, this induced growth promoting action by ovarian hormones in mammary gland is accompanied by an activation of DNA, RNA, and protein synthesis. Furthermore, the increased DNA polymerase activity associated with increased DNA synthesis in mammary tissue probably depends on estrogen and progesterone stimulation (9). Most studies regarding the macromolecular events of hormonal action during mammary development (mammogenesis) were centered around regulation of RNA synthesis. Recently it was found that both DNA synthesis and DNA polymerase activities are independent of ovarian hormones in precancerous HAN cells as compared with normal mammary tissue (9). RNA synthesis, as measured by 5-^{3}H-uridine incorporation shows that administration of 17β-estradiol-plus progesterone to intact or ovariectomized or adrenalectomized virgin BALB/c mouse mammary gland induces a sharp rise in rapidly labeled RNA similar to that of mammary tissue of pregnancy. The preneoplastic cells from the preneoplastic nodule synthesized rapidly labeled RNA, regardless of tumorigenic potential; this new rapidly labeled RNA includes both ribosomal precursor RNA and heterogeneous nuclear RNA. Ovariectomy and adrenalectomy or extended treatment with 17β-estradiol plus progesterone failed to alter the pattern of rapidly labeled RNA synthesis in the preneoplastic cells. Thus, RNA synthesis in preneoplastic cells remains unresponsive to the control of ovarian hormones. A similar unresponsiveness to hormonal control of rapidly labeled RNA synthesis in the mammary tumors deriving from these precancerous tissues was also demonstrated. Therefore, the preneoplastic cells exhibit an altered responsiveness to host hormonal control (8).

Effects of estrogens and antiestrogens on cell growth, DNA synthesis, and protein synthesis have been documented in hormonally responsive mammary cancer cells in tissue culture (53). Determination of net DNA synthesis with inorganic [^{32}P]ortophosphate can be more accurate than is commonly used [^{3}H]dThd in order to monitor DNA synthesis.

Estrogen administration increases the net DNA synthesis as compared with controls in MCF-7 human breast cancer cells in tissue culture. Stimulation is most evident after 36 hours of hormone treatment (2). It was previously reported that estrogens act in vivo by stimulating G_0 cells to reenter the cycle at G_1. Also, the estrogen addition of MCF-7 decreased the cell cycle time by shortening the length of the G_1 phase of the cell cycle. Since MCF-7 cells are a transformed cell line, the ability of estrogen hormones to influence cell growth and DNA synthesis in these systems seems to mimic the action of estrogens in vivo. Thus, the MCF-7 cell line, which represents a transformed cell, can provide a highly useful system for the investigation of hormones and antihormones on the regulation of growth and progression of precancerous and cancerous cells in vitro (2,44).

Scanning electron microscopic and TEM examination of human MCF-7 breast cancer cells in culture (75) recently showed that estradiol treatment between 2 and 11 days markedly modifies their cell surface morphology and induces a secretory activity. Thus, estradiol progressively increases the number and length of microvilli at the cell surface; the cells become more globular and less tightly attached to the surface of the dish. The cells exhibit an abundant RER, clear mitochondria, Golgi complexes, and several secretory granules, ultrastructurally defining them as secretory cells. These morphological and cell surface changes are induced only by estradiol in physiological concentrations. 5α-Dihydrotestosterone does not induce any changes, whereas progesterone completely inhibits the effect of estradiol on the microvilli and on secretory activity. Antiestrogens, such as tamoxifen or hydroxytamoxifen, were not observed to induce secretory activity, but did change the cell morphology relative to that of control cells. The effects of estradiol were seen only in estrogen receptor positive mammary cancer cells, but not in estrogen negative receptor cell lines.

It is possible that estrogens exert these drastic changes on cell morphology and secretory activity of human breast cancer cells by increasing the release of a specific and major glycoprotein with a molecular weight of approximately 50,000. It is not clear whether this glycoprotein-induced estradiol is secreted by exocytosis or whether it is a regular membrane constituent that is shed into the medium only in the presence of estrogens. Thus, the transformed cancer cells can be converted to secretory cells by this specific glycoprotein in the presence of estrogens (84). Marked ultrastructural changes of malignant cells (chondrocytes) were also detected in a transplantable swarm chondrosarcoma in rats after the administration of various hormones.

Marked atrophy of neoplastic cells occurred when this tumor was transplanted into hypophysectomized rats. Maximal restoration of neoplastic cell growth was achieved when cortisone, thyroxine (T_4), and growth hormone (GH) were given together. An intermediate degree of cell growth restoration was observed when cortisone and T_4 or GH alone were administered to tumor-bearing hypophysectomized rats. Cortisone and T_4 treatments were associated with increased RER and nucleolar enlargement, whereas GH treatment was associated with a marked dilatation of the endoplasmic reticulum (ER). When cortisone, GH, and T_4 were given in combination, a marked increase in exocytotic/pinocytotic vesicles and apparent deposition of cartilage matrix was observed.

These ultrastructural studies, combined with biochemical observations, demonstrate that malignant chondrocytes from a transplantable chondrosarcoma are hormonally controlled cancerous cells. Thus, cellular growth and differentiation of neoplastic chondrocytes are hormone responsive and hormone dependent. Growth hormone exerts dramatic effects on neoplastic cells; when GH, cortisone, and T_4 are administered together, these hormones have a synergistic effect on neoplastic cell growth and differentiation. However, in vivo administration of cortisone is associated with a reduction in number and size of chondrocytes in normal cartilage (62).

Hence, hormones can control the cell growth and differentiation of malignant cells (human breast cells and rat chondrocytes), both in vitro and in vivo (44,62). Combined administration of hormones and chemical carcinogens also alters the cell growth and differentiation of thyroid, mammary, and lung tumors. Thus, in female rats injected with carcinogen *N*-nitrosomethylurea (NMU), a slight hypothyroidism favors the development of mammary and lung tumors, while a severe hypothyroidism produces the opposite effect. Conversely, the combination of PTU treatment and the carcinogen induces malignant thyroid neoplasms (67). The significance of the response of cancerous cells to hormone administration or deprivation might therefore have important implications for understanding the regulating or modulating factors of neoplastic cell growth and differentiation.

Recently, selenium was found to provide a prophylaxis of mammary DMBA induced in rats. Selenium can inhibit both the initiation and promotion phases of mammary carcinogenesis. It can also inhibit the reappearance of mammary tumors that had regressed after ovariectomy. Thus, selenium can inhibit the progression of initiated or precancerous cells toward cancerous or malignant cells. This antitumorigenic effect of selenium is independent of the presence of prolactin and estrogens. It is possible that selenium exerts its anticarcinogenic role by protecting DNA against single-strand breakage and facilitation of the repair process. Thus, in hepatocarcinogenesis, namely during the initiation phase, selenium includes protection of liver DNA against single-strand breakage induced by AAF and facilitation of DNA repair (89). Selenium can therefore be used in an effort toward cancer prevention and in chemotherapy of mammary tumors.

Recent investigations also show that hormones control DNA synthesis and ornithine decarboxylase activity (ODC) in adult hepatocytes. Insulin and epidermal growth factor (EGF) were synergistic and induced a marked increase in DNA synthesis and ODC activity in primary cultures of adult rat hepatocytes.

Dexamethasone exerts a divergent effect, inducing ODC slightly and inhibiting DNA synthesis strongly, whereas asparagine and glutamine induce ODC activity but inhibit DNA synthesis. These results show that although there is some correlation between ODC induction and DNA synthesis, ODC is not essential for cell growth (79).

Hepatocytes treated with insulin and EGF show that the DNA content increases from 2N to 4N and to 8N in some cells. There are also reports regarding ODC induction in cultured cells, including hepatoma cells (14).

ODC induction in primary cultured liver cells by various hormones, including insulin, glucocorticoids, and glucagon, has also been reported (55).

Although dexamethasone, glutamine, and asparagine have been shown to inhibit DNA synthesis and induce ODC, their mechanisms are still unknown. It is possible that cell dispersion causes a shift of the cell cycle of hepatocytes from the G_0 phase to G_1 phase, but it is more likely that cell responsiveness to glucagon depends on as yet undefined conditions of cell preparations. Therefore, under present conditions in primary culture of adult rat hepatocytes, mature hepatocytes could enter G_2 phase through S phase, but could not enter M phase (79).

Interesting data regarding the role of hormones in controlling the preneoplastic and neoplastic cell populations were derived from the study of epidermal tumors in vivo. Thus, hormones and hormonelike substances (prostaglandins, epidermal growth factor, chalones) significantly change the evolution and morphology of initiated (preneoplastic) cells from mouse epidermis exposed to a single dose of 3-MCA. The initiated epidermal cells were observed for a long time (8 to 9 months) and the DNA, RNA, protein synthesis, and ultrastructural pattern were studied periodically. Light and electron microscopic autoradiography and isotope incorporation using ^{3}H-thymidine, ^{3}H-uridine, and ^{3}H-leucine for the synthesis of DNA, RNA, and proteins, respectively, were employed.

Quantitative evaluation of autoradiograms showed a marked increase in ^{3}H-thymidine, ^{3}H-uridine, and ^{3}H-leucine incorporation into the nuclear chromatin, nucleoli, and cytoplasm (polysomes and RER) after administration of PGE_2 and $PGF_{2\alpha}$ (prostaglandins E_2 and $F_{2\alpha}$), calcitonin, and T_4, followed by a moderate increase after estradiol and PGA_2 and a marked decrease after hydrocortisone and hypophysectomy.

Alterations in DNA, RNA, and protein synthesis are accompanied by significant changes in the ultrastructural pattern of precancerous epidermal cells, such as hypertrophied nuclei, prominent nucleoli, alterations of RER, tonofilaments, polysomes, surface changes (microvilli, ruffles, blebs), and occurrence of dark cells. Marked atrophic and degenerative changes, such as small nuclei and nucleoli, poor chromatin, reduced RER and polysome populations, and desmosomes.

Thus, hormones and hormonomimetic agents might act as cocarcinogens or tumor promoters by influencing DNA, RNA, and protein synthesis in precancerous cells (61). Hormones can also regulate the DNA synthesis of cancerous epidermal cells. Thus, hormones and hormonelike substances can modify DNA synthesis in the epidermal neoplastic cells of MCA-induced neoplasms.

It is well demonstrated that long-term application of 3-MCA on dorsal skin induces squamous cell carcinomas in mice and basal cell carcinomas in rats. In order to study DNA synthesis in cancerous cells, DNA labeling and light and electron microscopic autoradiography with ^{3}H-thymidine were used in mice-bearing squamous cell carcinomas and rats bearing basal cell carcinomas treated with T_4, glucagon, estradiol, cortisol, calcitonin, $PGF_{2\alpha}$, and PGA_2, or having a hormone deficiency (gonadectomy or hypophysectomy). Quantitative determination of autoradiograms shows that T_4 glucagon, $PGF_{2\alpha}$, calcitonin, and estradiol markedly enhance DNA synthesis in the nuclear chromatin of both squamous cancerous cells and basal cancerous cells, while a notable inhibition occurs after cortisol administration, hypophysectomy, and castration.

Light and electron microscopic autoradiograms also demonstrate interesting changes in ^{3}H-thymidine distribution in cancerous cells, and labeled nuclei are mostly located at the periphery of horn pearls of squamous cell carcinomas, whereas in the basal cell carcinomas the dark cells are heavily labeled (Fig. 3–16). Electron microscopic autoradiograms also show that most developed grains are located in the heterochromatin (genetic chromatin); no grains were shown to occur in the light or euchromatin (metabolic chromatin). Furthermore, estradiol induces a peculiar peripheral autoradiographic distribution, mainly on the nuclear envelope. Therefore, hormones and hormonomimetic agents influence primarily the S phase of the cell cycle of cancerous cells, regulating the homeostasis of epidermal cancerous cell

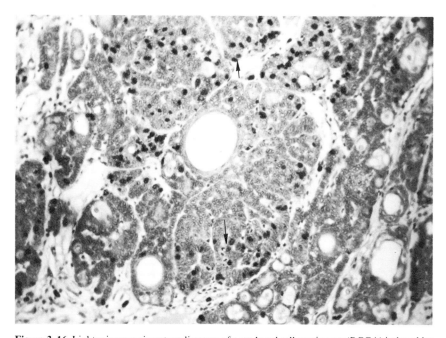

Figure 3–16 Light microscopic autoradiogram of a rat basal cell carcinoma (BCCA) induced by chemical carcinogen (MCA). Several dark cells disposed at the periphery of tumor mass (arrows). No light cells are labeled. Paraffin section, NTB_2 nuclear emulsion, hematoxylin & eosin stain, $\times 400$.

populations and subsequently modulating the carcinogenic process by interfering with DNA synthesis (57).

Most sex-steroid-mediated events shown to be involved in DNA synthesis and cell division are DNA polymerase and possibly nuclear transfer of specific receptor protein. However, other experimental models using cell cultures that have some advantages (homogeneity of cell type, absence of systemic effects, and control of the medium) over in vivo models in studying the effects of steroid hormones on cell proliferation show that the key event involves steroidal alteration of the probability of cells entering DNA synthesis.

In addition to these events, it seems likely that steroids regulate cell proliferation by synthesizing regulatory proteins. Also, the loss of responsiveness is related neither to receptor quantity nor to its intracellular distribution, but mostly to a postreceptor event, namely RNA and protein synthetic machinery. Biochemical comparison of androgen-deprived cells before and after their loss in androgen responsiveness suggests RNA or protein synthesis, or both, as the prime mechanism(s) (41). Thus, the loss of hormone responsiveness might be attributable to postreceptor events, namely changes in RNA and protein synthesis (20).

COMMENTS AND CONCLUSIONS

The major goal of this study is threefold: first, to define and identify the precancerous and cancerous cells; second, to determine the similarities and dissimilarities between these two cell populations, and third, to find the role of hormones or hormonomimetic agents in controlling the development of precancerous cells into cancerous or malignant cells.

However, it should be emphasized that precancerous cells from liver, skin, thyroid, lung, and mammary glands are all heterogeneous cell populations. These cells exhibit a different ultrastructural pattern, antigenicity, enzymatic alterations, autoradiographic distribution, and most importantly a different invasiveness and propensity to development into cancerous or malignant cells (12). Thus, only some precancerous cells, usually large cells with abundant SER, hypertrophic nuclei and prominent nucleoli, increased tonofilaments, abundant microvilli, and loss of desmosomes and histochemical alterations exhibit invasive capacity. These are phenotypically altered cells. Other precancerous cells can remain latent or even regress toward normal cells (61). Also, only those hyperplastic cells having invasive properties behave differently, losing their control, especially hormonal control. They are not more hormone responsive than their original or normal cells.

Only these are true precancerous cells, which finally evolve into cancerous or malignant cells. This situation raises a number of problems and difficulties regarding precancerous cells, resulting in conflicting reports. Some studies are still speculative. Inasmuch as both precancerous and cancerous cells are heterogeneous cell populations, it is sometimes difficult to make a sharp distinction between them on the basis of hormone responsiveness, antigenicity, autoradiographic capacity, cell surface, and even ultrastructural pattern. Most well-differentiated neoplastic cells behave like preneoplastic cells, exhibiting a high degree of hormone responsiveness owing to the presence of most hormone receptors (these cells still retain the same receptors found in normal and precancerous cells); having chiefly the same antigens, ability to incorporate isotopes, and manufacture the original hormones; as well as displaying a similar ultrastructural pattern.

Conversely, the poorly differentiated or undifferentiated neoplastic cells exhibit a partial or complete loss of their ultrastructural pattern, cell surface antigens, autoradiographic capacity, and their hormone receptors and subseqently a loss of hormone responsiveness. Thus, the cell biology and behavior of cancerous cells are heterogeneous, some being disposed in a more ordinate pattern, well differentiated and responsive to hormonal control, whereas others being poorly differentiated or undifferentiated, growing in more disorderly or chaotic pattern, with complete or partial loss of hormonal control and exhibiting a high degree of autonomy in regard to cell growth and differentiation.

The recognition of early precancerous changes specific to carcinogenesis in skin, liver, thyroid, stomach, or lung would be extremely helpful in the diagnosis of early premalignant or early malignant changes and consequently in early detection and treatment of precancerous diseases.

After prolonged exposure to chemical carcinogens and hormones, the first step undergone by certain cells is the occurrence of hyperplastic and hypertrophic cells (e.g., epidermal nodular hyperplasia, liver, thyroid, or lung hyperplasia), followed by metaplasia (or dysplasia), formation of benign neoplasm, and finally malignant neoplasms.

A body of recent evidence strongly suggests that chemical or hormonal carcinogenesis is a progressive or stepwise process. Through the use of such modern approaches as electron microscopy, SEM, high-resolution autoradiography, and various tumor markers, we were able to detect these precancerous or malignant lesions with greater accuracy, namely their hormonal control or lack of control, one of the most important criteria in distinguishing between precancerous and cancerous cells. Although there are some specific ultrastructural or cell surface changes for precancerous or cancerous cells that can differentiate these two cell populations, and some of these early changes are similar to those occurring with chemical irritants, wounds, or partial hepatectomy; some of these cell alterations are still indicative of specific morphological changes (e.g., the formation of epidermal pseudopodia, occurrence of microvilli, loss of desmosomes and cell junctions, increased polysome formation and abundant RER with a shift in predominance of SER for some precancerous stages in hepatocarcinogenesis and thyroid carcinomas. Hypertrophy of nuclei, prominent nucleoli, lysosome formation, and clumped tonofilaments are often seen in several experimental precancerous cells (mouse, rat, hamster) or human precancerous cells (Bowen's disease, carcinoma in situ, hepatic peliosis) (12,59,65).

Some workers assume that the early changes in epidermal–dermal junction, namely basal lamina, are characteristic of early stages (preneoplastic lesions); an enzymatic degradation of basement membrane collagen can be correlated with the metastatic potential (43,52). Also, an increase in microtubule formation was mentioned in the neoplastic transformed cells; however, we cannot find this microtubule increase or other changes in the cytoskeleton of transformed cells as a constant feature.

Further studies should center on specific morphology, cell kinetics, immunological cell surface changes, and tumor markers for precancerous cells, which will be of a tremendous advantage in the prevention and treatment of early stages of tumorigenesis. Such studies are still in the early stages. An important criterion is the use of tumor markers (antigens, hormone markers). Thus, assays for carcinoembryonic antigens (CEAs), α-fetoprotein (AFP), colon-specific antigens (CSA), thyroglobulin (TG), transferrin (TF), ferritin (FE), human T cell antigens (OKT$_3$, OKT$_4$, OKT$_5$), fibronectin (FN), and β_2-microglobulin were developed; determinations of these markers in several neoplasms were recently carried out (65,77,83). Biopsies from malignant skin lesions (basal cell carcinoma, malignant melanomas, and squamous cell carcinomas) and from patients with premalignant or benign skin lesions (Bowen's disease) by the use of the immunoperoxidase method showed a significant loss of β_2-microglobulin from the surface of cancerous cells compared with benign and a partial loss in the premalignant or precancerous conditions (83). This loss of β_2-microglobulin might be attributable either to great alterations in the cell surface of cancerous cells that can no longer synthesize and be available to specific antibody or to a rapid replication of change in the genetic material. These cancerous cells are no longer capable of synthesizing specific antigens. More recently, investigations regarding tumor markers in carcinoma and premalignant lesions of the stomach in humans showed a close similarity between the cells of adenocarcinoma and cells of intestinal metaplasia, but not to similar metaplastic cells in atrophic gastritis. It would also appear that there are two types of morphologically identical intestinal metaplasia: one related to cancer, the other not. Thus, cancerous cells of gastric carcinoma have a notably different tumor marker profile than that of normal cells and metaplastic cells of atrophic gastritis (77).

These data are of great importance to the pathologist and endocrinologist in determining whether a suspected malignant lesion should be completely excised or is still responsive to hormonal control and should thus be treated by systemic therapy. Although some premalignant cells show a tumor marker profile similar to that of cancer cells, others do not. It has also been reported that certain tumor markers (CEA, α-fetoprotein, HPL (human placental lactogen), and β-HCG) are found in a variety of cancers and premalignant conditions and do not distinguish between them (29). This could be attributable to the presence of a common cross-reacting substance.

Hence, there are no reliable markers for cancerous and precancerous cells. What tumor markers can reflect is chiefly a different or abnormal cellular phenotype as compared with that of normal differentiated cells, owing to incomplete differentiation. They do not provide accurate specificity for malignant or premalignant cells, however (29).

Also, differences between cell surface phenotypic antigens have been reported in human T lymphocytes in cutaneous T cell lymphoma. Thus, the mature T cell antigen phenotype of malignant T cells is identical for circulating and malignant skin T cells. By contrast, malignant skin T cells express the immature human T cell antigen Thy-1, surface membrane transferrin receptors, and Ia-like determinants, while circulating malignant T-cells do not express these antigens. T cells from benign (premalignant) dermatoses also express Thy-1 and Ia-like antigens. Hence, cancerous T cells express different phenotypic antigens, possibly because of their microenvironment (31).

Recent data regarding the cell growth, metastatic capacity, and biochemical characteristics of malignant cells in vitro from different types of cancers (rhabdomyosarcoma, fibrosarcoma, SV 40 transformed human lung fibroblasts and five cell lines derived from human dermatofibrosarcoma protuberans) have been reported. Cells that produce less FN show marked chemotactic migration. By contrast, no chemotactic migration has been noted in DFP cells that show a collagen and FN synthesis similar to that of normal cells. These data suggest that an increased level of FN and of collagen-derived peptides (CDPs) in the environment of malignant tumors has an important role in initiating the metastasizing process as well as in locating these metastases in connective tissue-rich organs (65). Interestingly, ultrastructural changes found in some metaplastic (premalignant) cells were similar to those in cancer cells.

Hence, clinical, experimental, and morphological evidence strongly suggest that precancerous lesions are composed of a heterogeneous cell population. Only some of these cells are transformed into cancer cells, others are not. This means that only some hyperplastic and nodular lesions (liver, skin, thyroid, lung, mammary gland, or stomach) exhibit similar ultrastructural alterations, cell surface changes, partial loss of antigenic capacity, and partial loss of hormone responsiveness. Only these cells exhibit a tumorigenic potential and can be considered truly preneoplastic or precancerous cells; others are merely hyperplastic cells that can regress to normal cells. Most ultrastructural features, cell surface antigens, cell kinetics, and hormone receptors of hyperplastic cells are similar to those of the normal cells from which they were derived, whereas ultrastructural characteristics, cell surface

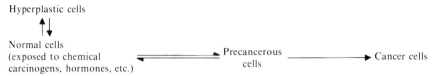

Figure 3-17 Normal cells, hyperplastic cells, precancerous cells, and cancerous cells.

antigens, cellular kinetics, and partial loss of hormone receptors of precancerous cells are similar or close to those of malignant cells. The schema in Figure 3–17 shows the relationship among normal cells, hyperplastic cells, precancerous cells, and cancerous cells.

Precancerous cells are thus transformed and phenotypically altered cells that exhibit a morphological–antigenic–tumor marker profile similar to that of cancer cells and accompanied by a partial loss of control. They also exhibit a greater tendency to chemotactic migration and metastatic capacity.

Hence, a distinction between hyperplastic cells and preneoplastic cells should always be made to avoid conflicting data and reports regarding the preneoplastic cells as a homogeneous cell population, as occurred in several instances.

Despite the new methods at our disposal, the identification of precancerous cells remains a difficult task. An experimental model for the study of premalignant lesions or so-called resistant hyperplastic nodules is yet to be developed.

Another intriguing question is: How do hormones control or regulate the homeostasis between precancerous and cancerous cell populations? The mechanism(s) by which hormones regulate and control the cell homeostasis are more complex and not yet fully understood. Although direct evidence of the ability of hormones to transform normal cells into precancerous and cancerous cells is lacking, and their mitogenic role remains controversial, there is ample evidence that hormones and hormonomimetic agents are potential factors in controlling cellular homeostasis, namely the progression of precancerous cells toward cancer cells. The mechanisms whereby hormones control cellular homeostasis and the precancerous and cancerous cell populations include the following possibilities:

1. Accelerating or delaying the rate of transformation of preneoplastic into neoplastic cells.
2. Interfering with DNA, RNA, and protein synthesis of precancerous cells.
3. Influencing cell differentiation and proliferation, and consequently the cell kinetics of precancerous and cancerous cells.
4. Inducing changes in cell surface, cytoskeleton, and cell mobility.
5. Increasing the selection of abnormal or phenotypically altered cells.

The nature of the molecular mechanisms of hormones and of their action on precancerous and cancerous cells is still obscure. It is generally contended that hormones exert profound effects on cell growth and differentiation. To express their action, glucocorticoids and sex steroid hormones (estrogens, androgens, progesterone) must enter the cell and bind to a cytoplasmic receptor. This steroid–receptor complex enters the nucleus, where it increases the rate of transcription, particularly the post-transcription phase, with a consequent increase in the messenger RNA (mRNA); consequently, hormones influence the gene expression. But just how hormones modulate gene expression, by turning the differential genes on and off in transformed cells, remains unclear.

Recently, an attractive model derived from bacteria and eukaryotic cells demonstrated that hormones might act on cloned genes put back into cells. Cloned genes, for example, globin and ovalbumin, have been placed in cells, where they are shown to function. Hormonal regulation of some cloned genes has recently been reported (17,46). It is postulated that the hormone–receptor complex interacts directly with sequences in or near the cloned genes, thereby modifying the gene sequences and gene expression in the transformed (i.e., preneoplastic and neoplastic) cells. If it works, this model will prove a satisfactory explanation of the hormonal regulation of gene expression in transformed or phenotypically altered cells.

It is possible that hormones and hormonelike substances have more than one means to control the progression of precancerous cells into cancerous cells. Our investigations have demonstrated that hormones interfere significantly with the DNA, RNA, and protein synthesis of precancerous and cancerous cells of epidermal tumors (57,61). Although the role of hormones in the first stage, that is, initiation of cells, or in the transformation of normal cells into precancerous cells is still controversial, it can certainly be said that hormones influence and modulate the later stages of progression of precancerous cells into cancer cells.

For clinical oncologists, it is of great importance to control and restrain the progression of precancerous cells into malignant cells and to maintain this cell population in a latent stage for as long as possible. A hormonal milieu or hormonal cell environment is required for preneoplastic cells of hormone-dependent cancers to progress to cancer cells. Also, this hormonal milieu might facilitate or restrain the cell progression in hormone-independent cancers. This possibility could explain the clinical observations of several premalignant lesions or carcinoma in situ (in such organs as stomach, mammary gland, uterus, thyroid, liver, skin, and lung), which can remain in this latent state for several years.

Experimental and clinical observations strongly suggest that a hormonal imbalance can accelerate the evolution of precancerous lesions in malignant tumors. It seems likely that hormones interfering with DNA, RNA, and protein synthesis influence cell differentiation and proliferation as well. Ultrastructural, cell surface, cell kinetics, and hormone-receptor studies indicate that when a cell is moving toward malignancy, it loses its differentiation by first becoming a poorly differentiated cell and then an undifferentiated cell. Hence, tumor progression and cellular differentiation are only two facets of the same process—neoplastic transformation.

The current focus of ultrastructural research on cancer has been the cancerous cell. Further studies regarding the progression of precancerous cells into cancer cells as well as their behavior cell events are needed. An emphasis on the stepwise events of cellular, biochemical, molecular, and immunological changes during carcinogenesis, together with studies of cancer and precancer cell populations, should open new perspectives for cancer research (24). Since most studies to date have been carried out in vitro on cells deprived of their natural microenvironment, it is difficult to relate such results to the in vivo situation—a major challenge of this vital research.

The increasing experimental and clinical observations demonstrating the ability of many precancerous cells to revert back to normal cells is fostering great interest in the use of interventions or agents that will either restrain or interrupt the process of transformation or increase the likelihood of regression. Hormones, hormonomimetic agents, vitamins, immunological, and dietary factors are being explored as possible means.

Hormones and hormonomimetic agents (hormonoids) are important factors in restraining or interrupting this process. Hormones might act as cocarcinogens, by altering the rate of transformation of precancerous to cancer cells. Although the mechanism(s) of action at cellular and macromolecular levels of many commonly used hormones, such as sex steroids, corticosteroids, thyroid hormones, insulin, and glucagon, in transformed cells is currently better understood, the role of such hormonelike substances as PG, GF, and thymus and pineal extracts in tumorigenesis is still unclear. More than 50 years ago, Engel observed that thymus extract (thymus opton) induced a marked and constant inhibition of mouse carcinoma (21); more recently, it was found that certain isolated thymic fractions either inhibit or retard embryonal development and the growth of tumor transplants and different chemically induced tumors (72).

Pineal extract also induces regression of spontaneous mammary carcinomas and Ehrlich carcinomas in mice (22). Tumors induced with benzopyrene in mice also respond to pineal extracts. Walker carcinosarcoma treated with pineal extract shows more extensive necrosis than occurs in untreated animals. Conversely, pinealectomy stimulates tumor spread (47). Both thymic and pineal extracts inhibit or mitigate metaplastic hepatobiliary estrogen-induced lesions in guinea pigs (56). It is possible that pineal and thymus extract act on cell division and proliferation, exhibiting an antiproliferative action. They can also interfere with host-immune resistance and with the pituitary gonadal or pituitary–hypothalamic axis.

Although we do not know the precise mechanism(s) of thymus and pineal extracts, or melatonin, there is a definite relationship between these extracts and the development of malignant tumors and metastasis formation (39). It is interesting that thymus and pineal gland can influence the growth and distribution of metastases. Thus, the formation of metastases from Yoshida sarcoma is significantly accelerated in rats undergoing a simultaneous thymectomy and pinealectomy. Pinealectomized animals were observed to have metastases primarily in the pancreas, whereas thymectomized rats were found to have metastases only in the liver; rats that had the double surgery developed metastases in the pancreas and in the liver (47).

Recently, it was found that virally transformed mouse cells exhibit great instability in gene expression. Gene expression can be regulated by DNA methylation (16). This instability in gene expression can lead to variation in clones of cells, with a new clone of cells emerging as an older clone declines, disappearing after proliferation. It is possible that hormones and hormonelike substances that interfere with DNA synthesis and gene expression might have a role in the formation of new clones and the decline of old clones of cells in cell subpopulations.

SUMMARY

Precancerous and cancerous cells are heterogeneous cell population that exhibit varying morphological, biochemical, antigenic, and hormone responsiveness. Both precancerous and cancerous cells emerge from normal cells exposed to chemical oncogens or hormones. These phenotypically altered cells still preserve some structural, antigenic, and hormone receptors from the normal cells from which they originate. Electron microscopy and SEM are useful in identifying not only various cell types, but subtypes in the same precancerous or cancer cell population, the progressive cell surface changes, and cell connections as well.

Homeostasis of precancerous and cancerous cells—the progression of precancerous cells to cancer cells—is a controllable process. Fortunately, both precancerous and cancer cells continue to be responsive cells, giving researchers a handle whereby hormones and hormonelike substances (hormonoids) can control the homeostasis and progression of precancerous cells to cancer cells. These substances can restrain this progression and maintain the precancerous cells in a latent state for years; conversely, they can stimulate this transformation. Hence, hormones are important cellular homeostatic factors.

REFERENCES

1. Adamson, R., Banerjee, M., and Medina, D.: Susceptibility of mammary tumor virus from BALB/c mouse mammary nodule outgrowth cells in DNA synthesis to 3-methylcholanthrene. *J. Natl. Cancer Inst. 46*:899–907 (1971).
2. Aitken, S., and Lippman, M.: Hormonal regulation of net DNA synthesis in MCF-7 human breast cancer cells in tissue culture. *Cancer Res. 42*:1727–1735 (1982).

3. Armelin, J.: Cell cycle regulation in mammalian cells: Hormones and commitment to DNA synthesis. *Arch. Biol. Med. Exp. (Santiago) 12*:319–324 (1979).

4. Asch, B., Medina, D., and Brinkley, B.: Microtubules and actin-containing filaments of normal, preneoplastic and neoplastic mouse mammary epithelial cells. *Cancer Res. 39*:893–907 (1979).

5. Asch, B., and Medina, D.: Concanavalin A induced agglutinability of normal, preneoplastic and neoplastic mouse mammary cells. *J. Natl. Cancer Inst. 61*: 1423–1430 (1978).

6. Asch, B., Medina, D., Mace, M., and Brinkley, B.: Modulation of concanavalin A mediated agglutination of normal and neoplastic mouse mammary epithelial cells. *J. Cell Biol. 79*:271a (1978).

7. Ashley, D.: A male–female differential in tumor incidence. *Br. J. Cancer 23*:21–25 (1969).

8. Banerjee, D., Banerjee, M., and Mehta, G.: Hormonal regulation of rapidly labeled RNA in normal, preneoplastic and neoplastic tissues of mouse mammary gland. *J. Natl. Cancer Inst. 51*:843–849 (1973).

9. Banerjee, M., Mehta, R., and Wagner, J.: DNA polymerase activity and DNA synthesis in preneoplastic nodule outgrowths of BALB/c and C₃H mouse mammary gland. *J. Natl. Cancer Inst. 50*:339–345 (1973).

10. Banerjee, D., and Rogers, F.: Stimulation of the synthesis of the macromolecules by ovarian hormones during early development of the mouse mammary gland. *J. Endocrinol. 49*:39–49 (1970).

11. Bertram, J., and Heidelberger, C.: Cell cycle dependency of oncogenic transformation induced by N-methyl-N′-nitro-N-nitro-soguanidine in culture. *Cancer Res. 34*:526–537 (1974).

12. Bibby, M.: The specificity of early changes in the skin during carcinogenesis. *Br. J. Dermatol. 104*:485–487 (1981).

13. Black, M., and Kwon, S.: Precancerous mastopathy: Structural and biological considerations. *Pathol. Res. Pract. 166*:491–514 (1980).

14. Canellakis, Z., and Theoharides, T.: Stimulation of ornithine decarboxylase synthesis and its control by polyamines in regenerating rat liver and cultured rat hepatoma cells. *J. Biol. Chem. 251*:4436–4441 (1976).

15. Cervenka, J.: Chromosomal changes associated with premalignancy and cancer. In McKinell, R., DiBerardino, M., Blumenfeld, M., and Bergad, R. (eds.): *Differentiation and Neoplasis.* (Berlin, Springer-Verlag, 1980), pp. 93–101.

16. Clough, D., Kunkel, L., and Davidson, R.: 5-Azacytidine induced reactivation of a herpes simplex thymidine kinase gene. *Science 216*:70–73 (1982).

17. Coffino, P.: Hormonal regulation of cloned genes. *Nature 292*:492–493 (1981).

18. Coman, D.: Reduction in cellular adhesiveness upon contact with a carcinogen. *Cancer Res. 20*:1202–1204 (1960).

19. DeGerlache, J., Land, M., Taper, H., and Roberfroid, M.: Separate isolation of cells from nodules and surrounding parenchyma of the same precancerous rat liver: Biochemical and cytochemical characterization. *Toxicology 18*: 225–232 (1980).

20. Edwards, D., Adams, D., and McGuire, W.: Estrogen regulation of growth and specific protein synthesis in human breast cancer cells in tissue culture. In Leavitt, W. (ed.): *Hormones and Cancer.* (New York, Plenum Press, 1982), pp. 133–149.

21. Engel, D.: Experimentalle studien über die Beeinflüssung des tumor wachstum mit abbauprodukten (Abderhaldenschen optonen) fon endokrinen drüsen bei maüsen. *Z. Krebsforsch. 19*:339–380 (1922).

22. Engel, P.: Über den Einfluss von hypophysen vorderlappen hormonen und epi-

physenhormon auf das wachstum von Impftumoren *Z. Krebsforsch. 41*: 281–291 (1934).

23. Farber, E.: The sequential analysis of liver cancer induction. *Biochem. Biophys. Acta 605*:149–166 (1980).

24. Farber, E.: Chemical carcinogenesis: A biologic perspective. *Am. J. Pathol. 106*: 271–296 (1982).

25. Fialkow, P.: Use of genetic markers to study cellular origin and development of tumors in human females. *Adv. Cancer Res. 15*:191–223 (1972).

26. Foulds, E.: *Neoplastic Development*, vols. 1 and 2. (New York, Academic Press, 1975).

27. Fujiwara, Y.: Effect of cyclohexamide on regulatory protein for initiating mammalian DNA replication at the nuclear membrane. *Cancer Res. 32*:2089–2095 (1972).

28. Gelfant, S.: A new concept of tissue and tumor cell proliferation. *Cancer Res. 40*: 1269–1273 (1980).

29. Goldengerg, D.: Oncofetal and other tumor associated antigens of the human digestive system. *Curr. Top. Pathol. 63*:289–342 (1976).

30. Grath, C., Prass, W., Maloney, T., and Jones, R.: Induction of endogenous mammary tumor virus expression during hormonal induction of mammary adenoacanthomas and carcinomas of BALB/c female mice. *J. Natl. Cancer Inst. 67*:841–850 (1981).

31. Haynes, B., Hensley, L., and Jegasothy, B.: Differentiation of human T lymphocytes. II. Phenotypic difference in skin and blood malignant T-cells in cutaneous T-cell lymphoma. *J. Invest. Dermatol. 78*:323–326 (1982).

32. Hicks, R.: Early carcinogenesis, differentiation and promotion. *Br. J. Cancer 41*: 661–663 (1980).

33. Highman, B., Greenman, D., Norvell, M., Farmer, J., and Shellenberger, T.: Neoplastic and preoplastic lesions induced in female C_3H mice by diets containing diethylstilbestrol or 17β-estradiol. *J. Environ. Pathol. Toxicol. 4*:81–95 (1980).

34. Waterhouse, J., Muir, C., Correa, P., and Powel, J. (eds.): *Cancer Incidence in Five Continents*, IARC Scientific Publication No. 15, vol. III. (Lyons, International Agency for Research on Cancer, 1976), pp. 109–412.

35. Ip, C.: Prophylaxis of mammary neoplasia by selenium supplementation in the initiation and promotion phases of chemical carcinogens. *Cancer Res. 41*: 4386–4390 (1981).

36. Iversen, V., Iversen, O., and Hennings, H.: Diurnal variation in susceptibility of mouse skin to the tumorigenic action of methylcholanthrene. *J. Natl. Cancer Inst. 45*:269–276 (1970).

37. Iyer, A., and Banerjee, M.: Sequential expression of preneoplastic and neoplastic characteristics of mouse mammary epithelial cells transformed in organ culture. *J. Natl. Cancer Inst. 66*:893–905 (1981).

38. Karasaki, S.: The fine structure of proliferating cells in preneoplastic rat livers during azo dye carcinogenesis. *J. Cell Biol. 40*:322–335 (1969).

39. Kerenyi, N.: Tumors of the pineal gland. In Kellen, J., and Hilf, R. (eds.): *Influences of Hormones in Tumor Development*, vol. I. (Boca Raton, CRC Press, 1979), pp. 155–165.

40. Kerr, J., Wyllie, A., and Currie, A.: Apoptosis, a basic biological phenomenon with wide ranging implication in tissue kinetics. *Br. J. Cancer 26*:239–256 (1972).

41. King, R.: Studies on the regulation of cell proliferation in culture by steroids. In Dumont, J., and Nunez, J. (eds.): *Hormones and Cell Regulation*, vol. 2. (Amsterdam, Elsevier/North-Holland, 1978), pp. 15–36.

42. Knudson, A.: Heredity and human cancer. *Am J. Pathol. 77*:77–84 (1974).
43. Komitowski, D.: Epidermal–dermal junction during experimental skin carcinogenesis and cocarcinogenesis as revealed by scanning electron microscopy. *J. Invest. Dermatol. 78*:395–401 (1982).
44. Korenman, S.: The endocrinology of breast cancer. *Cancer 46*:874–878 (1980).
45. Koss, L.: Precancerous lesions. In Fraumeni, J. (ed.): *Persons of High Risk of Cancer.* (New York, Academic Press, 1975), pp. 85–101.
46. Kurtz, D.: Hormonal inducibility of rat α_{2u} globulin genes in transfected mouse cells. *Nature 291*:629–631 (1981).
47. Lapin, V.: Influence of simultaneous pinealectomy and thymectomy on the growth and formation of metastases of the Yoshida sarcoma. *Exp. Pathol. 9:* 108–112 (1974).
48. Levan, A., Levan, G., and Mitelman, F.: Chromosomes and cancer. *Hereditas 86*:15–29 (1977).
49. Lewensohm, R., Ringbork, R., and Hansson, J.: Different activities of unscheduled DNA synthesis in human melanoma and bone marrow cells. *Cancer Res. 42*:84–88 (1982).
50. Lin, F., Banerjee, M., and Crump, L.: Cell cycle related hormone carcinogen interaction during chemical carcinogen induction of nodule like mammary lesions in organ culture. *Cancer Res. 36*:1607–1614 (1976).
51. Lingeman, C.: Hormones and hormono mimetic compounds in the etiology of cancer. In Lingeman, C. (ed.): *Recent Results in Cancer Research: Carcinogenic Hormones.* (Berlin, Springer-Verlag, 1979) pp. 1–48.
52. Liotta, L., Tryggvason, K., Garbissa, S., Hart, J., Foltz, C., and Shafie, S.: Metastatic potential correlates with enzymatic degradation of basement membrane collagen. *Nature 284*:67–68 (1980).
53. Lippman, M., and Bolan, G.: Estrogen responsive human breast cancer in long term tissue culture. *Nature 256*:592–593 (1975).
54. Lipsett, M.: Hormonal syndromes associated with neoplasia. *Adv. Metab. Disord. 3*:111–152 (1968).
55. Lumeng, L: Hormonal control of ornithine decarboxylase in isolated liver cells and the effect of ethanol oxidation. *Biochem. Biophys. Acta 587*:556–566 (1979).
56. Lupulescu, A.: *Hormonii steroizi [Steroid hormones].* (Bucharest, Edit. Med., 1958), pp. 230–233.
57. Lupulescu, A.: Hormonal regulation of DNA synthesis in cancerous epidermal cells, *J. Cell Biol. 87*:103 (1980).
58. Lupulescu, A.: Ultrastructural pathology of thyroid gland. In Motta, P. (ed.): *Electron Microscopy in Biology and Medicine: Ultrastructure of Endocrine Cells and Tissues.* (Hague-Boston, M. Nijhoff), in press.
59. Lupulescu, A., Mehregan, H., Rahbari, H., Pinkus, H., and Birmingham, D.: Veneral warts vs. Bowen disease. A histologic and ultrastructural study of five cases. *JAMA 237*:2520–2522 (1977).
60. Lupulescu, A., and Pinkus, H.: Electron microscopic observations on rat epidermis during experimental carcinogenesis. *Oncology 33*:24–28 (1976).
61. Lupulescu, A., Rogers, J., and Birmingham, D.: Hormonal control of preneoplastic cells during carcinogenesis in mice. *J. Cell Biol. 79*:187a (1978).
62. McCumbee, W., Lebowitz, H., and McCarty, K.: Hormone responsiveness of a transplantable rat chondrosarcoma. III. Ultrastructural evidence of in vivo hormone dependence. *Am. J. Pathol. 103*:56–69 (1981).
63. Medina, D.: Preneoplastic lesions in mouse mammary tumorigenesis. *Methods Cancer Res. 7*:3–53 (1973).
64. Medina, D., Oborn, C., and Asch, B.: Distinction between preneoplastic and

neoplastic mammary cell populations in vitro by cytochalasin B induced multinucleation. *Cancer Res. 40*:329–333 (1980).

65. Mensing, H., Albini, A., Krieg, T., Muller, P., Pontz, B., and Meigel, W.: Chemotactic properties and biochemical features of malignant cells in vitro. *J. Invest. Dermatol. 78*:331a (1982).

66. Miller, C., Fuseler, J., and Brinkley, B.: Cytoplasmic microtubules in transformed mouse and nontransformed human cell hybrids: Correlation with in vitro growth. *Cell 12*:319–331 (1977).

67. Milmore, J., Chandrasekeran, V., and Weisburger, J.: Effects of hypothyroidism on development of nitrosomethyl urea induced tumors of the mammary gland, thyroid gland and other tissues. *Proc. Soc. Exp. Biol. Med. 169*: 487–493 (1982).

68. Nagasawa, H., Yamai, R., Nakajima, Y., and Mori, J.: Effects of progesterone on normal and preneoplastic mammary development in mice in relation to prolactin and estrogen. *Eur. J. Cancer 16*:1069–1077 (1980).

69. Nishiya, I., Ishizaki, Y., and Sasaki, M.: Nuclear DNA content and the number of Barr bodies in premalignant and malignant lesions of the uterine cervix. *Acta Cytol. 25*:407–411 (1981).

70. Nowell, P.: The clonal evolution of tumor cell population. *Science 194*:23–28 (1976).

71. Pardee, A.: Restriction point for control of normal animal cell proliferation. *Proc. Natl. Acad. Sci USA 71*:1286–1290 (1974).

72. Potop, I., Biener, J., Bălăceanu, M., and Lupulescu, A.: Action de certains fractions isolées du thymus sur l'embryogénèse et sur le developpement des greffes tumorales dans l'oeuf. V. *International Congress of Biochemistry* (Oxford, Pergamon Press, 1961), p. 438a.

73. Prehn, R.: Tumor progression and homeostasis. *Adv. Cancer Res. 23*:203–236 (1976).

74. Raick, A.: Ultrastructural, histological and biochemical alterations produced by 12-0-tetradecanoyl-phorbol-13-acetate on mouse epidermis and their relevance to the skin tumor promotion. *Cancer Res. 33*:269–286 (1973).

75. Russo, J., Bradley, R., McGrath, C., and Russo, I.: Scanning and transmission electron microscopy study of a human breast carcinoma cell line (MCF-7) cultured in collagen-coated cellulose sponge. *Cancer Res. 37*:2004–2014 (1977).

76. Sabine, J.: Metabolic control mechanisms in precancerous liver. *CRC Crit. Rev. Toxicol. 7*:189–218 (1980).

77. Skinner, J., and Whitehead, R.: Tumor markers in carcinoma and premalignant states of the stomach in humans. *Eur. J. Cancer 18*:227–235 (1982).

78. Stout, D., and Becher, F.: Progressive DNA damages in hepatic nodules during 2-acetylaminofluorene carcinogenesis. *Cancer Res. 40*:1269–1273 (1980).

79. Tomita, Y., Nakamura, T., and Ichihara A.: Control of DNA synthesis and ornithine decarboxylase activity by hormones and amino acids in primary cultures of adult rat hepatocytes. *Exp. Cell Res. 135*:363–371 (1981).

80. Tripath, R., and Garner, A.: The ultrastructure of pre-invasive cancer of corneal epithelium. *Cancer Res. 32*:90–97 (1972).

81. Trump, B., Hestfield, B., Phelps, P., Sanefuji, H., and Shamsuddin, A.: Cell surface changes in preneoplastic and neoplastic epithelium. *Scan. Electr. Micr. 3*:43–60 (1980).

82. Tucker, R., Sanford, K., and Frankel, F.: Tubulin and actin in paired non-neoplastic and spontaneously transformed neoplastic cell lines in vitro: Fluorescent antibody studies. *Cell 13*:629–642 (1978).

83. Turbitt, M., and Mackie, R.: Loss of β_2 microblobulin from the cell surface of

cutaneous malignant and premalignant lesions. *Br. J. Dermatol. 104*:507–513 (1981).

84. Vic, P., Vignon, F., Derocq, D., and Rochefort, H.: Effect of estradiol on the ultrastructure of the MCF-7 human breast cancer cells in culture. *Cancer Res. 42*:667–673 (1982).

85. Wallach, D.: Cellular membranes and tumor behavior: A new hypothesis. *Proc. Natl. Acad. Sci USA 61*:868–874 (1968).

86. Wanson, J., Ridder, L., and Mosselmans, R.: Invasiveness of hyperplastic nodule cells from diethyl nitrosamine treated rat liver. *Cancer Res. 41*:5162–5175 (1981).

87. Weiss, H., Wildner, G., Gutz, H., Ebeling, K., Sternoff, G., and Tanneberger, S.: DNA distribution patterns of preneoplastic cells and their interpretation. *Oncology 38*:210–218 (1981).

88. Woods, D., and Smith, C.: Ultrastructure and development of epithelial cell pseudopodia in chemically induced premalignant lesions of the hamster cheek pouch. *Exp. Mol. Pathol. 12*:160–174 (1970).

89. Wortzman, M., Besbris, H., and Cohen, H.: Effect of dietary selenium on the interaction between 2-acetyl aminofluorene and rat liver DNA in vivo. *Cancer Res. 40*:2670–2676 (1980).

90. Yuspa, S., Hennings, H., and Saffiotti, U.: Cutaneous chemical carcinogenesis: Past, present and future. *J. Invest. Dermatol. 67*:199–208 (1976).

Chapter 4

ROLE OF HORMONES IN THE ETIOLOGY AND PATHOGENESIS OF CANCER

GENERAL CONSIDERATIONS AND PROSPECTS IN CARCINOGENESIS

At the end of the last century, the British surgeon Beatson, through his intuitive studies, made the assumption that hormones can play a cardinal role in the etiology of mammary cancers. In his paper on the treatment of

89

inoperable cases of the mamma, he wrote, "without the desire of being in any way dogmatic in the etiology of cancer . . . but the facts which I observed indicate a possibility in the direction of an altered condition of the ovary and testicle, that we are to look for the real exciting cause of cancer, and if so, the sooner we direct our energies into that channel the better. All I feel is that there are grounds for the belief that the etiology of cancer lies in an ovarian or testicular stimulus" (3). Hence, even before hormones were actually discovered, Beatson had believed an ovarian secretion to be an important controlling factor in the causation and development of human breast cancer. Thus the hormonal concept of carcinogenesis was originated.

Later, Lathrop and Loeb (47) showed the hormonal milieu of multiple pregnancies to predispose to carcinoma formation; these workers also observed that large numbers of ovariectomized mice failed to acquire mammary cancer (47). At the same time, similar observations regarding the role of an anterior pituitary extract on cancer development in mice were reported by White and Titcombe (105). However, important scientific achievements in this field were not made until the modern era of endocrinology a few years later, when hormones were being isolated and purified. Lacassagne was the first investigator to demonstrate the role of sex hormones (estrogens) in cancer development (44). In his original experiment, weekly injections of estrone benzoate induced mammary cancer in each of three male mice after 5 to 6 months of treatment; it was recognized that steroid hormones have a special ability to develop tumors in mammalian tissues. Since that initial experiment, the association between hormones and tumor development in different organs has been repeatedly demonstrated (5,6,25,27,35,46,50,54,56,74,76,89,100).

Epidemiological studies in the 1940s on highly inbred mouse strains led Bittner and co-workers (8,9) to the discovery of three factors in the etiology of spontaneous mammary carcinoma: genetic susceptibility, hormonal influences, and the famous milk factor, now identified as an oncornavirus.

The abundant investigations that followed reported that most of the chemical carcinogens, either alone or in combination with hormones, can induce several types of cancers in different laboratory animals (25,28,50, 56,102). In addition to chemical carcinogens, the hormones, viruses, and physical agents (e.g., radiation) have been shown to produce leukemic states and tumors in different organs (89). Thus, hormonal interactions with chemical, viral, or physical carcinogens became of broad interest in experimental carcinogenesis. By modifying the environment of cells, hormones and hormonelike substances can induce cell hyperplasia (premalignant changes) that can independently produce or be accelerated into benign, and later to autonomous or malignant tumors, by the addition of carcinogenic factors. These findings also demonstrated that endogenous carcinogenesis is an important concept as compared with environmental carcinogenesis (6,8,22,37).

Meantime, important investigations conducted by Huggins and associates showed hormones not only to be important etiological factors in the onset and development of tumors, but to be important in tumor regression and extinction as well (33,34,36). In studies of prostate cancer, Huggins demonstrated that changes in the hormonal environment can cause not only induction of cancers, but regression or extinction of these tumors as well. Injection of a synthetic estrogen (stilbestrol) profoundly decreases the size of benign and malignant prostate tumors in dogs. Extinction of experimental mammary cancer was also reported after administration of progesterone and androgens (35,78). Hormonal control is also applicable to far advanced prostatic carcinoma in human subjects. Testosterone accelerates the growth of human prostatic cancer, whereas orchiectomy or injection of natural or synthetic estrogens (stilbestrol) causes a dramatic regression of their tumors (33). Huggins assumed that hormones act by inducing a specific toxicity in the cancer cells, leaving the normal cells undamaged. These studies led to the concept of hormone-dependent and hormone-responsive tumors. Here, it was established that some cancers are hormone dependent and others hormone independent. Eight types of cancers are currently recognized as hormone responsive: cancers of the breast, prostate gland, thyroid, endometrium, kidney, and seminal vesicles, lymphomas and leukemia and carcinoma of scent glands (12,34).

Other investigations showed that experimental pulmonary, liver, thyroid, adrenal, and epidermal tumors (squamous cell carcinomas, basal cell carcinomas) are also drastically affected in onset and evolution by hormone administration (56–59,64,66). Hormones have been established as important etiological factors of hormone-dependent tumors and are also major controlling factors in the development of other types of cancers. Our present concept is that the etiology of tumors involves multiple factors, that is, cancers have a plurifactorial etiology (86). Among other factors (chemical carcinogens, viruses, physical carcinogens), hormones have an important role in the etiology and pathogenesis of neoplasia. In some types of cancers the role of hormones is essential, while in others it is only adjuvant.

It is important to note that many neoplastic cells induced by somatic mutations can remain in a latent stage of dormancy for several years, until some hormonal derangements (e.g., hormonal imbalance) stimulate them to multiply and form neoplasms. Immunological surveillance (14) is another important mechanism that controls neoplastic transformation. Thus, hormones are important endogenous factors in maintaining cell homeostasis (63,65,97). Neoplasia is the end result of the breaking up of these homeostatic cellular mechanisms. It was recently demonstrated that hormone effects are controlled by a basic feedback or thermostat mechanism. For example, thyroid, adrenal, or gonadal hormones are controlled by pituitary trophic or stimulating hormones; these in turn are controlled by hypothalamic releasing factors. These feedback mechanisms are crucial to hormonal carcinogenesis

(Fig. 4–1). In addition to hormones, some hormonelike substances (e.g., prostaglandins, epidermal growth factor) are also important etiological agents of cancers (64,85). In some types of cancers, hormones act directly, in others, indirectly. It is still debatable as to whether hormones can be classified as carcinogens per se, or only as cocarcinogens or modulator agents of carcinogenesis. Later in this section and in Chapter 6 the mechanism of hormone action is discussed in detail.

With the advancement of modern procedures, such as radioactive hormones, autoradiography, electron microscopy, and especially radio-immunoassay (109), it is possible to detect the incipient cellular changes, hormone receptors, and the initial hormonal disorders, in order to prevent neoplastic transformation in patients having high risk for cancer. During the preoperative stages, the high level of hormone receptors in the serum of the cancerous patient is an accurate indication that these cancers are responsive to such surgical procedures as ovariectomy, orchiectomy, and adrenalectomy. Mammary cancers that regress after ovariectomy always contain high levels of estradiol receptors that sediment with a peak at 8S on ultracentrifugation, whereas tumors that do not regress after ovariectomy have only a small number of 8S receptors in their cytosol (39).

Epidemiological studies and clinical observations show that the familiar risk for breast cancer in humans is always associated with elevated hormone levels (estrogens, prolactin, progesterone) (77,81,95). Many carcinomas induced by carcinogens, viruses, or radiation still require a specific hormone pattern for their growth. Elevation of these hormone levels increases susceptibility to carcinogens, decreases the latency period and increases the frequency of tumors. Thus the estriol/estradiol + estrone ratio is suggested as an accurate indicator in patients who have a high risk for breast cancer. A low ratio, which occurs frequently among caucasian women, indicates a high cancer risk, whereas a high ratio, which occurs more frequently among oriental women, suggests a low cancer risk (48,67). Modern methods show that cancerous cells are cells that can still respond to environmental factors, especially hormonal influences. Electron microscopic autoradiography can detect initial changes in the heterogeneous cell population, showing differences between the silent or dormant abnormal cells and those more active in neoplastic transformation. Thus it is possible to evaluate the chances that the tumor will remain in a benign stage and hormone responsive, or that it will move toward a malignant or autonomous stage and become hormone unresponsive or hormone independent. The use of these sensitive methods has brought new findings and has contributed to the elucidation of the role of hormones in etiology and pathogenesis of tumors.

Although a tremendous amount of literature concerning the role of hormones in experimental and human carcinogenesis has emerged during the past five decades, the role of hormones remains more clear in the etiology and pathogenesis of experimental tumors than in human cancers. For this

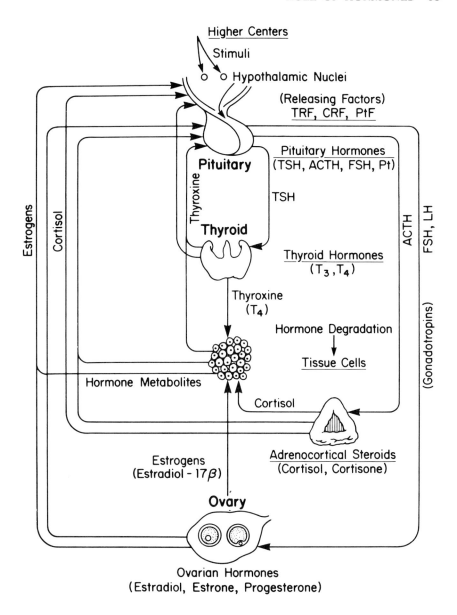

Figure 4–1 The basic feedback hormone mechanisms and their significance for carcinogenesis: hypothalamic–pituitary–thyroid axis, hypothalmic–pituitary axis, and hypothalamic–pituitary–ovarian axis.

reason, we will treat experimental carcinogenesis and human carcinogenesis separately.

ROLE OF HORMONES IN THE ETIOLOGY AND PATHOGENESIS OF EXPERIMENTAL CARCINOMAS

Hormones and hormonelike substances are implicated as etiological agents in spontaneous and experimental mammary carcinomas, endocrinological oncogenesis (pituitary tumors, thyroid tumors, ovarian, uterine, prostate, and adrenal tumors), liver tumors (hepatocarcinogenesis), pulmonary tumors, lymphoid tumors and leukemias, kidney tumors, bone tumors, and epidermal carcinomas.

Mammary Carcinomas

The most extensively studied and the first cancer in which hormonal control was demonstrated is mammary carcinoma. The growth and differentiation of normal mammary ductoalveolar epithelium are controlled by the presence of estrogens, progesterone, and prolactin (Fig. 4–2). From this hormonal cocktail (76,77), prolactin is the primary stimulus required for mammary growth and differentiation. Other stimuli have little or no effect in the absence of prolactin or mammotropic hormone (72). It is possible that estrogens and progesterone act by modifying the release of prolactin. In vitro studies show that glucocorticoid (cortisol), insulin, and thyroid hormones can induce a prolactin release from a mammary mouse cell suspension.

Of all the steroid hormones, estrogens possess the strongest ability to induce mammary cancer in different animal species, in doses 500 to 1000 times smaller than that of other steroids. The administration of naturally occurring estrogens (17B-estradiol and estrone) has induced cancers in many rodent species (44–46). The role of estrogens was first studied and well documented in mammary oncogenesis. Chronic administration of purified estrogens first induces hyperplastic alveolar nodules, and later true carcinomas. Because estrogen treatment often induces both mammary carcinomas and pituitary tumors, the emphasis has shifted to the anterior pituitary, primarily to prolactin and growth hormone. The role of hormones in the transformation of normal mammary ducts of alveolar epithelium to nodular formation and then to autonomous carcinomas has been investigated chiefly in C_3H mice. It is still uncertain as to whether estrogens alone can increase the rate of carcinoma formation from hyperplastic alveolar nodules. However, it is known that estrogens alone are critical to nodular induction and maintenence and that their transformation to carcinomas requires association with other hormones (prolactin, growth hormone, DOC, and cortisol).

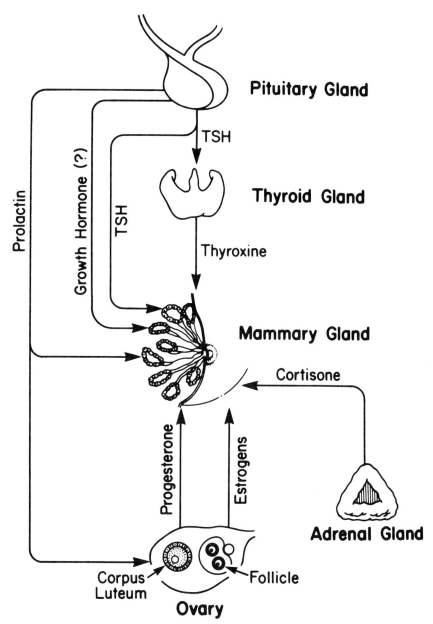

Figure 4-2 Hormonal control of mammary gland.

In recent years, other carcinogenic agents shown to be involved in mammary carcinogenesis are such chemical carcinogens as 3-methylcholanthrene (MCA), 7,12-dimethylbenzanthracene (DMBA), viruses, and physical agents (radiation). The role of hormones is significant in all types of cancers induced by these agents. For instance, inducement of mammary carcinomas in male mice by a chemical agent can be accelerated by administration of estrogens or by ovary transplantation. On the other hand, the rate of carcinoma formation is greatly reduced when the carcinogen is administered to ovariectomized female mice. Pregnancy, pseudopregnancy, and lactation increase the rate of chemically induced mammary carcinomas in mice, whereas a low rate is observed in virgin mice treated with the same chemicals (68).

Species differences in mammary responses to carcinogens and hormones are greater than those of any other target (or end) organs. Among laboratory animals, mammary cancers occur in mice and rats and in some strains of rabbits and dogs—almost exclusively in females. Mammary cancers rarely or never develop in pigs, hamsters, and monkeys. Original observations demonstrated that ovaries and their hormones have a cardinal role in the etiology of breast cancers. Ovariectomy reduces the incidence or prevents the occurrence of mammary cancer, whereas chronic treatment with estrogens is associated with a high incidence of mammary cancers (mostly fibroadenomas) in rats. Mammary carcinomas develop in both mice and rats in the form of adenocarcinomas, fibroadenomas, squamous carcinomas, or mixed tumors. The dose–response relationship is evidenced by rapid appearance of tumors with larger doses of hormone. Some tumors metastasize to the regional lymph nodes and lungs. The very low incidence of spontaneous mammary cancers in control rats as contrasted with their widespread appearance in response to large doses of estrogen, is a rather convincing piece of evidence for the carcinogenic action of estrogens. The development of mammary tumors depends on the presence of estrogens. Complete withdrawal of estrogens is followed by a complete tumor regression; estrogen reimplantation will then produce renewed tumor growth, proving that mammary tumors are indeed hormone dependent.

Furthermore, long-term administration of estrogen that induces mammary tumors in rats is usually associated with pituitary tumors; hypophysectomy will then bring about a complete regression of these neoplasms. These findings indicate that hormonal environment involves complex interactions (13,17,32,41). The presence of prolactin is of fundamental importance to the genesis of mammary cancer (24,72). Whereas estrogens can neither induce nor maintain the development of mammary tumors in the absence of prolactin, prolactin has demonstrated a limited capacity to induce and maintain tumor growth upon removal of either estrogen or the ovaries themselves. Hypothalamic lesions, pituitary grafts, or drugs (biogenic amines) that suppress the release of prolactin can either increase or inhibit the development of spontaneous or carcinogenic-induced breast tumors in C_3H/HeJ mice (103). Administration of testosterone propionate in adequate amounts significantly reduces the incidence of mammary tumors (78). Fewer tumors occur in testosterone-treated rats than in those that remain untreated. The administration of progesterone along with estrogens still produces inconclusive results regarding the incidence of mammary tumors.

These experiments provide evidence of the major role of estrogens in initiating mammary carcinogenesis and of the role of other hormones in maintaining tumor growth. Estrogen stimulates prolactin secretion and acts in conjunction with prolactin directly on the mammary epithelium to produce breast cancers (72,93). Hyperprolactinemia goes on to induce the development of mammary cancer.

These experimental investigations clearly underrate the major role of hormones in the etiology and pathogenesis of mammary cancer. It can be stated that without hormones breast cancer cannot occur (76). Mammary cancer has never been shown to occur in an undeveloped mammary gland either in animals or in human subjects. Clearly, of great importance in the genesis of mammary tumors are the presence and cooperative effect of estrogens, progesterone, and prolactin. An imbalance in the levels of these hormones can result in carcinogenesis. The risk to breast cancer appears to be greatly affected by the hormones of the pituitary–gonadal axis and their feedback mechanism. Ovariectomized mice and rats exhibit a decreased incidence of mammary cancer, whereas a moderate increase in the circulating estrogens, progesterone, and prolactin, by injection, transplantation, or interference with feedback mechanisms, has been shown to increase the incidence of mammary cancer in laboratory animals.

Hormones other than estrogens, progesterone, and prolactin, such as thyroid hormones, adrenal steroids, and growth hormone, as well as kidney secretions can interfere with mammary carcinogenesis (17,32,79,83). Hypophysectomy greatly reduces the occurrence of mammary cancer induced by chemical carcinogens (e.g., MCA or DMBA), by as much as 87 percent. When these same animals are then given pituitary grafts, tumor growth resumes.

Species differences have been demonstrated among hormone-responsive cancers (54). For example, spontaneous mammary cancer is common in the dog, mouse, and man. In the dog, breast cancer does not regress after ovariectomy or adrenalectomy (35). Also in various strains of mice having spontaneous mammary cancer in which a virus was demonstrable, cancer did not regress after ovariectomy, hypophysectomy, or administration of testosterone. Mammary cancer in the rat is the only hormone-dependent mammary cancer that can be induced by estrogens, ionizing radiation, and chemical carcinogens. Estrogen treatment of irradiated rats greatly increases the incidence of mammary carcinomas, probably by stimulation of prolactin secretions. Estrogen-induced mammary carcinomas in mice are generally adenocarcinomas. The earliest postirradiation mammary neoplasms in female rats tend to be adenocarcinomas but later, fibroadenomas appear (44,89). Fibroadenomas can be increased in neonatal rats with estrogens; testosterone decreases the incidence of carcinomas induced by DMBA and increases the incidence of fibroadenomas, whereas progesterone alone enhances cancer induction. These experiments suggest that hormones affect not only the onset and development of mammary carcinomas, but their nature or histological type as well. This role of hormones in differentiating histological type is even more apparent in other types of cancers, such as epidermal, liver, and thyroid.

The thyroid hormones and the state of the thyroid function are also important in mammary carcinogenesis. Hypothyroidism has been postulated to contribute to mammary cancer, since epidemiological studies show a higher incidence of breast cancer in women with goiters and low iodine intake (11). Hypothyroidism induced by propylthiouracil (PTU) administration reduces the carcinogenic capacity of DMBA to produce mammary adenocarcinomas in female rats. Hypothyroidism does not affect the initiation stage of mammary carcinogenesis, but it does interfere with the later stages of tumor growth by inhibiting its development (90). The incidence of DMBA-induced mammary tumors is also significantly reduced by surgical thyroidectomy (41).

Adrenal deficiency enhances mammary carcinogenesis in rats (73). The thyroid hormones thyroxine (T_4) and triiodothyronine (T_3) might change the sensitivity of mammary epithelium indirectly to hormonal stimulation. Conversely, hypothyroidism increases secretion of thyroid-stimulating hormone (TSH), thereby increasing the growth of mammary tissue and its response to prolactin. Experimental and clinical evidence indicates that the hypothalamic–pituitary–thyroid axis is important in the etiology and pathogenesis of breast cancer. Experiments in ovariectomized and thyroidectomized rats demonstrated that the mammotropic effect of prolactin is enhanced by thyroidectomy, and thus a suboptimal level of circulating thyroid hormones (T_4 and T_3) can sensitize the mammary epithelium to prolactin stimulation (73). Greater mammary development is seen in thyroidectomized–ovariectomized rats than in rats that were ovariectomized, but not thyroidectomized. This evidence suggests an important role for thyroid-prolactin balance in mammary carcinogenesis; alteration of this balance could increase neoplastic transformation. Additional data supporting the role of hypothalamic–pituitary–thyroid axis are presented below.

Endocrine Gland Carcinomas

In addition to mammary cancer, for which the causative and pathogenic role of hormones was most extensively studied, hormones and hormonelike substances were also found to play a major role in the neoplasms of other organs and tissues, such as endocrine glands (pituitary, thyroid, ovarian, uterine, adrenals, testicular, prostate), liver, lung, lymphoid organs, kidney bones, and skin.

Pituitary Tumors

Tumorigenesis of endocrine glands, especially of the pituitary gland, occurs primarily in laboratory rats and mice. These tumors generally begin with a moderate, slow-growing pituitary hyperplasia. They are not malignant. Most are chromophil (basophilic) or chromophobe adenomas. Several investigators have induced pituitary tumors in rats with administration of estrogen (estradiol, estrone, stilbestrol), and then found tumor regression after interrupting the administration of the estrogen. Interestingly, no regression was found in mice treated in the same manner. Pituitary tumors are transplantable in both rats and mice. Transplanted tumors grow only in estrogen-treated mice. Pituitary tumors can be prevented in estrogen-treated rats with administration of androgens. Progesterone can either increase or decrease tumor formation, depending on dose. The occurrence of pituitary tumors also depends on genetic influences, with certain strains of rats and mice. C57 mice are particularly susceptible to the development of pituitary tumors (chromophobe adenomas) in response to estrogen injection (26,27).

Recently, pituitary tumors were described in mice made hypothyroid either by the administration of large doses of radioiodine (^{131}I), by surgical removal of the thyroid, or by chronic iodine deficiency. These tumors are thyrotropic (TSH) tumors (7).

Thyroid Carcinomas

Thyroid tumors can be induced in mice and rats by long-term administration of a low-iodine diet; by long-term administration of goitrogens, that is, naturally occurring goitrogens or chemicals, such as methylthiouracil (MTU) or propythiouracil (PTU); by physical agents, such as external exposure to x-rays or intake of radioiodine (^{131}I); by such chemicals as 2-acetylamino-fluorene (AAF); by long-term administration of TSH; or by a combination of any these procedures. Of these means of tumor induction, the most important, from an etiological point of view, is the low-iodine, or chronic iodine-deficient diet. In rodents (mice, rats, hamsters) chronically exposed to a low-iodine diet, a wide range of thyroidal changes developed, beginning with moderate to extensive hyperplasia, then parenchymatous or colloid goiter, later thyroid adenomas, and finally carcinomas. These slow-growing tumors are hormone dependent during the early stages. They can metastasize to the lungs and lymph nodes, but they are not autonomous. Administration of TSH markedly increases the incidence and development of thyroid tumor in all species, including humans, whereas hypophysectomy inhibits neoplastic transformation. Some thyroid tumors, after several passages in animals, lose their hormone dependence but not their hormone responsiveness. Other thyroid tumors lose their organoid and follicular structures and become spindle and anaplastic carcinomas. The etiological role of a low-iodine diet and TSH in the incidence and pathogenesis of thyroid tumors has been emphasized in several independent investigational studies (1,7,25,59,110).

The use of electron microscopy and autoradiography has aided in our understanding of the histogenetic mechanism and hormone responsiveness of thyroid tumors, most of which are follicular or papillary adenomas and carcinomas. For example, benign tumors (adenomas) exhibit only a few nuclear or cytoplasmic abnormalities and normally incorporate ^{131}I and secrete T_4 and T_3; they are always hormonally dependent on TSH. Later stages of tumor development display large nuclear abnormalities and a high degree of dedifferentiation toward spindle or round cells, less incorporation of ^{131}I, and less responsiveness to TSH. These considerable differences between hormone-dependent thyroid nodules (or adenomas) and thyroid cancers, as depicted by electron microscopy and autoradiography, demonstrate that thyroid nodularity does not necessarily indicate a stage in thyroid carcinogenesis. These techniques point up a great similarity between experimentally induced thyroid tumors and human thyroid cancers in regard to both histogenetic mechanism and hormone responsiveness (59). The role of hormones in the pathogenesis of thyroid tumors should be regarded as biphasic: the early stages (i.e., benign tumors) display notable hormone dependency, while the later stages (i.e., malignant tumors) are characterized by hormone independence. Similar evidence has been obtained in thyroid tumors induced by goitrogens, chemical carcinogens, external x-irradiation, or radio-iodine. Tumors appear earlier and in greater numbers when the x-ray or ^{131}I is followed by administration of goitrogens of TSH. The combined treatment is much more carcinogenic than is the iodine-deficient diet or goitrogens alone. Radiation alone can also produce thyroid adenomas and carcinomas (20). Thus, TSH secretion might act as a promoting factor in the development of thyroid tumors (25,71,110). By reducing TSH secretion with a T_4-enriched diet, we can control the early stages of thyroid tumor formation.

These data on hormone dependency are indispensable to the therapy of human thyroid cancers. Electron microscopic evaluation and autoradiographic analysis are essential to the thyroidologist's and oncologist's ability to detect the early, hormone-dependent, stages of thyroid tumors and to study the sequential stages from thyroid hyperplasia, to goitrogenesis, to carcinogenesis.

Ovarian Tumors

Experimental studies show that ovarian tumors can be produced by radiation; by certain carcinogens such as DMBA; and by a hormonal imbalance (at the pituitary–ovarian axis) caused by a break in the feedback mechanism of gonadotropic–ovarian hormones.

X-Irradiation of mice often induces ovarian tumors. Some of these tumors are steroid-secreting tumors—either granulosa cell or luteinic cell tumors. Granulosa cell tumors of the mouse ovary can also be induced by DMBA administration. In both irradiated and DMBA-induced ovarian tumors, the gonadotropic pituitary hormones are necessary for both tumor induction and development. Initially, autonomous tumors are produced by the direct carcinogenic effect of DMBA on ovarian cells; this carcinogenic effect is later modified by the action of gonadotropins (27,81). Gonadotropic hormones usually enhance ovarian tumor formation. Both radiation- and chemically induced ovarian carcinomas are hormonally mediated. However, the most useful procedure for producing ovarian tumors and for following the sequential stages for hyperplasia, hormone-dependent tumors, and autonomous tumors is that of intrasplenic ovarian graft in castrated rats (8), a typical carcinogenesis caused by a hormone imbalance. For example, when ovarian hormones are destroyed by the liver, a massive increase in the level of gonadotropic hormones occurs, subsequently inducing ovarian tumors (Fig. 4–3). But when the ovaries are implanted subcutaneously, or when the ovarian tissue is grafted, induction of ovarian tumors does not occur. The primary

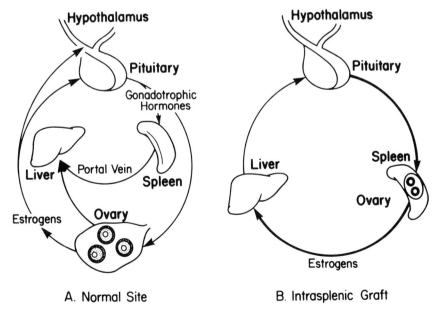

A. Normal Site   B. Intrasplenic Graft

Figure 4-3 Induction of ovarian tumor by disruption of hypothalamic–pituitary–ovarian axis: *a.* ovary into its normal site, *b.* intrasplenic graft.

ovarian tumors induced by transplantation of ovaries into the spleen are transplantable tumors. A high frequency of ovarian carcinomas (granulosa cell, luteomas, or mixed) appear among gonadectomized mice, guinea pigs, and rabbits bearing intrasplenic or intrapancreatic ovarian grafts. The pathogenesis of these ovarian tumors is attributable to hypersecretion of the gonadotropic hormones follicle-stimulating hormone (FSH) and luteinizing hormone due to decreased gonadal function. Other hormones, namely thyroid hormones (T_3 and T_4) and growth hormone (GH), can affect ovarian carcinogenesis. For example, hyperthyroid and gonadectomized mice with intrasplenic ovarian grafts were observed to have fewer ovarian carcinomas than were found in hypothyroid (thiouracil induced) mice or control mice. Induction of ovarian tumors (cystadenomas) by prolonged treatment with GH was also reported in rats (74). Ovarian tumors can be therefore produced by a direct effect of irradiation, by a chemical carcinogen, or by an indirect effect of a hormone imbalance (a break in the feedback mechanism between estrogens and gonadotropins).

Recently, progestational compounds were found to induce ovarian tumors in some strains of mice. Subcutaneous implantation of 19-norprogesterone or norethindrone pellets was shown to induce ovarian tumors (granulosa cell tumors) in BALB/c mice. Lipschütz and co-workers induced ovarian granulosa cell tumors in mice (BALB/c) by prolonged administration of both progesterone and 19-norcontraceptive (norethindrone or norethynodrel) (51). In ovarian tumorigenesis, as in mammary tumorigenesis, genetic factors can explain why some strains are more susceptible than others.

Uterine Tumors (Endometrial Cancers)

Estrogen administration often induces fibromyomas in guinea pigs (27,50). Also, neoplastic responses can be seen in mice, rats, and rabbits. Prolonged estrogen administration induces tumors of the uterine cervix in mice and an abnormal hyperplasia in monkeys. These tumors always remain benign, however, never becoming malignant, even after long periods of estrogen administration, and regressing after estrogen withdrawal. It is interesting that uterine cervical tumors can occur after subcutaneous testosterone implantation in mice. These tumors can be transplanted into other mice only under androgen administration (99). Uterine adenomatose hyperplasia, endometriosis, and endometrial carcinomas have been induced in mice, rats, and rabbits by prolonged estrogen, progesterone, and 19-norcontraceptive administration. The uterine tumors were hormonally dependent (52).

Adrenal Gland Tumors

Adrenal cortex tumors have been frequently produced in the dbs strain of mice, members of which were ovariectomized immediately after birth. These postcastration adrenocortical tumors secrete sex hormones; hypophysectomy, ovarian grafts, and the administration of estrogens and androgens can prevent the occurrence of postcastration adrenal tumors (107). Adrenal tumors can also be produced in rats by prolonged administration of estrogen (79) or pituitary GH (75). Prolactin can enhance adrenal tumorigenesis. Estrogen administration induces only adrenal hyperplasia, not adrenal tumors. Species differences can alter adrenal tumorigenesis and the effect of hormones.

Prolonged administration of estrogens (e.g., estradiol propionate) can induce adrenal medullary hyperplasia and sometimes pheochromocytomas in rats (57). These experimental pheochromocytomas secrete catecholamines. Concomitant administration of estrogens and GH increases the incidence of pheochromocytomas in rats and guinea pigs. Also, aldosterone, reserpine, and glucagon administration modify the catecholamine content and the evolution of chromaffin hyperplasia in guinea pigs (58). Genetic factors also affect the susceptibility to adrenal tumor formation.

Testicular Tumors

Chronic administration of estrogens can induce hyperplasia of interstitial cells and eventually cause tumor formation in BALB/c male mice. Both natural and synthetic estrogens can induce testicular tumors. These tumors are mostly seminoma and Leydig cell tumors; they can be transplanted only under estrogen stimulation, and not in non-estrogen-treated rats. These tumors can secrete large amounts of androstanediol and 11-deoxycorticosterone. Leydig cell tumors can secrete both estrogens and androgens and are hormone-dependent. Testicular tumor development depends on estrogen administration; when estrogens are withdrawn, tumor growth ceases. Certain chemical carcinogens can induce testicular tumors. There are also great species differences in tumor development, influenced by genetic factors.

Prostate Gland Tumors

The study of spontaneous canine prostate tumors led Huggins to the concept of hormone-dependent tumors. Injections of synthetic estrogens (stilbestrol) markedly decreased the size of benign and malignant tumors in dogs, whereas androgens were found to stimulate their growth, thereby establishing hormonal control of tumor growth. Experimental prostate tumors (adenocarcinomas) can also be induced in rats. Castration or administration of diethylstilbestrol (DES) prevents the formation of these tumors (33,34,36). Hormone dependence and hormone independence were correlated with the presence or absence of steroid (or androgen) receptors on these cells. Although androgens are known to exert an important role in the etiology of prostate carcinoma and hypertrophy, there is no direct evidence that these tumors are actually caused by hormones. However, the growth and development of tumors of the prostate gland and of the prostate exhibit strong hormonal influences (Fig. 4-4). Recently, the induction of prostatic adeno-

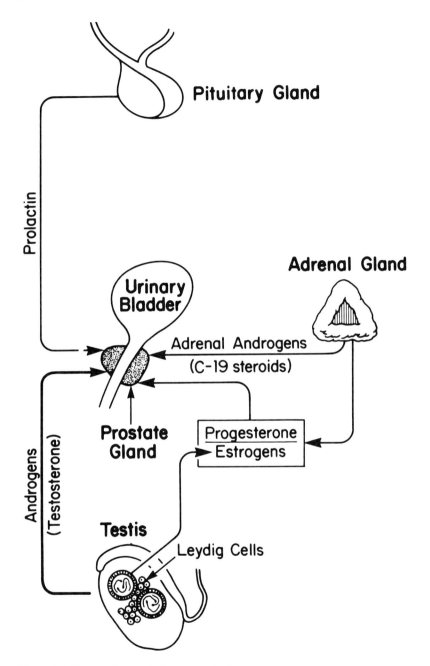

Figure 4-4 Hormonal control of prostate gland.

carcinoma was reported in NB rats after prolonged treatment with testosterone propionate pellets (80), emphasizing the possible hormonal etiology of prostate cancer in male patients.

Liver Tumors (Hepatocarcinogenesis)

Liver tumors have been induced in several animal species (rats, guinea pigs, mice, trout, ducks, ferrets, sheep, and monkeys) with various chemical carcinogens, particularly aflatoxin G_1, N-nitroso compounds (dimethylnitrosoamine), and AAF. Mice are usually resistant to the carcinogenic action of aflatoxin; however, both mice and rats are highly susceptible to carcinogenic action during early life, particularly neonates. In addition to chemical carcinogens, studies using sex steroids show slight but uncertain evidence of increased incidence of liver cell tumors in mice. In rats, combined treatment of progestagens (norethisterone and estrogens) stimulates the development of liver tumors. In the dog and monkey, there is no clear evidence that steroid hormones are associated with liver tumor formation, but liver adenomas have been induced in Beagle bitches subjected to prolonged treatment with progesterone and medroxyprogesterone. In guinea pigs, induction of biliary adenocarcinomas after prolonged administration of estrogen was previously reported. These estrogen-induced liver and biliary tumors and hyperplasia can be prevented or made to regress by administration of progesterone, testosterone, cortisone, thymic hormones, and deoxycorticosterone. Administration of GH promotes liver cancer formation, whereas hypophysectomy inhibits it (56). These studies show the important role of the liver in steroid homeostasis, which by degradatation and metabolization, possibly produces more active carcinogenic metabolites. Also, some liver tumors are hormone responsive, particularly in the early stages. Several investigators have noted a higher incidence of hepatomas in male than in female mice. Castration reduces the incidence of liver tumors among the males. However, the incidence of hepatomas is shown to increase in estrogen-treated C_3H male mice; administration of testosterone propionate does not increase this incidence in female mice. Liver tumors can also be induced by a strong carcinogen, such as AAF. Administration of goitrogens can then reduce AAF-induced hepatocarcinogenesis.

Chemical liver carcinogenesis is strongly influenced by endocrine factors. Thus, male rats are more sensitive than females; hypophysectomy or thyroidectomy inhibits liver carcinogenesis, but extrahepatic carcinogenesis does ensue. In rats treated with the active AAF metabolite and implanted with secreting pituitary tumors (ACTH, GH, and prolactin), the hepatomas appear earlier and with a higher incidence (102). Of these pituitary hormones, ACTH was active in hepatocarcinogenesis.

Experiments in male rats painted with AAF showed the determining role of endocrine factors in the susceptibility of the liver to carcinogens. Thus, in rats treated with carcinogens alone, hepatomas predominate, with only few adenomas and cholangiomas. Thyroidectomy and adrenalectomy completely block the hepatocarcinogenesis at the initiation stage. In thyroidectomized rats treated with GH or cortisone, there is only a slight inhibition of liver tumorigenesis with a moderate predominance of adenomas and cholangiomas (29). Thus, an alteration of the endocrine constellation can drastically affect the development and onset of liver tumors in carcinogen-treated animals.

Pulmonary Tumors

Lung adenomas can be induced in rats by the administration of chemical carcinogens, such as urethane or ethyl carbamate. In recent years, liver and lung adenomas were also induced by the application of organic particulates obtained from atmospheric pollution as well as by some N-nitroso compounds, particularly ethylnitrosourea given to newborn mice (100). Some hormones have been shown to be involved in the induction and development of lung tumors. For example, repeated injections of purified GH over a period of 485 days induced the occurrence of lymphosarcomas of the lung in female rats. Histological studies have shown that lymphosarcomas arise from the transformation of peribronchial lymphoid hyperplasia (74). It has also been demonstrated that after several months repeated injections of estradiol propionate to female guinea pigs can induce the occurrence of lung adenomas. The onset and development of pulmonary estrogen-induced adenomas are strongly affected by endocrine factors. Thus, concomitant administration of deoxycorticosterone (DOC), cortisone, progesterone, and testosterone can prevent estrogen-induced lung tumorigenesis in guinea pigs—progesterone being the most active and testosterone the least active counteragent. Administration of GH enhances the development of lung tumors, whereas hypophysectomy markedly inhibits it. These studies demonstrate that lung tumors can be induced by hormones (e.g., GH and estrogens) and chemical carcinogens (e.g., urethane, air pollutants). Estrogen-induced lung tumors in female guinea pigs are hormone-responsive tumors (56).

Genetic influences can explain the different susceptibilities among different species. Thus, hormonally induced lung tumors occur most often in rats and guinea pigs and very seldom in mice, dogs, or hamsters. A spontaneous pulmonary adenomatosis observed in laboratory mice could have been caused by *Mycoplasma*.

Lymphoid Tumors and Leukemias

A high incidence of lymphoid tumors was reported in some strains of mice exposed to estrogens, chemical carcinogens, or x-irradiation. A high frequency of leukemia is also observed in mice treated similarly. The lymphomagenic action of estrogens is inhibited by testosterone propionate, but not by cortisone. However, both testosterone and cortisone inhibit the lymphomagenic effects of x-rays in mice. In some strains of mice, the incidence was shown to be about 30 times higher than in non-estrogen-treated mice of the same strain. Also, the lymphoid tumors were found to occur earlier in estrogen-treated mice (45). These transplantable tumors occur in the thymus and in all lymphoid tissues. Concomitant administration of testosterone propionate reduces the incidence of lymphomas. Estrogens decrease the incidence of lymphomas in irradiated male mice and androgens reduce the incidence in irradiated female mice (27).

Lymphoid tumors also occur in mice treated with chemical carcinogens, such as DMBA and methylcholanthrene, as well as in estrogen-treated rats, involving chiefly the mesenteric nodes. It is possible that estrogen action is mediated by the adrenal cortex. For example, adrenalectomized mice show an increased incidence of lymphoid tumors after irradiation. Cortisone inhibits lymphoid tumor development in irradiated mice but has no effect on the lymphoid tumors of estrogen-treated mice.

Kidney Tumors

Renal cortical carcinomas (RCCs) have been induced by synthetic estrogens (stilbestrol) in male hamsters and castrated female hamsters; when estrogen treatment is stopped, the tumors regress. These neoplasms arise from multiple foci in both the renal cortex and pelvis, attain a huge size, and are histologically malignant, yet do not metastasize. They do not appear in intact female hamsters or other species treated similarly. They are specific to hamsters and are frequently associated with pituitary pars intermedial tumors (42). However, they can be induced in intact female hamsters when progesterone secretion is low, such as at early age or if testosterone was injected immediately after birth. Also, simultaneous administration of progesterone prevents the occurrence of renal tumors in estrogen-treated male hamsters. Testosterone and DOC exert similar inhibitory effects on renal carcinomas. Androgens can cause renal hypertrophy in rats and mice, however. These renal carcinomas, despite their histological malignancy, are hormone dependent. The fact that these tumors occur only in the male hamster kidney could be attributable to histological differences (such as a higher number of cuboidal or columnar cells in the epithelium of Bowman's capsule) or to enzymatic differences specific to this organ. In addition to hormones, genetic factors might explain their species specificity (27,28).

Carcinomas and papillomas of the bladder, primarily associated with urinary calculi, have been observed in some strains of rats after the subcutaneous implantation of stilbestrol pellets. Neither occurs in mice.

Bone Tumors

Bone, or osteogenic, tumors have been induced more often in female mice (77 percent) than in males (29 percent) of the same strain. These tumors are estrogenic; they arise mostly from the periosteum and have a multifocal origin. Possible slight histological differences of bone periosteum and different strain and species, such as less structural organization of osteoblasts, could explain the high susceptibility of some strains to these tumors (27).

Epidermal Carcinomas: Squamous and Basal Cell

Mouse skin is an ideal system for the study of different chemical carcinogens, since it possesses mostly activating properties and has only a limited detoxifying capacity. Many standard carcinogens are tested on mouse or rat skin. Skin tumorigenesis provides some advantages over liver or lung tumorigenesis, because the tumors are visible and their onset and development or regression can be easily monitored. Thus, the curves of tumorigenesis are more accurate. In mice, most skin tumors are papillomas and squamous cell carcinomas, whereas rats have a predominance of basal cell carcinomas after exposure to the same carcinogenic agent (3-MCA). Although the skin is not a hormone-dependent organ, the onset and development of epidermal tumors are markedly modified by hormone administration.

Some investigations have shown important sex- and age-based differences among different strains of mice in response to the same carcinogen. The modifying role of sex on the incidence and development of liver and skin tumors in mice was previously reported, showing the sex of the animals to be an important modifying factor in the occurrence and distribution of liver tumors, lung tumors, lymphomas, and ovarian and mammary gland carcinogenesis. Male mice from some hybrid strains were observed to have more lung tumors, while hybrid females were more susceptible to liver lymphomas, ovarian, and mammary tumors when exposed to ethylnitrosourea, a short-acting carcinogen (100). Also, sex in certain strains of mice affects susceptibility to skin tumorigenesis. Male Swiss mice in which skin tumorigenesis was initiated by small doses of DMBA and then promoted by croton oil, had more papillomas than did females. It is interesting to note that skin tumorigenesis is also influenced by the estrous cycle and castration. Female mice exposed to carcinogens during diestrus, when the estrogen level is low, had a greater incidence of tumors than did females exposed in other stages of the cycle. Castration before application of DMBA decreased tumor incidence in male mice, but increased tumor incidence in females (2). These observations demonstrate that the incidence and multiplicity of both liver and skin tumors are indeed modified by sex hormones.

Our investigation explored the effects of a broad spectrum of hormones (thyroxine, estradiol, hydrocortisone, calcitonin, insulin, glucagon), hormonelike substances (prostaglandins E_1 and F_2 plus their metabolities U-46619 and U-44069), reserpine, vitamin A, and endocrine deprivation (hypophysectomy, gonadectomy, and thyroidectomy) on the incidence, development, and regression of epidermal tumors (squamous cell carcinomas and basal cell carcinomas).

Since skin tumors are the only visible tumors, their onset, development, and regression are easier to monitor, thereby establishing more accurate curves of tumorigenesis. Such new techniques as electron microscopy; isotope studies in DNA, RNA, and protein synthesis; SEM, and autoradiography have been used to study the effect of these hormones on neoplastic transformation and cellular evolution in order to detect their initial changes at cellular and molecular levels. These findings can provide us with a better understanding of the intrinsic mechanism of action of hormones and carcinogens and elucidate the role of hormones in the causation and development of experimental and human cancers. Since these tumors are histologically and ultrastructurally similar to human cancers, most of these data can be extrapolated to carcinogenesis in humans. In an interesting study involving the local application of the standard and potent carcinogen MCA on the dorsal and shaved areas of mouse and rat skin, two different types of cancers were induced: squamous cell carcinomas in mice and basal cell carcinomas in rats (64,66,111). Fibrosarcomas, sarcomas, and mammary and lung tumors are only occasionally found in these animals. The tumors usually become visible after a latency period of 5 to 6 months in mice and of 8 to 10 months in rats. These tumors are usually found in the painted area or surrounding it, but are sometimes found far from the application point, such as in the eye, stomach, or muscles. Carcinogen 3-MCA was applied in a concentration of 0.3 to 0.4 percent in acetone solution, three times weekly by pipetting and gently rubbing into the skin. Combined treatment with hormones, such as thyroxine, estradiol, hydrocortisone, calcitonin, glucagon, and insulin and with hormonelike substances, that is, PGE_2, $PGF_{2\alpha}$, and their new endoperoxides U-46619 (15(s)-hydroxy-11α,9α-(epoxy methano)prosta-5z, 13E-dienoic acid) and U-44069 (15(s)hydroxy-9α,11α-epoxymethanoprosta-5z, 13E-dienoic acid), were used at the initiation period and throughout carcinogenesis.

For comparison purposes, groups in which carcinogen was similarly applied on their dorsal skin after the endocrine glands were removed by hypophysectomy, castration, or thyroidectomy were also studied. Multiple large, keratinized tumors coalescing and occupying the entire dorsal area are seen in mice. These are squamous cell carcinomas. Different types of tumors developed in rats. These tumors occur later (mostly at 8 months) as pinkish, pearly nodules. These basal cell carcinomas grow slowly and then centrally ulcerate and coalesce, forming clusters of tumors. Both squamous and basal cell carcinomas are locally invasive tumors that rarely metastasize. Their onset and development are markedly affected by hormones, hormonelike substances, and endocrine deprivation. The incidence and multiplicity of tumors in animals treated with carcinogens and hormones, with carcinogens alone, and with hormones alone and in endocrine-deprived animals were recorded at different time intervals (3, 6, 9, 12, and 16 months) in an effort to follow their onset, development, and regression under the influence or absence of various endocrine factors. Since epidermal tumors are visible tumors, their onset and development can be easily determined; in this way, the influence of hormones on carcinomas can be more accurately demonstrated. The incidence and development of carcinomas were markedly affected by hormone treatments

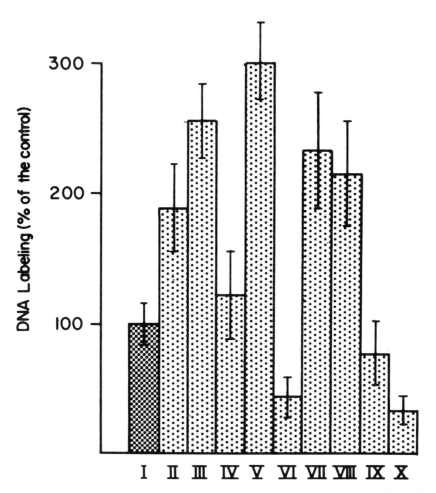

Figure 4-5 DNA labeling in squamous cell carcinomas: I. controls (taken as 100); II. MCA; III. MCA and $PGF_{2\alpha}$; IV. MCA and PGA_2; V. MCA and thyroxine; VI. MCA and hydrocortisone; VII. MCA and estradiol: VIII. MCA and calcitonin; IX. MCA and castration; X. MCA and hypophysectomy.

and by endocrine deprivation. Thus thyroxine, prostaglandins ($PGF_{2\alpha}$ and PGE_2), estradiol, glucagon, and calcitonin markedly enhanced the occurrence and development of carcinomas, whereas PGA_2 and the new metabolites of the prostaglandin series, U-46619 and U-44069, had only a moderately enhancing effect. Treatment with insulin and reserpine induced moderate inhibition, whereas hydrocortisone, hypophysectomy, thyroidectomy, and gonadectomy markedly inhibited the induction and development of carcinomas. From these tumorigenic curves it can be seen that hormones significantly affect the onset and development of carcinomas.

Studies with radioactive amino acids such as ^{3}H-thymidine, ^{3}H-leucine, and ^{3}H-uridine and DNA labeling methods (43) show that hormones profoundly interfere with DNA, RNA, and protein synthesis in cancerous cells (Fig. 4–5). Light microscopic autoradiography on Bouin-fixed and paraffin-embedded tissue from carcinomas show that ^{3}H-thymidine in the nuclei and ^{3}H-leucine in the cytoplasm of neoplastic cells are significantly affected by hormone administration.

Quantitative analysis of autoradiograms demonstrates that hormones significantly influence DNA synthesis in the cancerous cells. The number and percentage of labeled cells are much higher or more sharply reduced in different experimental groups treated with hormones as compared with either animals treated with carcinogens alone or with control animals (Fig. 4–6). The autoradiographic distribution shows that some cellular compartments of neoplastic transformations are more active than others, which can remain in a silent or dormant stage. Thus, most of the labeled cells are found in the basal initial proliferative compartments. A focal distribution of labeled cells and nuclei is seen as well.

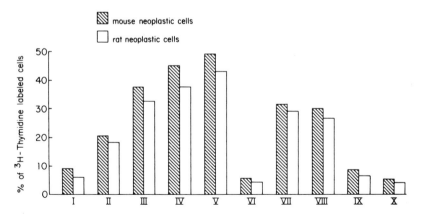

Figure 4-6 Distribution of labeled neoplastic cells between different experimental groups: I. control; II. carcinogen and diluent; III. carcinogen and $PGF_{2\alpha}$; IV. carcinogen and glucagon; V. carcinogen and estradiol; VI. carcinogen and hydrocortisone; VII. carcinogen and estradiol; VIII. carcinogen and calcitonin; IX. carcinogen and castration; X. carcinogen and hypophysectomy.

Light microscopic autoradiography is useful in detecting the events and stages of neoplastic transformation under the influence of hormones. The autoradiographic distribution is more homogeneous during the initial hyperplastic stages or benign tumors than in the more advanced, malignant, or autonomous tumors, in which the distribution becomes more heterogeneous.

Electron microscopic autoradiography is a more sensitive method for studying DNA synthesis and its replication, as well as RNA and the site(s) of protein synthesis in cancerous cells. Thus, we can better visualize the intracellular kinetics of the isotope and its specific location. Thin sections (600 to 900 Å) containing embedded material were obtained from plastic (Epon/Araldite) with an ultrotome-LKB III, then were mounted on grids and covered with a thin layer of Ilford L₄ Nuclear Emulsion using a wire loop procedure. The sections were exposed for a period of 2 to 4 months, then developed and stained briefly with uranyl acetate and lead citrate (15). The radioisotopes appeared either as coiled filaments or were marked by grains and were located primarily in specific areas, such as in the nuclear chromatin for ³H-thymidine, nucleoli for ³H-uridine, and in the ribosomes or endoplasmic reticulum cisternae for ³H-leucine. In the nuclear chromatin of neoplastic cells, incorporation of ³H-thymidine as developed grains takes place mostly in the dense chromatin, heterochromatin, or the genetic chromatin from which the chromosomes and their genes originate; no isotope incorporation is seen in the loose chromatin, or euchromatin (metabolic chromatin). Electron micrographic autoradiography displayed interesting findings regarding the site(s) of DNA synthesis and its replication in the neoplastic cells after the administration of hormones. Thus, some hormones induce a marked incorporation over the squamous or basal neoplastic cells, whereas others, such as hydrocortisone, significantly decrease or inhibit it. Some hormones change the distribution of the isotopes; for instance, estradiol administration induces a predominant location of developed grains on the nuclear membrane. Both light and electron microscopic autoradiography show interesting data regarding DNA synthesis, cell division, and differentiation during neoplastic transformation. Thus, some cell compartments are more proliferative than others. Also, some cells are active, while others remain in a silent or dormant stage, indicating that cancerous cells are a heterogeneous population, with some cells in a benign stage and others having become malignant with a tendency to metastasize.

Electron microscopic evaluation in combination with light microscopy has proved the most valuable tool in the diagnosis and classification of these neoplasms. The cellular evolution and neoplastic transformation of cells from hyperplastic to benign and later to malignant or autonomous cancer cells can also be studied more accurately with the aid of electron microscopy. Hormone responsiveness in differentiated and undifferentiated cells can be evaluated with electron microscopy, high-resolution autoradiography, and SEM. These methods can provide data regarding the initial cellular changes, their later transformation to benign (still hormone-responsive), and malignant or cancerous cells (unresponsive, or autonomous).

Tumor histopathology shows interesting findings regarding the cellular pattern, cell growth and differentation, cell atypicality, and invasiveness under various hormonal treatments. Thus, typical and well-differentiated squamous cell carcinomas, with characteristic epithelial pearl formation and a mild dermal infiltration, occur predominantly in MCA-treated mice, whereas mainly basal cell carcinomas are composed of small basophilic cells with large nuclei. Increased tumor invasiveness and atypicality with several mitoses occur after combined administration of MCA and prostaglandins (especially $PGF_{2\alpha}$), thyroxine, glucagon, estradiol, and calcitonin, whereas a marked inhibition occurs after hydrocortisone administration, hypophysectomy, gonadectomy, and thyroidectomy. Invasive squamous cell carcinomas with the formation of several epithelial or horn pearls is frequently seen in mice treated with MCA and $PGF_{2\alpha}$. Basal cell carcinomas induced by MCA and $PGF_{2\alpha}$ exhibit two distinct cellular compartments, that is, dark cells alternating with clear cells. Hormones can also change the cellular pattern. In mice, thyroxine-induced tumors composed of cellular cords with undifferentiated or anaplastic cells with several mitoses are seen. An intense stimulation of neoplastic cell growth is also observed in rats treated concomitantly with MCA and thyroxine. The solid basal cell carcinomas are composed predominantly of anastomosed cellular cords with small hyperchromatic cells and large nuclei; multinucleated and atypical cells are visible as well.

A fasciculate pattern similar to that in the adrenal gland or organoid (similar to liver) is occasionally seen after thyroxine or glucagon administration. Hormones can also shift the cellular pattern from more invasive tumors to keratinized tumors or sclerotic neoplasms. Thus estradiol and insulin administration increase the incidence of keratotic tumors, in which the tumor masses are replaced by keratin layers. More frequently, calcitonin and testosterone have been shown to induce the occurrence of sclerotic neoplasms in which large areas of tumor cells are replaced and fragmented by advanced sclerosis. Moderate inhibition of cell growth occurs in castrated mice and rats. Marked tumor regression or inhibition is frequently observed in hydrocortisone- and MCA-treated mice and rats after hypophysectomy or thyroidectomy. In such cases, no neoplasms occur, but a moderate epidermal hyperplasia with few proliferative cells, which are acanthotic and vacuolated, is seen (Fig. 4-7). Thus, hormones can markedly increase or decrease tumor growth, differentiation, and invasiveness. Hormones can change the cellular pattern to a more benign or malignant type of neoplasm and to keratotic or sclerotic cancers.

The ultrastructural pathology of carcinomas demonstrates some interesting features of neoplastic cells and their organelle distribution, as well as the cell biology of cancer cells after hormone administration. Some specific

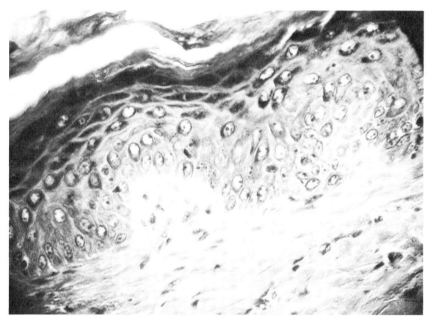

Figure 4-7 A marked inhibition of tumor development can be seen in a mouse treated with carcinogen and hydrocortisone; only a mild epidermal hyperplasia occurred. H & E stain, ×800.

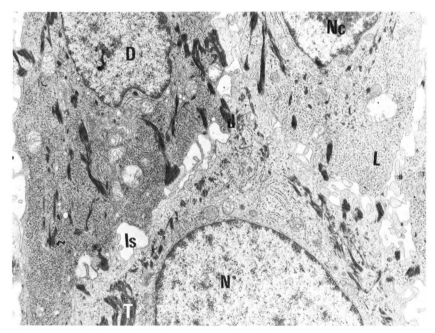

Figure 4-8 Distinct dark (D) and light (L) neoplastic cells in a mouse squamous cell carcinoma, separated by enlarged intercellular spaces (Is) with few desmosomes (d); enlarged nuclei (N) with nucleoli (Nc) and tonofilaments (T). Uranyl acetate and lead citrate stain, ×8,000.

effects of hormones on mitochondria, lysosomes, endoplasmic reticulum, and its membranous system, which can indicate the important role of hormones in controlling the precancerous and cancerous cell populatons, are also shown.

Electron microscopic examination of neoplastic cells highlights distinct ultrastructural characteristics for each type of carcinoma, thus permitting a more accurate diagnosis. For instance, in squamous cell carcinoma (Fig. 4-8), we note the typical dark and light neoplastic cells, enlarged intercellular spaces, large nuclei and nucleoli, several tonofilaments, few desmosomes, and an abundant population of polysomes. This ultrastructural pattern is quite characteristic of squamous cell carcinomas. Figure 4-9 shows the smaller, dark, basophilic cells, abundant rough endoplasmic reticulum, several free ribosomes, dense droplets, dentated nuclei, and the fat droplets that occur predominantly in basal cell carcinomas. Although the basement membrane is still intact, several cytoplasmic protrusions through it can be seen.

The appearance of dark and light cells in both cancers might indicate some similarities in the epidermal cells undergoing neoplastic transformation. It is possible that dark and light cells represent two different clones of cells having different behavior regarding their invasiveness. Ultrastructurally, more tonofilaments, a more condensed endoplasmic reticulum, and attached

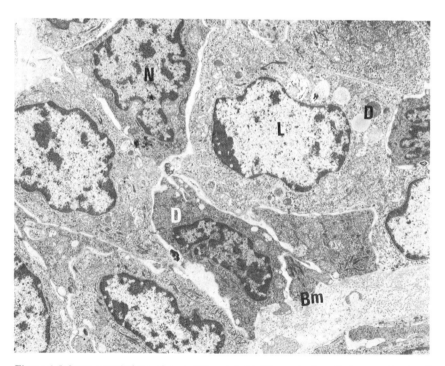

Figure 4-9 Large populations of dark (D) and light (L) neoplastic cells in a rat basal cell carcinoma which are smaller and contain dentated nuclei (N) and several dense droplets (D), basement membrane (Bm). Uranyl acetate and lead citrate stain, ×8,000.

ribosomes predominate in the dark cells, as compared with light cells. The nuclei are hyperchromatic in the dark cells, while the light cells contain more loose chromatin. The dark cell population increases during neoplastic transformation; however, we do not know with certainty whether the light and dark cells are two distinct cellular compartments or whether they are simply two different cellular phases during carcinogenesis. A more heterogeneous cell population and nuclear and mitochondrial abnormalities are more frequently seen in the squamous cell carcinomas as compared with a more homogeneous cell population and fewer nuclear and mitochondrial abnormalities in the basal cell carcinomas. These ultrastructural differences might suggest the differences between these two cancers in regard to the ability of each to invade and metastasize.

Hormones can also change the cellular differentiation (benign, malignant, or undifferentiated), migration, and responsiveness of neoplastic cells. Thus, such hormones as T_4, $PGF_{2\alpha}$, PGE_2 and estradiol enhance cellular differentiation and division, whereas other hormones, such as glucagon, calcitonin, and insulin, induce more undifferentiated or anaplastic patterns. Hydrocortisone, hypophysectomy, and castration induce a marked inhibition of cell growth and differentiation.

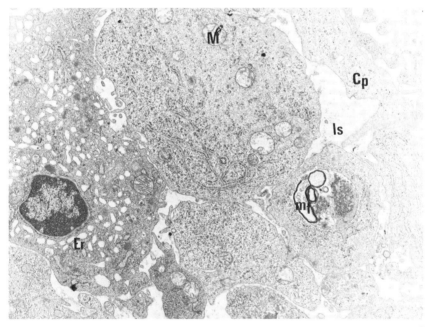

Figure 4–10 Heterogenous neoplastic cellular pattern is predominant in a mouse squamous cell carcinoma following thyroxine administration. Cells are dispersed, separated by enlarged intercellular spaces (Is) with cytoplasmic projections (Cp), vacuolated endoplasmic reticulum (Er), mitochondria (M), and myelin figures (Mf). Uranyl acetate and lead citrate stain, ×15,000.

A heterogeneous pattern with neoplastic cells containing tumefied or ballooned mitochondria, a large population of polysomes, conglomerated lysosomes, and myelin figures, encircled by a fine membrane and a dilated or vacuolar endoplasmic reticulum is predominantly visible in squamous cell carcinomas after thyroxine administration (Fig. 4-10). Several mitoses with large chromosomes in metaphase or anaphase can also be seen. In rats, a predominance of vacuolated cells with large vacuoles (or lumina) can be seen in the neoplastic cells of basal cell carcinomas after thyroxine administration (Fig. 4-11). A more differentiated, cystoid vascular pattern with large and well differentiated cells containing enlarged nuclei, mitochondria, a large population of free ribosomes, and narrow intercellular spaces can be seen in squamous cell carcinomas in glucagon-treated mice (Figs. 4-12, 4-13 and 4-14). An enhancement of cell growth and proliferation with a predominance of dark and light neoplastic cells containing enlarged nuclei with intranuclear vesicles and several lysosomes and phagolysosomes with disrupted membranes, as well as small dense granules can be seen in basal cell and squamous cell carinomas following insulin treatment (Figs. 4-14, 4-15, 4-16). Estradiol induces moderate stimulation of cell growth and proliferation in squamous cell carcinomas along with the occurrence of several large intramitochondrial

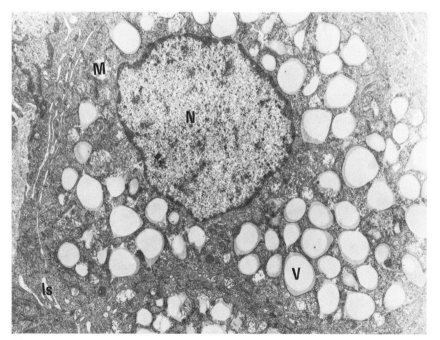

Figure 4-11 Several large vacuoles (V) can be seen in neoplastic cells of a rat basal cell carcinoma following thyroxine administration. Enlarged intercellular spaces (Is), nuclei (N) and mitochondria (M). Uranyl acetate and lead citrate stain, ×11,000.

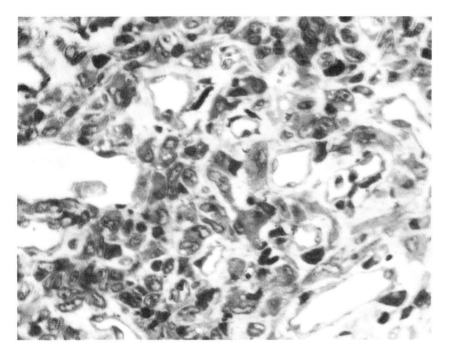

Figure 4-12 Cystoid-vascular squamous cell carcinomas with atypical cells and nuclei. Invasive and multinucleated cells are seen in mouse treated with MCA and glucagon. Epon section (~1μ); stained with toluidine blue, ×400.

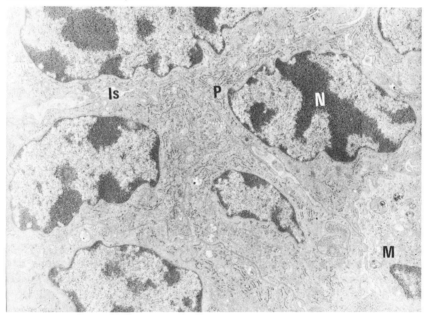

Figure 4-13 Anaplastic cellular pattern with several differentiated and/or poorly differentiated cells in a mouse squamous cell carcinoma following glucagon administration. Large nuclei (N) with dispersed chromatin, several free polysomes (P), mitochondria (M) and narrow intercellular spaces (Is) can be seen. Uranyl acetate and lead citrate stain, ×8,000.

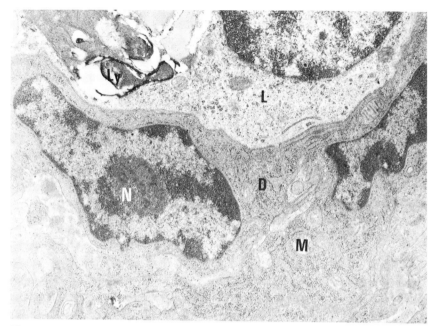

Figure 4-14 More differentiated dark (D) and light (L) cells with enlarged nuclei (N), agglomerated lysosomes (Ly) and disrupted membranes, tumefied mitochondria (M) are seen in a mouse squamous cell carcinoma after glucagon. Uranyl acetate and lead citrate stain, ×15,000.

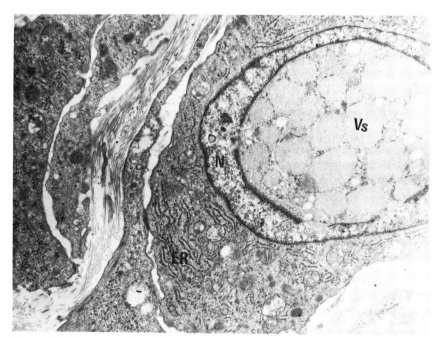

Figure 4-15 Neoplastic cells exhibiting a large population of intranuclear vesicles (Vs), nucleus (N) and abundant endoplasmic reticulum (ER) can be seen in a rat with basal cell carcinoma after insulin treatment. Uranyl acetate and lead citrate stain, ×11,000.

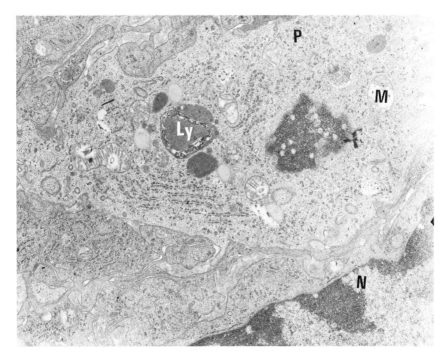

Figure 4–16 Several lysosomes (Ly) can be seen in the neoplastic cells of squamous cell carcinoma following insulin administration. Nucleus (N), swollen mitochondria (M) and polysomes (P). Uranyl acetate and lead citrate stain, ×22,000.

granules that occupy almost the entire mitochondrion; these granules appear mostly near the nucleus, but can also be seen elsewhere in the cytoplasm. Small tubular nuclear inclusions and the protrusion of some nuclear chromatin into the cytoplasm is also occasionally visible. It can be postulated that this protrusion of nuclear chromatin is related to an increase in the transcription–translation phenomenon (Fig. 4–17). Calcitonin treatment induces poor cell growth and differentiation with a marked increase in tonofilament population and sclerosis.

By contrast, hydrocortisone and dexamethasone administration, hypophysectomy, gonadectomy, and thyroidectomy induce a marked inhibition of neoplastic cell growth and differentiation in both mouse and rat carcinomas (88). Only a moderate hyperplasia is observed in these cases; the cells are inhibited in their neoplastic transformation. Marked inhibition of cell growth and differentiation occurs in hydrocortisone-treated mice and rats with carcinomas; only slightly hyperplastic cells with enlarged intercellular spaces and cell extensions can be seen (Figs. 4–18 and 4–19).

Scanning electron microscopy can exhibit important aspects of the cytoarchitecture, orientation, and cell surface changes in carcinomas. Hor-

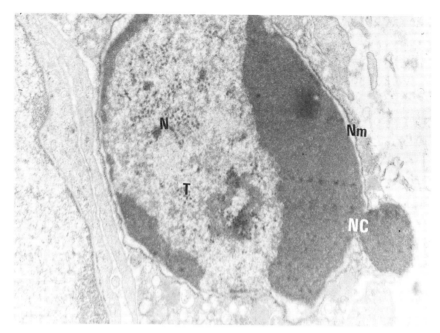

Figure 4-17 Neoplastic cells from a mouse squamous cell carcinoma following estradiol treatment. Small tubular inclusions (T) within nucleus (N) and a large protrusion of nuclear chromatin (NC) penetrating through the nuclear membrane (Nm) into cytoplasm can be seen. Epon, uranyl acetate, and lead citrate stain, ×22,000.

mones can induce significant changes in the cell growth and proliferation during neoplastic transformation. Each type of neoplastic cell exhibits characteristics of its cell surface and orientation. Squamous neoplastic cells of mice are elongated, are sometimes pear shaped or polyhedral with cell extensions, and exhibit several microvilli on their surface after thyroxine administration (Fig. 4–20).

A different cellular pattern appears in basal cell carcinomas of rats, in which most cells are round or oval and separated by intercellular spaces with a large network of cell extensions. Sometimes these neoplastic cells are more polymorphic and elongated and exhibit several blebs and microvilli along their surface. The cells emit long extensions that are interwoven. Red blood cells are visible on their surface (Fig. 4–21). Marked cell surface changes with shrunken cells and flat surfaces can be observed in hypophysectomized rats treated with carcinogens (Fig. 4–22).

Thus, SEM is useful in detecting the early effect of hormones on neoplastic cells and studying cell–cell interactions. Scanning electron microscopy is also used to classify and diagnose human cancers of the lung, thyroid and skin (61,62,66). This technique affords an opportunity to learn more about tumor growth and its propagation. For example, when cell growth loses

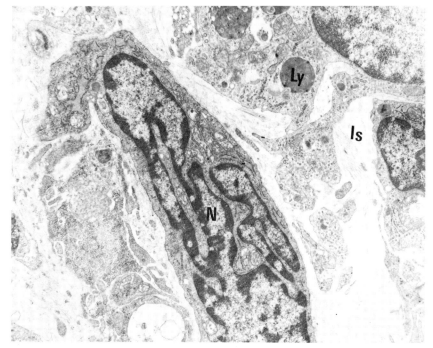

Figure 4-18 Marked inhibition of neoplastic transformation in a mouse similarly treated with MCA and hydrocortisone. Few atrophic cells with atypical nuclei (N), lysosomes (Ly), and enlarged intercellular spaces (Is). Epon, uranyl acetate and lead citrate stain, ×11,000.

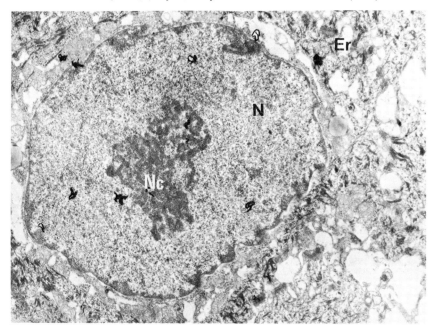

Figure 4-19 Marked inhibition of ³H-thymidine incorporation in the nuclear chromatin (N) of epidermal cells of a mouse treated with carcinogen and hydrocortisone. Nucleolus (Nc) and enlarged endoplasmic reticulum (Er). Ilford L₄ nuclear emulsion, exposed for 3 months, developed with microdol-X and slightly stained with uranyl acetate and lead citrate, ×11,000.

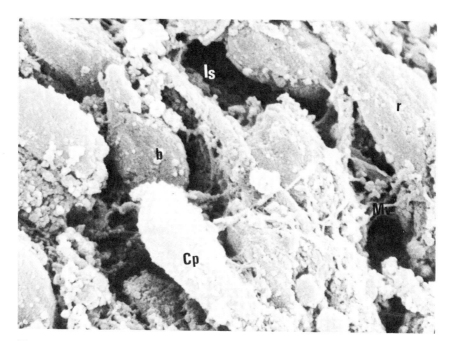

Figure 4-20 SEM of squamous cell carcinoma showing the organization and cell surfaces of cancer cells following thyroxine administration. The neoplastic cells (Cp) are elongated as pears (pyriformis). Several ridges (R) and blebs (b) are visible. Cells are separated by microvilli (Mv) and enlarged intercellular spaces (Is). Critical point method and gold coating, ×8,000.

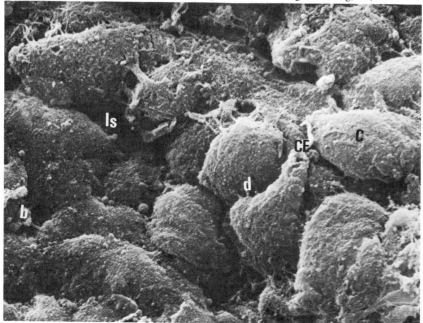

Figure 4-21 Neoplastic cells are differently organized in a rat with basal cell carcinoma following thyroxine administration. Many cells are oval or elongated (C) with cell extensions (CE). Blebs (b) can be seen and also intercellular spaces (Is) and a few desmosomes (d). Critical point method and gold coating, ×8,000.

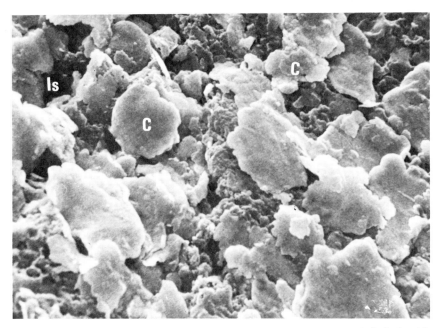

Figure 4–22 Marked cell surface changes in a hypophysectomized rat treated similarly with carcinogen. Neoplastic cells (C) are shrunken and irregular with a flat surface; they are randomly organized and separated by narrow intercellular space (Is). Neoplastic transformation is arrested in its initial stage. Critical point method and gold coating, ×8,000.

its organized, differentiated pattern, encountered mainly in the benign tumors or adenomas, its growth becomes disorganized or more chaotic, through the loss of intercellular connections. This pattern is predominant in autonomous or malignant tumors. The transitional stages between so-called nodules or benign tumors and carcinomas can be better visualized with SEM. This stage of nodularity is very important in many experimentally induced as well as human cancers. Some of these nodules, called cold nodules, have a tendency to become malignant and to become autonomous, or hormone independent, whereas hot nodules are benign and can remain as such for several years, continuing to be hormone responsive. The nodular thyroid and lungs are among the most common diseases with which the pathologists and oncologists are confronted.

Electron microscopy, high-resolution autoradiography, and SEM give us more valid data regarding tumor organization, growth, propagation, and hormone dependence.

ROLE OF HORMONES IN THE ETIOLOGY AND PATHOGENESIS OF HUMAN CANCERS

Although the hormones and hormonelike substances are crucial to the induction, development, and regression of several types of experimental carcinomas in target tissues and in other organs (liver, lung, skin, lymphoid tissue, kidney, and bones), their role in the etiology and pathogenesis of human cancers has not as yet been demonstrated.

The hormones have a definite role in the etiology and pathogenesis of experimental carcinomas, whereas they have only a presumptive role in the etiology and pathogenesis of human cancers. Several pieces of clinical evidence prove the existence of hormone-responsive and hormone-dependent human cancers. Seven human cancers (carcinoma of breast, lymphosarcoma and leukemia, carcinoma of prostate, carcinoma of kidney, carcinoma of thyroid, carcinoma of endometrium, and carcinoma of seminal vesicles) are known to be hormone responsive (34), the first four of which are common to humans and animals.

Breast Cancer

The etiological role of hormones in human breast cancer was clearly foreseen by the empirical observation of Beatson several years before the hormones were discovered. Beatson described the beneficial effects of ovariectomy in the advanced breast cancer of two women. Later, it was found the orchiectomy has similar beneficial effects on breast cancer in men (23). Since hormones are crucial to the development of mammary glands in animals as well as in humans, it has often been stated that hormones are essential factors in the etiology of breast cancer and that without hormones no breast cancer can occur (76).

First, the role of sex steroids (estrogen and progesterone) was believed to be the most important in the induction of breast cancer; later the balance was shifted to prolactin, glucocorticoids, and thyroid hormones. A hormonal imbalance among these hormones is considered crucial. However, methodological difficulties, especially case-control studies, make it difficult to demonstrate this hormonal imbalance in humans; many reports regarding the levels of estrogens (estradiol, estrone, estriol) and prolactin are conflicting.

A different epidemiological approach demonstrated that the daughters of patients with breast cancer are at greater familial risk of breast cancer as compared with controls (83). According to this approach, the estriol/estradiol + estrone ratio is also indicated as a means for detecting those women who are at greater risk for breast cancer, that is, a low estriol concentration predisposes to breast cancer, whereas a high concentration is protective (48). This risk ratio is supported by the low concentration of estriol found in caucasian women, who have a high incidence of breast cancer, as compared with the high estriol quotient and low incidence among Japanese women. This simple association is not confirmed by other investigators in case-control studies, however. Hormonal imbalance as well as genetic and environmental factors might explain these differences. The carcinogenic potential of estriol is not significantly different from that of the other two estrogens, estradiol and estrone, to account for a hormone–risk association. Estriol is a weak carcinogen because it is not strongly bound to the nuclear receptors and is rapidly lost.

Recent studies are better designed. Several cohort studies of women in the United States who had used estrogens for the relief of menopausal symptoms show an increased risk of breast cancer among these women. Also, an increased risk of breast cancer has been observed among women who had used oral contraceptives for 2 to 4 years, especially in women older than 25 years who had had previous pregnancies or benign breast disease. Estriol, progesterone, and androgens are postulated to exert modulating effects on the carcinogenic action of estrogens, and consequently on the development of breast cancer (81,92,108).

Other studies emphasize the major role of prolactin in the etiology and pathogenesis of breast cancer (95), chiefly on the basis of experimental data. Although no consistently high level of prolactin has been reported in patients with breast cancer, an elevated level of prolactin has been found in patients who have a high risk of breast cancer. It is possible that estrogens function as carcinogens by increasing the release of prolactin. Several studies are under way to explore this possibility. Hypophysectomy, which decreases the circulating prolactin, does induce a regression in human breast cancer. Furthermore, administration of reserpine or related drugs that increase prolactin secretion increase by three- to fivefold the risk for breast cancer. However, drugs that inhibit prolactin secretion (L-DOPA) only rarely produce a regression in the development of breast cancer. These findings still await confirmation. One possibility is that prolactin intervenes in the occurrence and growth of human breast cancer through its receptors, since human breast tumors were found to contain prolactin receptors (18), in addition to estrogen and insulin receptors (21,39,69). Another possibility is that insulin exerts a permissive role regarding the actions of other hormones; for example, epidemiological studies show a distribution of breast cancer similar to that for iodine-deficient goiter.

The exploration of the hypothalamic–pituitary–thyroid axis in patients with breast cancer shows a low thyroid function compared with that found in women without breast cancer (91). The state of a person's thyroid function might affect the evolution of breast cancer by altering the steroid hormone production.

Prostaglandins might also have an important role in the causation and development of human breast cancer. Specimens from human malignant breast tumors contain and synthesize more prostaglandins than do benign neoplasms or normal breast tissue from the same patients. The tendency to metastasize is always found to be associated with an increase in prostaglandins from the F series (PGF) (4,38,96).

These investigations along different lines all appear to indicate that estrogens and prolactin might have a direct role in the etiology and pathogenesis of human mammary carcinogenesis, while androgens, progesterone, glucocorticoids, thyroid hormones, and insulin seem to have only a permissive or indirect role.

Prostate Cancer

Spontaneous prostate tumors occur only in dogs and humans. Huggins demonstrated that the prostate cancer that occurs in dogs is similar to that seen in male patients and that it is hormone dependent. In experimenting with endocrine manipulation, either by castration or by estrogen administration, Huggins proved that the occurrence and growth of prostatic carcinomas can be controlled by hormones. Prostate neoplasms occur in dogs as well as in men only when the testis is present; therefore, a continuous supply of androgen is necessary. Prostatic tumors have never been reported either in castrated dogs or in eunuchs. It was soon observed that orchidectomy or estrogen administration causes a rapid shrinkage of prostate tumors in dogs as well as in humans. It was, therefore, established that orchiectomy and estrogen administration induce a significant regression of cancer in human prostate, whereas testosterone enhances the growth of these neoplasms in untreated cases. Stilbestrol was the first synthetic estrogen used in the treatment of these tumors, heralding the chemotherapy of malignant diseases (33–36). The prostate is a target organ for androgens; its growth, maintenance, and functional activity are largely dependent on the androgen secreted by testis (Fig. 4–4). The gland atrophies after castration and regains its growth after androgen administration.

Despite considerable work regarding the role of hormones in controlling the development and regression of prostatic cancer, there is little direct evidence regarding the role of hormones in the causation of these neoplasms (30). In addition to sex steroids (e.g., androgens and estrogens), which play an important role in pathogenesis, and possibly in the etiology of human prostate neoplasms (Fig. 4–23), other hormones (i.e., progestins, prolactin, LH, and corticosterone) figure in the growth and maintenance of prostate gland as well as in the development and treatment of prostatic cancer. Thus, greater atrophy of the prostate gland was found after combined hypophysectomy and castration than after castration alone.

Conflicting reports and discrepancies are reflected in the question of which hormones are active. Some find that GH and ACTH are active; others find prolactin, FSH, and LH active (55). Evidence that these hormones directly intervene in controlling the development of the prostate gland is lacking, but it is possible that they interfere with and alter the androgen and estrogen balance. Both steroid and protein receptors were found on human prostatic cancers; the therapeutic value and prognosis can be somewhat correlated with the presence of androgen and estrogen receptors.

In conclusion, most of the clinical and experimental evidence has clearly demonstrated the role of hormones, especially of androgens and estrogens, in

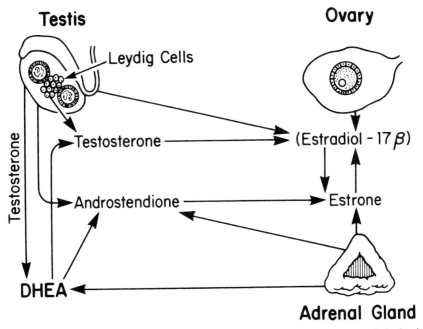

Figure 4-23 Major pathways of sex steroid metabolism in humans (DHEA: Dehydrepiandrosterone).

the pathogenesis and therapy of human prostate cancers. Further investigations are needed to demonstrate whether these hormones exert a direct role in the causation or etiology of these neoplasms.

Uterine (Endometrial) Cancer

Cancer of the breast, endometrium, ovary, and vagina have been shown to represent approximately 50 percent of all cancers afflicting women (81). Yet studies indicate that long-term administration of estrogens, progesterone, and 19-norcontraceptives can induce such marked pathological changes in the uterus of mice, rats, and rabbits as endometriosis, adenomatous hyperplasia, and tumors of endometrial stroma (fibrosarcoma, sarcoma) (52). Their role is still poorly understood in the etiology of human endometrial cancer. The appearance of the endometrial tumors is fundamentally hormone dependent in animals, depending both on the dose of the administered steroid and on the duration of the administration. It is important to note that these are hormone-dependent tumors, which appear during the postmenopausal part of a woman's life, when these organs are either involuting or atrophic. This is strong evidence that estrogens given for the relief of menopausal symptoms can increase the risk of endometrial carcinoma. Several epidemiological studies in the United States as well as elsewhere indicate a considerable increase in the incidence of endometrial cancer with the use of exogenous estrogens. These studies show a strong association between the use of exogenous estrogens for menopausal symptoms and the increase in the risk for endometrial carcinoma. A similar incidence was found among women treated with DES for gonadal dysgenesis. Case-control studies show that the cyclic use of estrogens induces a lower incidence of endometrial cancer than does continuous use (98). Although there is still conflicting evidence, a dramatic increase of four- to eightfold in the risk of endometrial cancer is associated with the use of estrogens, for climacterium, especially in the last decade (1970–1980), in the United States. There are also indications of a positive dose-response relationship involving the strength of medication and the duration of its use (81). A recent cohort study shows a decline in the incidence of endometrial carcinoma for 1979–1980, coincidental with the reduction in the use of estrogens for the symptoms of the climacteric (40). There is also some evidence that the use of oral contraceptives increases neoplastic changes and the incidence of endometrial carcinoma. In addition to endometrial carcinoma, inconclusive data show that oral contraceptives increase the incidence of liver cancer (hepatocellular adenomas), malignant melanoma, and pituitary tumors, while decreasing the risk of ovarian cancer. Therefore, perhaps only the long-term use of contraceptives increases the risk of cervical dysplasia and endometrial carcinoma, but we lack sufficient evidence to make a definite conclusion.

Also, endogenous hormones (estrogens, progesterone, androgens, and prolactin) can play an important role in the causation and development of endometrial carcinomas. More sensitive techniques, such as radioimmuno-assays and the use of radioactive hormones labeled with ^{3}H or ^{125}I indicate a strong association between the high estrogen production in the absence of ovulation and an increased risk for endometrial cancer. Thus, increased estrone production is always associated with an increased risk for the development of endometrial cancer.

There are two different routes in the etiology and pathogenesis of endometrial carcinoma. One route involves adult women before menopause, in whom 17β-estradiol is continuously secreted from the ovary, later producing uterine hyperplasia, atypical hyperplasia, and carcinoma in some cases. The second, more frequent route involves postmenopausal women, in whom excess estrone has a more significant role. The high production of estrone might result from the extraglandular conversion of androstendione. When the production of estrone is increased by any process, the risk for endometrial carcinoma is greatly increased (81). Also, the frequent incidence of adenomatous uterine hyperplasia and true endometrial cancer among women with granulosa–theca cell tumors of the ovary, which are estrogen-secreting tumors, supports this view (31). It has also been shown that estriol and progesterone exert modulating effects on the carcinogenic action of 17β-estradiol on the human endometrium by increasing the ability of the endometrium to inactivate the estradiol (108). This increasing ability results either from increased dehydrogenase activity or from decreased numbers of uterine receptors for estradiol. There is a strong association between the increased level of endogenous or exogenous administration of estrogens and contraceptives and the risk for endometrial cancer, but the demonstration of a carcinogenic role will require more conclusive evidence (81,92).

Thyroid Cancer

Although there is ample experimental evidence that TSH or chronic iodine deficiency alone can induce benign or even malignant thyroid tumors in animals (7,20,59), this is not well demonstrated in human thyroid cancers. Transitional structural changes of thyroid cells during their neoplastic transformation can be clearly visualized by electron microscopy, autoradiography, and SEM. The thyroid cancer of experimental animals bears a great resemblance to that of humans (59,60,62,110). Therefore, since no thyroid neoplasms occur in hypophysectomized animals, the role of TSH is considered crucial to experimentally induced thyroid cancers. Experimental evidence suggests the existence of thyroid cancer on a preexisting goiter. There is also a strong association between the incidence of thyroid and breast cancers and goiter belts, indicating that iodine deficiency might play an important causative and pathogenic role in human thyroid carcinogenesis. Concomitant administration of other cocarcinogens, such as chemical agents or ionizing radiation, greatly increases the occurrence of thyroid neoplasms in such goiters. However, the role of TSH and cocarcinogens is not always clear in the etiology and development of human thyroid cancers (71). Endemic goiter is not always associated with an increased incidence of thyroid cancer despite an increased incidence of follicular and anaplastic thyroid carcinomas in some endemic goiters (101). Hence, the hypersecretion of TSH alone is not an indispensable factor in the occurrence and development of human thyroid cancer, since many thyroid cancers can occur in a nonpreexisting goitrous thyroid.

However, a major investigative etiological factor in thyroid neoplasms in childhood, as well as in adult life, is ionizing radiation. Retrospective case studies on a large scale show that about 80 percent of thyroid carcinomas arising in childhood were preceded by x-ray exposure of the thyroid gland, especially thymic x-ray treatment; this incidence has shown a marked decrease with the discontinuance of this therapy (106). An increased incidence of thyroid carcinoma was also reported after exposure to x-irradiation, whether external, as in an atomic bomb explosion, or internal, as in radioiodine. The risk is greater with external radiation (82). Thyroid radiation in adults can also produce thyroid carcinomas, but at a slower incidence than occurs in children. Most radiation-induced thyroid carcinomas are of the follicular-papillary type. Ultrastructural, immunological, autoradiographic, and SEM studies indicate that most human thyroid carcinomas are of either follicular of papillary type and are similar, regardless of the original carcinogenic agent: abnormal thyroglobulin synthesis is observed with a predominant slow-sedimenting component (iodinated serum globulins) and decreasing 19S-thyroglobulin, already reported in human thyroid cancers. These abnormalities can be related to the influence of mRNA (messenger RNA) (59). Most benign thyroid neoplasms are hormone-responsive, hormone-dependent tumors; treatment with thyroid hormones (e.g., thyroxine, triiodothyronine) significantly reduces their growth and ability to metastasize. However, only a few malignant or autonomous thyroid carcinomas preserve their hormone dependence and responsiveness to thyroid hormone administration, most of which remain hormone independent.

Liver Cancer

Solid experimental evidence shows that hormones exert an important role in hepatocarcinogenesis (29,56,102). Sex hormones (estrogens, androgens) enhance the production of hepatomas; adrenalectomy inhibits the tumor induction by DAB. Adrenalectomy, deoxycorticosterone, and prednisolone inhibit hepatoma induction as well as the bile duct proliferation that occurs after afloatoxin administration. Thyroidectomy prevents tumorigenesis during the initiation stage, while hypophysectomy completely suppresses the induction of hepatomas by AAF. In general, the hormonal responsiveness of liver tumors is affected by the aging process; the carcinogenic process is slower in older animals (84).

An increasing number of hepatocellular adenomas was recently reported in young women using oral contraceptives (49)—(by 1977, 172 cases of liver cancer were reported). Although it can be said that this number is small, compared with the large number of women taking oral contraceptives, the incidence of liver tumors might actually be much higher, because it is difficult to detect the occult small nodules. Liver tumors appear only after prolonged exposure to oral contraceptives. Thus, a strong association between the occurrence of liver tumors and the prolonged use of oral contraceptives, especially combinations containing mestranol and ethynilestradiol, does exist. A liver scan with radioisotopes, ultrasound, and liver biopsies provide the possibility of detecting these tumors and preventing their development and metastases.

Lymphoid Cancers and Leukemias

Laboratory studies show that lymphoid tumors and leukemias can be induced in different strains of mice and rats by chemical agents, radiation, and hormones. Both chemical- and radiation-induced leukemias and lymphomas are hormone responsive. It was reported earlier that lymphoid hyperplasia is one of the clinical manifestations of adrenal insufficiency (Addison's disease), while the administration of glucocorticoids and ACTH suppresses the lymphocyte function and decreases their number by cytolysis. The cytolytic effect of glucocorticoids was demonstrated in both experimental and human leukemic lymphocytes; they are slower in humans than in rats. The cytolytic effects of glucocorticoids on lymphocytes, mainly the T lymphocyte cell population, can be explained by decreased glucose uptake and by suppression of transcription and translation (70). These effects made glucocorticoids a cornerstone in today's therapeutic use of hormones in human leukemias, especially in acute lymphocytic leukemia (ALL) of children, in whom they often produce long remissions. The effectiveness of glucocorticoids depends on the presence or lack of receptors on the lymphocytic cells (87). Despite these beneficial therapeutic effects, there is no conclusive evidence that hormones play a significant role in the causation and development of human lymphoid tumors or leukemias.

Malignant Melanoma and Renal Cell Carcinoma

The possible hormone dependence of malignant melanoma and renal cell carcinoma is a subject that has been open for speculation for many years. Recently, experimental and clinical data have suggested that some melanomas and renal cell carcinomas might be hormonally sensitive to steroid hormones. Steroid hormone receptors were only found in a limited number of patients with malignant melanoma or renal cell carcinoma. However, the presence (or absence) of steroid receptors cannot be correlated with hormonal therapy responses (in vivo and in vitro), even though the prognosis for females with malignant melanomas is always better than for males, at least in the first stages of tumor development. Preexisting melanomas are reportedly exacerbated during pregnancy, yet show regression postpartum (104). Also, a beneficial effect was reported in some patients after treatment with DES. Although renal carcinomas are easily induced by hormones in Syrian hamsters, thereby suggesting the hormone dependence of these cancers, this experimental model is not directly applicable to the human situation. Although hormones might influence the growth of these tumors, there is no direct evidence that hormones play a determining role in the etiology of human malignant and renal cell carcinoma.

POSSIBLE PATHOGENETIC MECHANISM(S) OF HORMONES IN CARCINOGENESIS

The mechanism(s) by which hormones intervene in carcinogenesis and affect the development of tumors is still unknown. How do hormones act on the cells of target tissues, as well as of nontarget tissues, eliciting so great a variety of benign and malignant tumors? Are hormones carcinogenic per se, acting in a similar manner to that of the well-known chemical, viral, or physical carcinogens? Or are hormones only cocarcinogens, promoters, or modulators of neoplastic transformations? Although the mechanism of action of hormones in carcinogenesis is fully discussed in Chapter 6, it is important to review their effects as well as the possible mechanism(s) for a better understanding of their role in the causation and development of cancers.

Hormones as Carcinogenic Agents

Although it is difficult to prove a direct carcinogenic effect of hormones stricto senso, and many investigators incline toward a permissive or indirect role of hormones that elicits only the preneoplastic changes of a chemical, viral, or physical carcinogen, there are enough situations in which hormones alone have induced hyperplastic changes that can later develop into benign or malignant (autonomous) growth, to support a direct effect. Cells are still responsive or hormonally controlled in the first stages as well as in the latent but not in fully autonomous tumors. In association with other carcinogens, hormones always enhance or accelerate the incidence and development of cancers. In my opinion, hormones and hormonelike substances can intervene and affect the occurrence and development of cancers in several ways, by:

1. Activating the oncogenic virus production (e.g., mammary tumor virus in mice).
2. Increasing or decreasing the metabolic activation of chemical carcinogens.
3. Influencing the rate of transformation of preneoplastic cells to neoplastic cells.
4. Intervening in DNA synthesis and stimulating cell division and proliferation.
5. Influencing tumor occurrence and development through immuno-suppressive action.
6. Inducing preneoplastic changes, required as a background for neoplastic transformation.
7. Acting only as modulators of carcinogenesis, by rendering the cells more susceptible or resistant to the effect(s) of chemical, viral or physical carcinogens.

Some of these hypotheses are still incomplete and in part speculative.

Hormones As Cocarcinogens

By accelerating the rate of proliferation of abnormal cells and shortening the latent period (latency or dormant stage), hormones might behave as cocarcinogens. The effect of hormones on preneoplastic and neoplastic cells and the elicitation of tumor development are complex and still poorly understood (5). There is no one valid explanation; hormones can act in one or usually in two or three different ways, such as enhancing the progression of the preneoplastic cells to neoplastic cells, stimulating DNA synthesis, or shortening the latent period. Previous investigations using electron microscopy, high-resolution autoradiography, and SEM show hormones to be important factors in controlling the preneoplastic cell population and their progression to cancerous cells (63). Thus, thyroxine, $PGF_{2\alpha}$, calcitonin, and estradiol stimulate the progression of preneoplastic epidermal cells to neoplastic cells, whereas hydrocortisone and hypophysectomy suppress this transformation. Hormones also markedly affect DNA synthesis in neoplastic epidermal cells induced by a chemical carcinogen (3-MCA). Thyroxine, $PGF_{2\alpha}$, calcitonin, and estradiol markedly enhance DNA synthesis in the nuclei of cancerous cells, whereas hydrocortisone, hypophysectomy, and castration inhibit it. These findings strongly suggest that precancerous and cancerous cell populations are still in a controllable state responsive to environmental factors.

Hormones as Modulators or Modifiers of Carcinogenesis

The progression of preneoplastic cells to neoplastic cells is not an irreversible process determined by genetic factors alone; it can be modulated and modified by hormones and hormonelike substances as well. Cancerous cells are less responsive to hormones than are preneoplastic cells. These data suggest that hormones act on cancerous cells by a specific modus operandi, different from other chemical, viral, or physical carcinogens. Most carcinogens are mutagenic, while hormones are mutagenic on only a few occasions. Sex hormones and glucocorticoids occasionally display teratogenic effects.

Modern and accurate methods afford a better understanding of the role of hormones in controlling the cell biology of cancerous cells, the cornerstone of carcinogenesis.

Comments and Conclusions

Although the role of hormones in the etiology and pathogenesis of cancer was suspected for a long time (3,47,54,105), not until 1932 was it demonstrated that the inoculation of estrone could induce mammary adenocarcinomas in male mice (44). Current experimental and clinical findings clearly demonstrate that hormones drastically affect the occurrence, development, and regression of several types of cancers in laboratory animals as well as in humans. Hence, hormones play an important role in tumor formation and behavior. This role is still more evident in experimental carcinomas than in human cancers. In some cancers hormones exert a direct etiological and pathogenic role; in others their role is only presumed or indirect. Three common human cancers—of the breast, prostate, and endometrium—are fundamentally regulated in their growth and function by hormones. In other human cancers, hormones can also play an important role in onset, development, and regression.

Despite the ample evidence that hormones are major factors in the development and function of several types of cancer, there is little support for hormones per se as primary carcinogens. There are similarities between hormones and carcinogens. For example, both can induce tumors with a similar histological pattern; these tumors can be benign and malignant and can also metastasize. Yet hormones induce carcinomas mostly in target organs whose growth and maintenance depends fundamentally on the presence of specific hormones. Also, prolonged exposure to hormones is required before cancer occurs, whereas a single injection or application of a chemical carcinogen can induce cancer. In addition, almost all carcinogens are mutagenic, whereas hormones are not. Therefore, the main question—Are hormones primary carcinogens?—remains unsolved because their mechanism(s) of action at a cellular or molecular level is still poorly understood. Recent data indicate that hormones are important physiological factors in controlling cell division and proliferation; in this way, they play a major role in homeostatic cellular mechanism. Cell homeostasis is the basic mechanism for normal growth and function; abnormal growth is almost synonymous with carcinogenesis. Modern methods, such as high-resolution autoradiography, electron microscopy, and SEM show that the neoplastic transformation is always a sequential process, from initiation, to promotion, to progression. Carcinogens affect the first step, primarily because of changes induced in DNA synthesis, producing abnormal somatic mutations and the occurrence of abnormal cells; hormones act mostly on the second and third steps of neoplastic transformation by controlling the preneoplastic cell population and its progression to neoplastic or cancerous cells. Using these procedures it is also possible to estimate more accurately the nuclear grade (anaplasia and nuclear monstrosities) and correlate it with the presence of hormone receptors, to establish hormone dependence or responsiveness.

It has also been postulated that hormones exert a preparative action, rendering cells more susceptible to the effect of a known chemical, viral, or physical agent. Here, their role is more permissive, acting mainly as tumor promoters or cocarcinogens. When hormonal imbalances occur, they are accompanied by great risk for development of cancer. The study of the induction and development of experimental carcinomas, in many cases cytologically similar or identical to those occurring in humans, elucidates the role of hormones in human carcinogenesis (16). However, it is still more difficult to demonstrate this role in human cancer than in experimental animals because a longer period (20 to 30 years) is required before human cancers occur and because methodological difficulties interfere with case-control studies. Experimental and clinical evidence clearly demonstrates that an increase in exogenous or endogenous hormones greatly increases the risk of cancer development. Thus, a relationship between tumor etiology and the endocrine status was established for some cancers. The etiology and pathogenesis of cancers appear to be of a plurifactorial origin, among which hormones are important factors. There is ample evidence in humans that hormones play a direct etiological and pathogenic role in hormone-dependent cancers. There is no breast, endometrial, or prostate cancer in the absence of hormones; for example, no breast cancer has been reported in ovariectomized women, no endometrial cancer in women with gonadal dysgenesis, and no prostate cancer in eunuchs. After hormonal replacement by exogenous hormones takes place, the growth and development of these cancers resume.

Several other cancers involve hormones or hormonelike substances that can accelerate or delay their onset and development, such as liver cancer, thyroid, skin, lung, ovarian, kidney, lymphoid tumors, and leukemias. A hormonal milieu, similar to the *milieu interieur* of the French physiologist Claude Bernard, is critical to growth and cell homeostasis in hormone-responsive or target tissues. This is also important for other tissues, since a wide range of tumors can be induced, enhanced, or suppressed by hormone administration. Therefore, the hormonal environment or hormonal milieu is important to etiology and tumor pathogenesis. It is also important to prevent the occurrence of cancers by detecting the hormonal imbalance earlier through the use of such sensitive methods as radioimmunoassays. Thus abnormalities in hormone metabolism (estrogens and C_{-19} steroids) were frequently associated with breast cancer.

Using a variety of hormones, our investigations show that the incidence, development, and multiplicity of carcinomas, even in nontarget tissues (liver, lung, skin) and thyroid, are markedly affected by hormone administration or an endocrine deficiency (hypophysectomy, gonadectomy, thyroidectomy). These findings provide an endocrinological basis for the cell biology of cancers.

In addition to the role of hormones in the causation and development of tumors, they can play an important role in cellular evolution, by interfering with cellular differentiation and dedifferentiation. Hormone administration can shift the cellular pattern toward more benign or malignant types of neoplasms. They can reduce or enhance the malignancy of neoplasms as well as their metastasizing capacity. For instance, in the liver, hormones can increase the incidence of hepatomas versus cholangiomas; in the skin, they increase the predominance of more keratotic (keratoacanthomas), sclerotic, solid, or trabecular (hepatoid) patterns; in the thyroid, in addition to more adenomas or carcinomas, they can increase the occurrence of a spindle cell or anaplastic carcinoma.

The study of the hormonal control of epidermal neoplasms provides us with interesting findings regarding the differentiation of neoplastic cells. Ultrastructural studies revealed that epidermal cells are pluripotential cells with a capacity for endocrine and neuro-endocrine differentiation. Thus the cells from squamous cell carcinomas in mice and basal cell carcinomas in rats occasionally exhibit a large population of membrane-bound electron dense or endocrine-like granules. Some of these cells resemble argyrophilic cells and "oat cell" carcinomas.

The occurrence of argyrophilic cells with distinct morphologic granules were recently reported in human basal cell carcinomas. Some of these basal cell carcinomas exhibit an endocrine differentiation or a neuro-endocrine differentiation with the presence of calcitonin, insulin glucagon, somatostatin and ACTH which were detected by using immunohistochemical methods. Also endocrine tumors such as oat cell carcinoma can be intermingled in the esophagus with a squamous cell carcinoma. These findings illustrate that neoplastic epithelial cells possess a great potential for multidirectional differentiation and hormones or hormone-like substances can markedly orientate the cytodifferentiation of epidermal neoplastic cells. Hormones are used in this study in order to manipulate this pluripotential of neoplastic epidermal cells. The APUD cells previously reported in basal cell carcinomas can derive from pluripotential epidermal cells, as it was suggested. Occurrence of endocrine cells has also been reported in a transplantable rat adenocarcinoma of the colon and it is concluded that endocrine cells are derived from endoderm.

An increased risk for human cancers (endometrial, ovarian, breast, and liver) was reported in the last decade (1970–1980) owing to the increased use of exogenous estrogens as replacement therapy for climacterium. Increased incidence of these tumors in women taking oral contraceptives was similarly reported. A decrease of these cancers was reported during the last two to three years, when hormonal treatment was decreased or forbidden. Therefore, there is a direct relationship between hormone administration and a greater risk of cancer. Recent experimental and clinical evidence indicates that hormonelike substances (prostaglandins, epidermal growth factor) might also have an important role in the causation and development of cancers (4,64–66,85,94). There is a great difference in the susceptibility to cancer among different species, as well as among different strains of the same species. Therefore, genetic factors are also important in the etiology and pathogenesis of tumors. Genes can make cells susceptible to hormonal action or to the virus. Interactions of hormones, drugs, and nutritional factors can also play an important role in the etiology of cancers (53). The fact that hormones exert an important role in the etiology and pathogenesis of cancers does not always imply that hormones are carcinogenic per se. They can exert a critical role in preparing and rendering the cells more susceptible to an unknown carcinogenic agent, making them cocarcinogens, tumor promoters, and tumor modifiers. All these actions can be explained by the important effects of hormones in the homeostatic cellular mechanism(s) by regulating the preneoplastic cells and their progression to neoplastic cells, cell division of normal and abnormal cells, DNA synthesis, and cell differentiation. Both steroid and protein hormones can play an important role in the etiology and pathogenesis of cancers. In addition to hormone-dependent cancers in which the hormones play a determining role in their etiology and pathogenesis, in other cancers, such as liver, lung, skin, kidney, bone, and thyroid, hormones can drastically affect the neoplasm growth, multiplicity, and regression, exerting a more adjuvant, indirect, or permissive role. This will be a promising field for future research. In spite of well-demonstrated cases in experimental carcinogenesis, there are still no conclusive data on the role of hormones in human carcinogenesis, except for the three hormone-dependent cancers, perhaps because of longer duration of latency in the induction and occurrence of cancers in humans (20 to 30 years in some cases), as well as a deficiency in epidemiological case-control studies. Cell environment, and especially hormonal milieu, are of crucial importance to cellular homeostasis.

Several recent studies report on the synthesis of ectopic hormones or hormones secreted by nonendocrine tissues. Some cancers (lung, kidney, thyroid) can secrete ACTH, TSH, PTH, FSH, or MSH. All these hormones are similar to those synthesized by the endocrine cells and are immunoreactive with the antihormonal serum (109). This indicates that during neoplastic transformation, cellular dedifferentiation permits nonendocrine tissues to manufacture hormones. These ectopic hormones can play an important pathogenetic role, inducing such clinical manifestations as Cushingoid syndrome and Graves disease, similar to those of the true clinical syndromes. Immunological factors are also important in the incidence and development of cancers. Hormones can act by modifying the immunological surveillance, being immunosuppressors. We can thus speak of immunological surveillance as well as hormonal surveillance mechanism(s) in carcinogenesis.

SUMMARY

Hormones can be said to be major factors in the etiology and pathogenesis of cancers. In hormone-dependent cancers, they exert a direct or determinant role; in hormone-responsive cancers, they exert a permissive or adjuvant role. Their mechanism of action on normal cells as well as on transformed cells (preneoplastic and neoplastic) is more complex and can be exerted in their own way or according to a specific modus operandi. The hormonal milieu and its feedback mechanism(s) are important in the causation and development of cancers: hypothalamic–pituitary–ovarian axis; hypothalamic–pituitary–thyroid axis; hypothalamic–pituitary–adrenal axis, etc. Many of the so-called spontaneous tumors should be considered endogenously induced tumors. With the introduction and employment of new methods, our knowledge will advance a better understanding and elucidation of the cell biology of cancer cells and its controlling factors. Neoplastic transformation is not always an irreversible process synonymous with death; rather, it can be stopped or regressed, so that hormones are important governing factors of tumor induction and development.

REFERENCES

1. Axelrad, A., and Leblond, C.: Induction of thyroid tumors in rats by a low iodine diet. *Cancer 8*:339–367 (1955).
2. Bates, R.: Sex hormones and skin tumorigenesis I. Effect of the estrous cycle and castration on tumorigenesis by 7,12-dimethylbenz(a)anthracene. *J. Natl. Cancer Inst. 41*:559–563 (1968).
3. Beatson, G.: On the treatment of inoperable cases of carcinoma of the mamma: Suggestions for a new method of treatment with illustrative cases. *Lancet 2*:104–162 (1896).
4. Bennett, A., Simpson, J., McDonald, A., and Stamford, I.: Breast cancer, prostaglandins and bone metastases. *Lancet 1*:1218–1220 (1975).
5. Berenblum, I.: Established principles and unresolved problems in carcinogenesis. *J. Nat. Cancer Inst. 60*:723–726 (1978).
6. Bielschowsky, F.: Neoplasia and internal environment. *Br. J. Cancer 9*:80–116 (1955).
7. Bielschowsky, F.: Chronic iodine deficiency as cause of neoplasia in thyroid and pituitary of aged rats. *Br. J. Cancer 7*:203–213 (1953).
8. Biskind, M., and Biskind, G.: Development of tumors in the rat ovary after transplantation into the spleen. *Proc. Soc. Exp. Biol. Med. 55*:176–179 (1944).
9. Bittner, J.: Possible relationship of the estrogenic hormones, genetic susceptibility and milk influence in the production of mammary cancer in mice. *Cancer Res. 2*:710–721 (1942).
10. Bittner, J.: The cause and control of mammary cancer in mice. *Harvey Lect. 42*:221–246 (1946).
11. Bogardus, G., and Finley, J.: Breast cancer and thyroid disease. *Surgery 49*:461–468 (1961).
12. Boyland, E.: Human hormone-dependent tumors. *Prog. Exp. Tumor Res. 2*:145–157 (1961).
13. Bulbrook, R.: Hormonal factors in the etiology and treatment of breast cancer. *Proc. Can. Cancer Conf. 6*:36–49 (1966).
14. Burnet, F.: *Immunological Surveillance*. Pergamon Press, Sydney, 1970.
15. Caro, L., and Tubergen, R.: High resolution autoradiography methods. *J. Cell Biol. 15*:173–188 (1962).
16. Carter, R.: Experimental tumors and their counterparts in man: Some similarities and differences. *Br. J. Cancer 41*:494 (1980).
17. Clifton, K., and Sridharan, R.: Endocrine factors and tumor growth. In Becker, F. (ed.): *Cancer*, vol. 3. New York, Plenum Press, 1975, pp. 249–285.
18. Costlow, M., and McGuire, W.: Prolactin receptors and hormone dependence in mammary carcinoma. In Sharma, R., and Criss, W. (eds.): *Endocrine Control of Neoplasia*. New York, Raven Press, 1978, pp. 121–150.
19. Curtis-Prior, P.: Cancer and prostaglandins. In *Prostaglandins: An Introduction to Their Biochemistry, Physiology and Pharmacology*. Amsterdam, Elsevier-North Holland, 1976, pp. 145–149.
20. Doniach, I.: Experimental induction of tumors of the thyroid by radiation. *Br. Med. Bull. 14*:181–183 (1958).
21. Engelsman, E., Persijn, J., Dorsten, C., and Cleton, F.: Oestrogen receptor in human breast cancer tissue and response to endocrine therapy. *Br. Med. J. 2*:750–752 (1973).

22. Epstein, S., Joshi, S., Andrea, J., Mantel, N., Sawicki, E., and Stanley, T: Carcinogenicity of organic particulate pollutants in urban air after administration of trace quantities to neonatal mice. *Nature 212*:1305–1307 (1966).

23. Farrow, J., and Adair, F.: Effect of orchidectomy on skeletal metastases from cancer of the male breast. *Science 95*:654 (1942).

24. Furth, J.: The role of prolactin in mammary carcinogenesis. In Pasteels, J., and Robyn, C. (eds.): *Human Prolactin, Proceedings of the International Symposium on Human Prolactin.* New York, American Elsevier, 1973, pp. 233–248.

25. Furth, J.: Vistas in the etiology and pathogenesis of tumors. *Fed. Proc. 20*:865–873 (1961).

26. Furth, J., and Clifton, K.: Experimental pituitary tumors. In Harris, G., and Donavan, B. (eds.): *The Pituitary Gland*, vol. 2 pp. 460–498. (London, Butterworths, 1966).

27. Gardner, W.: Hormonal aspects of experimental tumorigenesis. In Greenstein, J., and Haddow, A. (eds.): *Advances in Cancer Research*, vol. 1. (New York, Academic Press, 1953), pp. 173–232.

28. Gardner, W., Pfeiffer, C., and Trentin, J.: Hormonal factors in experimental carcinogenesis. In Homburger, F. (ed.): *The Physiopathology of Cancer*, 2nd ed.: (New York, Harper & Row, 1959), pp. 152–237.

29. Goodall, C.: Endocrine factors as determinants of the susceptibility of the liver to carcinogenic agents. *N.Z. Med J. 67*:32–43 (1968).

30. Griffiths, K., Davies, P., Harper, M., Peeling, W., and Pierrepon, C.: The etiology and endocrinology of prostatic cancer. Rose, D. (ed.): *Endocrinology of Cancer*, vol. 2. (Boca Raton, FL., CRC Press, 1979), pp. 1–55.

31. Gusberg, S.: Hormonal relations of endometrial cancer. In Clark, R., and Stanley, W. (eds.): *Proceedings of the Seventh National Cancer Conference.* (Philadelphia, J. B. Lippincott, 1973), pp. 213–216.

32. Hilf, R., Harmon, J., Matusik, R., and Ringler, M.: Hormonal control of mammary cancer. In Criss, W., Ono, T., and Sabine, R. (eds.): *Control Mechanisms in Cancer.* (New York, Raven Press, 1974), pp. 1–24.

33. Huggins, C.: Control of cancers of man by endocrinologic methods. *Cancer Res. 17*:467–472 (1957).

34. Huggins, C.: Endocrine-induced regression of cancers. *Science 156*:1050–1054, (1967).

35. Huggins, C., Briziarelli, G., and Sutton, H.: Rapid induction of mammary carcinoma in the rat and the influence of hormones on the tumors. *J. Exp. Med. 109*:25–42 (1959).

36. Huggins, C.: Two principles in endocrine therapy of cancers: Hormone deprival and hormone interference. In Sharma, R., and Criss, W. (eds.): *Endocrine Control in Neoplasia.* (New York, Raven Press, 1978), pp. 1–9.

37. Huseby, R.: Hormonal factors in relation to cancer. In *Environment and Cancer, M.D. Anderson Symposium.* (Baltimore, Williams & Wilkins, 1972), pp. 372–393.

38. Jaffe, B.: Prostaglandins and cancer. An update. *Prostaglandins 6*:453–461, 1974.

39. Jensen, E., Block, G., Smith, S., Kyser, K., and DeSombre, E.: Estrogen receptors and hormone dependency. In Dao, T. (ed.): *Estrogen Target Tissues and Neoplasia.* (Chicago, University of Chicago Press, 1972), pp. 23–57.

40. Jick, H., Watkins, R., Hunter, J., Dinau, B., Madson, S., Rothman, R., and

Walker, A.: Replacement estrogens and endometrial cancer. *N. Engl. J. Med. 300*:218–221 (1979).

41. Jull, J.: Hormonal mechanisms in carcinogenesis. In *Proceedings of the Canadian Cancer Conference.* (Toronto, Pergamon Press, 1966), pp. 109–123.

42. Kirkman, H., and Bacon, R.: Malignant renal tumors in male hamsters (Cricetus auratus) treated with estrogen. *Cancer Res. 10*:122–123 (1950).

43. Kreig, L., Kühlmann, I., and Marks, F.: Effect of tumor-promoting phorbol esters and of acetic acid on mechanisms controlling DNA synthesis and mitosis (chalones) on the biosynthesis of histidine-rich protein in mouse epidermis. *Cancer Res. 34*:3135–3146 (1974).

44. Lacassagne, A.: Apparition de cancers de la mammelle chez la souris mâle soumise à des injections de folliculine. *Compt. Rendu Acad. Sci. (Paris) 195*:630–632 (1932).

45. Lacassagne, A.: Relationship of hormones and mammary adenocarcinoma in the mouse. *Am. J. Cancer 37*:414–424 (1939).

46. Lacassagne, A.: Hormones and their relation to cancer. *Schweiz. Med. Wschr. 78*:705–708 (1948).

47. Lathrop, A., and Loeb, L.: The influence of pregnancies on the incidence of cancer in mice. *Proc. Soc. Exp. Biol. Med. 11*:38–40 (1913).

48. Lemon, H.: Endocrine influences on human mammary cancer formation. A critique. *Cancer 23*:781–790 (1969).

49. Letoublon, C., Champetier, J., Benbassa, A., Durand, A., Labond, Y., and Pasquier, D.: Tumeurs bénignes du foie et contraceptifs oraux [Benign liver tumors and oral contraceptives]. *Lyon Chir. 74*:121–124 (1978).

50. Lipschütz, A.: *Steroid Hormones and Tumors.* (Baltimore, Williams & Wilkins, 1950).

51. Lipschütz, A., Iglesias, R., Panasevich, V., and Salinas, S.: Granulosa cell tumor induced in mice by progesterone. *Br. J. Cancer 21*:144–152 (1967).

52. Lipschütz, A., Iglesias, R., Panasevich, V., and Salinas, S.: Pathological changes induced in the uterus of mice with prolonged administration of progesterone and 19-nor-contraceptives. *Br. J. Cancer 21*:160–165 (1967).

53. Lipsett, M.: Interactions of drugs, hormones and nutrition in the causes of cancer. *Cancer 43*:1967–1981 (1979).

54. Loeb, L.: Further investigations on the origin of tumors in mice: Internal secretion as a factor in the origin of tumors. *J. Med. Res. 40*:477–496 (1919).

55. Lostroh, A., and Li, C.H.: Stimulation of the sex accesories of hypophysectomized male rats by non-gonadotrophic hormones of the pituitary gland. *Acta Endocrinol. 25*:1–16 (1957).

56. Lupulescu, A.: *Hormonii Steroizi [Steroid Hormones].* (Bucharest, Medical Publications House, 1958).

57. Lupulescu, A.: Experimental pheochromocytomas. *Ann. Endocrinol. 22*: 459–468 (1961).

58. Lupulescu, A., Chivu, V., and Petrovici, A.: Effect of aldosterone, glucagon and growth hormone on the catecholamine content and the evolution of chromaffin hyperplasia in guinea pigs. *Experientia 22*:222–223, 1966.

59. Lupulescu, A., and Petrovici, A.: *Ultrastructure of the Thyroid Gland.* (Baltimore, Williams & Wilkins, 1969).

60. Lupulescu, A., Andreani, D., Monaco, F., and Andreoli, M.: Ultrastructure and soluble iodoproteins in human thyroid cancer. *J. Clin. Endocrinol. Metab. 28*:1257–1268 (1968).

61. Lupulescu, A., and Boyd, C.: Lung cancer: A transmission and scanning

electron microscopic study. Cancer 29:1530–1538 (1972).

62. Lupulescu, A., and Boyd, C.: Follicular adenomas: An ultrastructural and scanning electron microscopic study. *Arch Pathol. 93*:492–502 (1972).

63. Lupulescu, A., Roger, J., and Birmingham, D.: Hormonal control of preneoplastic epidermal cells during carcinogenesis in mice. (abstract) *J. Cell Biol. 79*:187 (1978).

64. Lupulescu, A.: Enhancement of carcinogenesis by prostaglandins in male albino swiss mice. *J. Natl. Cancer Inst. 61*:97–106 (1978).

65. Lupulescu, A.: Hormonal regulation of DNA synthesis in cancerous epidermal cells. (abstract) *J. Cell Biol. 87*:103 (1980).

66. Lupulescu, A.: Hormonal regulation of epidermal tumor development. *J. Invest. Dermatol. 77*:186–195 (1981).

67. MacMahon, B., Cole, P., and Brown, J.: Etiology of human breast cancer. A review. *J. Natl. Cancer Inst. 50*:21–42 (1973).

68. Marchant, J.: Chemical induction of breast tumors in mice of C$_{57}$B$_1$ strain. The influence of pseudopregnancy, pregnancy and lactation in induction by methylcholanthrene. *Br. J. Cancer 15*:568–573 (1961).

69. McGuire, W., and DeLagarza, M.: Similarity of the estrogen receptor in human and rat mammary carcinoma. *J. Clin. Endocrinol. Metab. 37*:986–989 (1973).

70. Medewar, P., and Sparrow, E.: The effects of adrenocortical hormone and pregnancy on skin transplantation immunity in mice. *J. Endocrinol. 14*:240–256 (1956).

71. Meissner, W.: Thyroid tumors. In Werner, S., and Ingbar, S. (eds.): *The Thyroid.* (Hagerstown, Md., Harper & Row, 1978), pp. 451–457.

72. Meites, J.: Relation of prolactin and estrogens to mammary tumorigenesis in the rat. *J. Natl. Cancer Inst. 48*:1217–1224 (1972).

73. Mittra, I., and Haywar, J.: Hypothalamic–pituitary–thyroid axis in breast cancer. *Lancet 1*:885–888 (1974).

74. Moon, H., Simpson, M., Li, C.H., and Evans, H.: Neoplasms in rats treated with pituitary growth hormone. I. Pulmonary and lymphatic tissue. *Cancer Res. 10*:297–308 (1950).

75. Moon, H., Simpson, M., Li, C.H., and Evans, H.: Neoplasms in rats treated with pituitary growth hormone. II. Adrenal glands. *Cancer Res. 10*:364–371 (1950).

76. Muhlbock, O.: Role of hormones in the etiology of breast cancer. *J. Natl. Cancer Inst. 48*:1213–1216 (1972).

77. Nandi, S.: Comparison of the tumorigenic effects of chemical carcinogens and hormones. *J. Anim. Sci. 40*:1263–1266 (1975).

78. Nathanson, I., and Andervont, H.: Effect of testosterone propionate on development and growth of mammary carcinoma in female mice. *Proc. Soc. Exp. Biol. Med. 40*:421–422 (1939).

79. Noble, R.: Hormonal regulation of tumor growth. *Pharmacol. Rev. 9*:367–426 (1957).

80. Noble, R.: The development of prostatic carcinoma in Nb rats following prolonged sex hormone administration. *Cancer Res. 37*:1929–1933 (1977).

81. *Oestrogens and Progestins in Relation to Human Cancer* Vol. 21: part II: *Sex Hormones. IARC Monographs.* (Lyons, International Agency for Research on Cancer, 1979), pp. 83–129.

82. Parker, L., Belsky, N., Yamamoto, T., Kavamoto, S., and Keehn, R.: Thyroid carcinoma after exposure to atomic radiation: A continuing survey of a fixed population, Hiroshima and Nagasaki. *Ann. Intern. Med. 80*:600–604 (1974).

83. Pike, M., Gerkins, V., Casagrande, J., Gray, J., Brown, J., and Henderson, B.: The hormonal basis of breast cancer. In *Natl. Cancer Inst. Monograph 53.* Bethesda, MD, 1979, pp. 187–193.

84. Pitot, H.: Carcinogenesis and Aging—Two related phenomena? *Am. J. Pathol. 87*:444–472 (1977).

85. Rose, S., Stahn, R., Passavoy, D., and Hernschman, H.: Epidermal growth factor enhancement of skin tumor induction. *Experientia 32*:913–915 (1976).

86. Rous, P.: The nearer causes of cancer. *JAMA 122*:373–381 (1944).

87. Schmidt, T., and Thompson, E.: Glucocorticoid receptor function in leukemic cells. In Sharma, R., and Criss, W. (eds.): *Endocrine Control of Neoplasia.* New York, Raven Press, 1978, pp. 263–290.

88. Scribner, J., and Slaga, T.: Multiple effects of dexamethasone on protein synthesis and hyperplasia caused by a tumor promoter. *Cancer Res. 33*:542–546 (1973).

89. Segaloff, A., and Maxfield, W.: The synergism between radiation and estrogen in the production of mammary cancer in the rat. *Cancer Res. 31*:166–168 (1971).

90. Shellaberger, C.: Hypothroidism and DMBA rat mammary carcinogenesis. *Proc. Am. Assoc. Cancer Res. 10*:79 (1969).

91. Sicher, K., and Waterhouse, J.: Thyroid activity in relation to prognosis in mammary cancer. *Br. J. Cancer 41*:512–518 (1967).

92. Süteri, P., Nisker, J., and Hammond, G.: Hormonal basis of risk factors for breast and endometrial cancer. In Iacobelli, S., King, R., Lindner, H., and Lippman, M. (eds): *Hormones and Cancer.* (New York, Raven Press, 1980), 499–505.

93. Sinha, D., Cooper, D., and Dao, T.: The nature of estrogen and prolactin effect on mammary tumorigenesis. *Cancer Res. 33*:411–414 (1973).

94. Smithline, F., Sherman, L., and Kolodny, H.: Prolactin and breast carcinoma. *N. Engl. J. Med. 292*:184–192 (1975).

95. Smythies, J.: Prostaglandins and Cancer. In *Psychoneuroendocrinology* 4: 177–189 (1979).

96. Spencer, J.: The influence of the thyroid in malignant disease. *Br. J. Cancer 8*:393–411 (1954).

97. Takizawa, S., Furth, J.J., and Furth, J.: DNA synthesis in autonomous and hormone responsive mammary tumors. *Cancer Res. 30*:206–211 (1970).

98. Thomas, D.: Role of exogenous female hormones in altering the risk of benign and malignant neoplasms in humans. *Cancer Res. 38*:3991–4000 (1978).

99. Van Nie, R., Benedetti, E., and Mühlbock, O.: A carcinogenic action of testosterone provoking uterine tumors in mice. *Nature 192*:1303 (1961).

100. Vesselinovitch, S., Rao, K., Mihailovich, N., Rice, J., and Lombard, L.: Development of broad spectrum of tumors by ethylnitrosourea and the modifying role of age, sex and strain. *Cancer Res. 34*:2530–2538 (1974).

101. Wahner, H., Cuello, C., Correa, P., Uribe, L., and Gaitan, E.: Thyroid carcinoma in an endemic goiter area, Cali, Columbia. *Am. J. Med. 40*:58–66 (1966).

102. Weisburger, J.: Hormones, chemicals and liver cancer. *N.Z. Med. J. 67*:44–56 (1968).

103. Welsch, C., and Gribler, C.: Prophylaxis of spontaneously developing mammary carcinoma in C_3H/HeJ female mice by suppression of prolactin. *Cancer Res. 33*:2939–2946 (1973).

104. White, L.: Studies on melanoma: II. Sex and survival in human melanoma. *N. Engl. J. Med. 260*:789–797 (1959).

105. White, C., and Titcombe, R.: The action of pituitary (anterior lobe) extract on cancer in mice. *Med. Chron. (Manchester) 9*:73–79 (1914–1915).

106. Winship, T., and Rosvoli, R.: Thyroid carcinoma in children: final report on a 20 year study. *Clin Proc. Children's Hosp. Wash. D.C. 26*:327–348 (1979).

107. Woolley, G.: Cortisone, related steroids and transplanted tumors of the mouse. *Cancer Res. 11*:291 (1951).

108. Wotiz, H., Shane, J., Vigersky, R., and Brecher, P.: The regulatory role of estriol in the proliferative action of oestradiol. In Forrest, A., and Kunkler, P. (eds.): *Prognostic Factors in Breast Cancer* (London, Livingstone, 1968), pp. 368–384.

109. Yalow, R.: Heterogeneity of peptide hormones. *Rec. Prog. Horm. Res. 30*:597–633 (1974).

110. Young, S., and Inman, R. (eds.): *Thyroid Neoplasia.* (London, Academic Press, 1968).

111. Zackheim, H., Simpson, W., and Lange, L.: Basal cell epitheliomas and other skin tumors produced in rats and mice by anthramine and methylcholanthrene. *J. Invest. Dermatol. 33*:385–402 (1959).

Chapter 5

HORMONE-DEPENDENT CANCERS—OVERVIEW

Early clinical and experimental observations demonstrated that some tumors originate in the target tissue and are unable to grow, develop, and propagate in the absence of certain hormones. These tumors were described as hormone-dependent tumors (HDTs). Thus, the induction, development, and regression of these cancers is hormone dependent. Regardless of their origin—spontaneous, chemical, viral, or hormonal—these tumors fail to grow and survive; they immediately shrink and regress when the respective hormone is removed. Moreover, these tumors cannot be transplanted in endocrine-deprived hosts. When the respective hormone is supplemented, however, these tumors begin to develop and progress, sometimes reaching huge proportions. They can also metastasize and be serially transplanted when this hormone is added.

Thus, a new term, hormone dependency, was coined for one type of tumor, as opposed to other cancers that can grow, develop, and survive and

145

also be transplanted regardless of the presence of hormone, generally described as hormone-independent tumors (HITs) or hormone-independent cancers.

Hence, the presence of hormones is obligatory for the induction, development, invasion, or regression of HDTs, but is irrelevant for HITs. Hormones play a cardinal role in the etiology and pathogenesis of hormone-dependent cancers (HDCs), but exert only an adjuvant role in the development of hormone-independent cancers (HICs). This was a significant advancement in the carcinogenic process, which can be modified or modulated by hormones. All HDCs can be therapeutically manipulated by hormones; and endocrine therapy—ablative or hormone therapy—has become a major therapeutic method with promising results.

In addition to cancers that originate and develop in target tissue, such as mammary gland, thyroid, prostate gland, uterus, ovary, adrenal gland, and testis, a large number of tumors that originate in nonendocrine organs (e.g., kidney, colon, lung, liver) can become hormone dependent in evolution; thus the notion of HDCs has expanded significantly in recent years (10,36,62). These cancers are usually described as estrogen-dependent, androgen-dependent, progesterone-dependent, TSH-dependent, or insulin-dependent tumors.

In several recent clinical and experimental investigations of mammary carcinoma, thyroid cancer, prostate tumors, ovarian tumors, uterine adenocarcinoma, and renal cell carcinoma, significant achievements were made with regard to their pathogenetic mechanisms and therapeutic procedures. Endocrine-induced regression or remission after castration, adrenalectomy, or hypophysectomy was reported at the beginning of this century. More recently, a large number of hormones or their antagonists (hormone antagonists) have been used alone or in combination with chemotherapeutic drugs, radiation therapy, or immune therapy, with encouraging results in patients with HDCs. Appropriate endocrine modifications often produce spectacular results; sometimes, the neoplastic lesions can regress or completely disappear in most HDCs.

CLASSIFICATION OF HORMONE-CONTROLLED CANCERS

There are eight HDCs, some of which are common to human subjects and laboratory animals (36): mammary carcinoma (human and rat); prostate carcinoma (human and rat); thyroid carcinoma (human and rat); lymphosarcoma; leukemia (human and mouse); carcinoma of endometrium (human); carcinoma of seminal vesicles (human); carcinoma of scent glands (hamster and dog) and carcinoma of the kidneys (human and hamster) (Table 5-1).

In addition to these eight HDCs, a broad spectrum of tumors were reported by different laboratories, including ours during the past decade, that

**Table 5-1. HORMONE-DEPENDENT CANCERS
OF HUMANS AND ANIMALS**

Mammary carcinoma	Human (female, male); rat
Prostate carcinoma	Human; rat
Thyroid carcinoma	Human; rat
Lymphosarcoma, leukemia	Mouse; human
Carcinoma of endometrium	Human
Carcinoma of kidney	Hamster; human
Carcinoma of seminal vesicles	Man
Carcinoma of scent glands	Hamster; dog

occur in nontarget tissues, the development and regression of which can be facilitated by hormones; these tumors are also partially or completely hormone responsive. This new category of hormone-responsive tumors (HRTs) includes skin tumors, tumors of the pancreas, colon carcinoma, and some lung cancers. Hormone receptors similar or identical to those of HDCs were found in some of these cancers (2,57,59). The clinical oncologist should always thoroughly estimate the hormone responsiveness of tumors before making any therapeutic decision. Thus, the endocrine status, or hormonal milieu is of crucial significance not only for the development and propagation of HDCs, but for their regression as well. This phenomenon of hormone dependency proves that the carcinogenic process is not necessarily an autonomous and self-perpetuating process; its growth and progression can be restrained or markedly reduced by hormone deprivation. Thus, when the hormonal milieu is altered by hormone administration, the rate of HDC growth is markedly enhanced; by contrast, when hormone deficiency is altered by removal of the endocrine source, regression, shrinkage, and sometimes tumor disappearance can occur.

Hormones are essential factors that can govern the incidence, development, and regression of HDCs. Recently, the use of more sensitive methods, such as electron microscopy, autoradiography for DNA, messenger RNA and protein synthesis, and hormone-receptor estimation, indicate that HDTs exhibit heterogeneous cell populations. The tumor is therefore a mosaic or mixture of neoplastic cells containing some cells that are more hormone responsive than others, which are only partially hormone dependent or that even develop a tendency for hormone independency or autonomy. The hormone-responsive cells are generally well-differentiated, highly dividing cells with a marked ^{3}H-thymidine labeling index, containing a high percentage of hormone receptors; in vitro they exhibit a tendency to adhere and form colonies by increased cell adhesiveness. Their cell surfaces are more regular, and generally these cells are more homogeneous, whereas the less hormone-responsive or hormone-independent cells exhibit a bizarre morphology with very irregular cell surfaces and a tendency to disperse. They are more polymorphic cells when examined by scanning electron microscopy (SEM), are poorly differentiated or even anaplastic cells, and contain a low percentage of hormone receptors. Thus, tumor behavior and its hormone responsiveness are largely dependent on the predominance of hormone-responsive cells or vice versa.

Hence, by gross morphologic examination we cannot distinguish between HDCs and HICs; we should always use more accurate methods to detect the earlier stages of hormone dependence or its loss for greater accuracy in making therapeutic predictions.

It is possible that the hormone-sensitive and hormone-insensitive cells differ from each other in chromosomal aberrations as well, with a higher rate of somatic mutations. Some visible chromosomal changes were reported in many malignant tumors, but these findings are not specific for one particular type of tumor. It seems likely that these heterogeneous cell populations or cell sublines arise in a tumor as a result of its tendency to undergo more mutations; thus cancerous cell populations are more unstable as compared with normal cells. These cell sublines display a different hormone sensitivity and also a different drug sensitivity. Therefore, it is important to institute a combined therapy—hormonotherapy with chemotherapy or hormonotherapy with radiotherapy. Thus, cells that survive hormone effects will be killed by chemotherapeutic drugs or by radiation therapy. One unanswered question in terms of normal physiology and carcinogenesis is: Why do only certain tissues (target tissues) respond to various steroid hormones by developing tumors, despite the fact that essentially all tissue cells contain the same genetic complement? And why do these target tissues develop tumors that can grow, survive, and propagate only in the presence of hormones and regress or die when the respective hormone is lacking? Thus neoplastic cells retain the same hormone dependency of normal cells. Advances in knowledge of the endocrine control of neoplastic transformation stem directly from advances in techniques that specifically visualize the binding of the hormone to target cells and thus provide more precise information regarding the tumor hormone-dependency. In addition to light and electron microscopic auto-radiography, which visualize the intracellular binding of steroid or protein hormones in the target cells, the estimation of hormone receptors by immuno-cytologic endocrinology provides more accurate data with regard to the intrinsic mechanism(s) of hormone-dependent carcinogenesis. However, not all mechanisms can be explained by hormone receptors (60). Not all positive receptor cells are hormone-responsive cells, and vice versa. The absence of a specific receptor, which is sometimes exceedingly difficult to prove, is not the only reason for hormone unresponsiveness. It seems likely that hormones also work through mechanisms that do not involve receptor molecules or hormone–receptor complexes, but that induce other biochemical aberrations or the occurrence of potential antihormones. Determination of hormone metabolites in patients with HDCs such as breast cancer and prostate cancers were also extensively used, but the correlation was not sufficient to influence therapy decisions. Thus the mechanisms of hormone dependency are more complex.

Another puzzling situation is that a HDC (mammary carcinoma, prostate tumors) can be dependent on one or more hormones or be independent of all hormones. Some neoplastic cells possess more than one hormone receptor (androgen, estrogen, or insulin) or are negative hormone receptors. Since nearly one-fourth (90,000) of deaths out of an estimated total number of 350,000 cancer deaths in the United States per year are caused by hormone-controlled cancers, the study of HDTs is an important part of carcinogenesis. Some HDCs are common to laboratory animals and humans, others are not.

EXPERIMENTAL HORMONE-DEPENDENT TUMORS

Hormone-dependent tumors that can occur spontaneously or be chemically, virally, or physically induced in laboratory animals are mammary carcinoma, prostate tumors, lymphosarcoma, leukemia, carcinoma of the thyroid, carcinoma of kidney, and carcinoma of scent glands. Some HDTs, such as mammary carcinoma, occur more frequently in rats; carcinoma of the kidney occurs mostly in hamsters, and prostate tumors in dogs.

Mammary Carcinoma

Spontaneous mammary carcinomas are common in mouse, dog, and humans. However, mammary carcinomas of mouse and dog differ from human mammary carcinoma, in that they are generally not hormone-responsive tumors. Thus, mouse and dog mammary carcinomas do not regress or shrink after ovariectomy, adrenalectomy, hypophysectomy, or testosterone administration, and in mouse they became hormone independent when a tumor reaches a palpable size (36,37).

Although the first hormone-induced mammary carcinoma was described in male mice, this species is not a suitable model for hormone-dependent breast cancer. The only suitable experimental model for the study of hormone-dependent mammary carcinoma is the rat, since only in this species are mammary carcinomas hormone dependent. Thus, the rat has a remarkable propensity to develop mammary tumors after exposure to estrogens, aromatic hydrocarbons, or ionizing radiation.

Estrogen-Induced Mammary Carcinomas

Long-term exposure of rats to large doses of estrogens alone, or combined with other sex steroids, leads to a high incidence of benign mammary tumors and in some cases of adenocarcinomas. However, this method is slow and inconsistent; the mammary cancers occur only in some estrogen-treated rats, while others never develop cancers. Combination of estrogens and progesterone may increase the incidence of mammary carcinomas in rats. However, the results are still conflicting and there is no valid evidence that estrogens are carcinogenic per se in rats or other laboratory animals. It is certain that the steroid hormones markedly enhance the incidence and development of mammary carcinomas in rats as compared with controls, by modifying their cell environment.

In dogs, however, administration of progestins (17α-hydroxyprogesterone) can induce and promote mammary tumorigenesis. Benign and malignant extensive mammary tumors are developing following progestins and these tumors are time and dose related. Thus, the progestins play an important role in dog mammary carcinogenesis, suggesting a great difference in the sensitivity between different species and also between different strains of the same species. In addition to sex steroids, other hormones, such as glucocorticoids, thyroid hormones, pituitary hormones (mainly prolactin), and recently insulin, are directly or indirectly involved in the induction and growth of breast cancers. Their role in the etiology and pathogenesis of mammary cancer was already studied (see Chapter 4).

More recently, it was found that mammary carcinomas can be enhanced by administration of insulin; insulin-dependent mammary tumors were reported in some species, including rat. Insulin receptors were described in experimental mammary cancers as well as in human breast cancer. The incidence of spontaneous mammary carcinomas in C_3H/HeN mice is also significantly influenced by triiodo-L-thyronine. However, tumor growth rate, tumor labeling, and mitotic indices are not significantly changed. Also, the histologic pattern is quite similar in both controls and triiodothyronine-treated mice. Since mammary tumorigenesis was increased in T_3-treated mice in spite of lower levels of serum prolactin, this suggest a direct role of T_3 on mammary tumor promotion (73).

Aromatic Hydrocarbon-Induced Mammary Carcinoma

Rat is a species with a remarkable propensity to develop mammary carcinoma after exposure to aromatics. Several aromatics are carcinogenic in rats: 3-methylcholanthrene (3-MCA), 2-acetylaminofluorene (2-AAF), and mostly 7,12-dimethylbenz(a)anthracen (7,12-IMBA), all of which act rapidly and can induce palpable tumors within 1 month; however, 7,12-DMBA is nearly 10 times more active than the others. Thus, after painting the skin of the mice and rats with 3-MCA for several months, we found palpable adenocarcinoma of mammary glands within 4 months, in addition to the development of skin tumors. A single dose of DMBA consistently and rapidly induces mammary carcinomas in rats. These tumors are invasive locally, reach tremendous size, but only seldom metastasize. Most of these mammary carcinomas are HDTs, and their evolution is markedly influenced by hormonal changes. Thus, an acceleration of growth rate in mammary carcinomas occurs in pregnancy, pseudopregnancy, or progesterone administration (37). Regression, and sometimes tumor extinction, can occur after hypophysectomy, ovariectomy, and testosterone/progesterone administration. Some mammary cancers do not regress after hypophysectomy and ovariectomy. It is possible that these tumors have a different histologic structure, yet do not contain estrogen receptors (83). It is interesting that mammary carcinoma induced by aromatics in rats are not always affected by hormones and sometimes behave as HICs. Thus, a strong correlation between estrogen receptors (ERs) and response of DMBA-induced mammary carcinomas to ovariectomy cannot be established. Hence, some investigators found that the concentrations of ER and prolactin receptors in DMBA-induced tumors are better correlated with endocrine ablation (ovariectomy, adrenalectomy, hypophysectomy), whereas others found no correlation between hormone receptors and tumor response (21,64). Progesterone receptors (PgRs) were also demonstrated in DMBA-induced mammary tumors. In addition to ovarian and pituitary hormones, some DMBA-induced mammary tumors are also insulin dependent. However, not all these tumors are insulin dependent. Experiments in vitro and in vivo indicate that insulin plays a role in DMBA mammary carcinogenesis in rats and has to be considered an important factor in hormone dependency. It is possible that insulin exerts its permissive role by influencing the levels of estrogen and prolactin receptors (28). The role of hormone receptors is very important in maintaining the hormone dependency of experimental as well as human mammary cancers. Recently, it has been suggested that mammary tumors contain a mixed population of cells or mosaic cell subpopulations; some of these neoplastic cells display hormone receptors and are thus hormone responsive, whereas others do not contain hormone receptors and are hormone-insensitive cells. The degree of hormone dependency or progression toward autonomous evolution depends largely on the presence or absence of hormone-receptor-containing cells. The autonomous mammary tumors contain a lower concentration of ER and PgR receptors than do the tumors, which are hormone dependent.

There is a difference in susceptibility of different strains of rats in regard to the development of mammary carcinomas. Thus, Nb rats are quite susceptible to estrogenization with induction of mammary tumors. A higher incidence of mammary tumors was observed in both sexes following subcutaneous implantation of estrogen pellets. Irrespective of the induction of carcinogensis (chemical, hormonal), the growth of HDTs was not irreversible, but was controlled by exogenous estrogens.

It is interesting that hormone dependency of mammary carcinomas can be elicited after a long period of dormancy or silence, if the estrogen is administered. Thus, hormone dependency is independent of tumor progression and can be retained in slow-growing or even in nongrowing tumors (62).

Ionizing Radiation-Induced Mammary Carcinomas

Rats are less sensitive to ionizing radiation in regard to mammary tumor induction as compared with aromatics or hormones. Thus, a single dose of radioactive isotopes, x-rays, or γ-rays elicits mammary tumors in rats. A single injection of ^{211}astatine (^{211}At) or a single-body irradiation with γ-rays from a ^{60}Co irradiator induces mammary carcinomas in female rats. In young female rats, mammary tumors can be induced by single and total-body x-irradiation. Despite that, the incidence of mammary tumor can be high in some rat strains (Sprague-Dawley female rats), and not all irradiated series develop mammary carcinomas (19). Histologically, these tumors are adeno-carcinomas and fibroadenomas. Recently, a synergism of estrogens and x-rays in mammary carcinoma formation was reported. Thus, irradiation of the body by x-rays associated with estrogen (diethylstilbestrol, DES, or 17-ethinylestradiol, EE_2) markedly increased the mammary carcinogenesis in female AC I rats. A high incidence of mammary carcinomas was observed in rats treated with DES or EE_2 and x-rays, whereas no significant number of tumors was observed in rats treated with estrogens or x-rays alone. Also, an earlier incidence of tumors was observed in rats treated with estrogens and x-rays (34).

Although DMBA-induced mammary tumors are easy reproducible and exhibit a high frequency of hormone dependency, they regress after ovariectomy and grow with marked increases in DNA synthesis and RNA synthesis. Mammary tumors induced by radiation exhibit a lesser degree of hormone dependency.

Thus, DMBA-induced mammary carcinoma is an ideal experimental model for the study of hormone dependency; most data from animal breast cancer studies can be extrapolated to human breast cancer and improve our knowledge of the hormone-dependent mechanism(s) of mammary cancers. Also, this model can be used for testing and screening the potential therapeutic drugs for breast cancer. It has also been found that rat DMBA-induced mammary carcinomas that regress after ovariectomy contain a specific cytoplasmic 17β-estradiol binding protein, whereas carcinomas that do not regress and that continue to grow after ovariectomy have a markedly reduced amount or lack of this cytoplasmic protein. Thus the hormonal dependency of breast tumors is due to the presence of this protein, whereas hormonal independence or tumor autonomy is due to a lack of this estradiol binding protein (55). It was recently demonstrated that 70 percent of DMBA-induced mammary tumors regress when Sprague-Dawley female rats were made diabetic after treatment with streptozotocin. This mammary tumor regression due to diabetes and thus insulin dependency or insulin-independency of mammary carcinomas involves the cAMP system and protein kinase activity; the sequence of events is similar to that observed during regression after ovariectomy (74). There has been a recent interest in the use of rat mammary carcinoma induced by N-nitrosomethylurea (NMU) as an experimental model for HDTs and for human breast cancer, because the hormone dependence of NMU-induced rat mammary carcinomas is more closely related to that of human breast cancer than to the DMBA model. Thus, the effects of hypophysectomy and prolactin were compared as to the growth of mammary-induced tumors in Sprague-Dawley rats, using NMU and DMBA. Unlike DMBA-induced rat mammary tumors, carcinomas obtained with NMU require estrogens for their growth, rather than being predominantly prolactin dependent. Hypophysectomy induces regression in both groups in a similar manner. Estradiol replacement frequently prevents tumor regression after hypophysectomy. The influence of ovine prolactin and growth hormone (GH) was also studied on NMU-induced mammary carcinomas revealing that these HDTs are more akin to human breast cancer; estrogens, prolactin, and growth hormone are involved in their optimal growth and hormone dependency (70). Studies on hormone receptors of DMBA- and NMU-induced rat mammary carcinomas show that neoplastic cells contain negligible amounts of (ER) and no PgR, but contain high amounts of androgen (Ra) and glucocorticoid receptors (Rgs). Thus these neoplastic cells are mostly responsive to glucocorticoids (32). Recently it was shown that DMBA-induced rat mammary carcinomas are dependent not only on sex steroids and estrogens, but on cAMP as well. Thus, estrogens stimulate, whereas ovariectomy, cyclic adenosine $3',5'$ monophosphate (cAMP), and dibutyrl cAMP arrest the growth of these tumors. Hence, cAMP-binding proteins may play a role in the regression stage of hormone-dependent mammary tumors, whereas estrogens may promote their growth (7).

Prostate Carcinoma

Earlier observations of Huggins and associates showed the occurrence of spontaneous prostate tumors in aged dogs to be somewhat similar to that occurring in humans (36). Because these tumors always regress after orchidectomy and estrogen therapy and are stimulated by androgen administration, they serve as a model for the study of human hormone-dependent prostate carcinoma. Canine prostate tumors can be benign (e.g., hyperplasia, adenomas, cystadenomas) or malignant (e.g., adenocarcinomas). Castration also prevents the occurrence of benign prostatic hyperplasia in dogs treated long term with androgens (testosterone or dehydrotestosterone). Castrated dogs treated with a combination of DHT and estrogens or androstanediol with estrogen for 1 year developed a massive prostate hypertrophy as compared with dogs treated with androstanediol alone (82). Thus androgen deficiency, androgen excess, and estrogen imbalance all play an important role in genesis of prostatic benign tumors and hyperplasia. Prostatic carcinoma is induced in mice and rats by steroid treatment with difficulty and only by direct application of the chemical carcinogen.

Recently, the induction of prostatic adenocarcinoma was reported in the Nb strain of rats by prolonged administration of androgens (testosterone propionate pellets). A combination of androgens with estrogens results in higher incidence of malignant tumors at a younger age. Pretreatment of Nb rats with estrogens for some months decreases the tumor response to subsequent treatment with testosterone (63). These data suggest a possible hormonal etiology and dependency of prostate tumors. However, a stronger evidence for hormone dependency of prostatic adenocarcinoma is that occurring in the inbred strain of Dunning R 3327 rats. This tumor fulfills all criteria needed for an animal model to be related to human hormone-dependent prostatic adenocarcinoma.

Thus, it arises spontaneously in rat prostate, exhibits histologic and biologic similarities to human prostatic adenocarcinoma, metastasizes in bones and lymph nodes, and is hormone dependent (i.e., responds to androgens and regresses after castration and estrogens). This tumor can be transplanted for several generations in the same inbred line of rats. Histologically, this is a well-differentiated prostatic adenocarcinoma similar to that found in humans. This rat prostatic adenocarcinoma exhibits an interesting hormone dependency. Thus, the tumor reaches a large size in the the presence of androgens and significantly regresses in castrated rats. Administration of testosterone to castrated animals induces a tumor growth similar to that of intact rats. Administration of diethylstilbestrol or antiandrogens (flutamide) prevents or inhibits the tumor growth (76). However, not all tumors are hormone dependent; some are hormone independent. Cell kinetic studies indicate that Dunning R 3327 transplantable rat adenocarcinoma contains a heterogeneous cell population, namely 70 to 90 percent of the total tumor cells are hormone sensitive and a subpopulation of 8 to 30 percent are hormone insensitive. The therapeutic relapse due to androgen deprivation represents the growth of the clone of cells, which are hormone insensitive, similar to that observed in human prostatic cancer. Also, during the serial passages of transplanted and HDT lines, HIT or even anaplastic tumors (AT) can develop, which suggests that not all neoplastic cells are hormone sensitive, that some of them (approximately 29 percent) are hormone insensitive, and explains why some tumors do not regress after castration and have lost their androgen dependency.

The estimation of steroid receptors in Dunning R 3327 rat prostatic carcinoma is a good criterion for distinguishing HDT from HIT. Thus both AR and ER concentrations are higher in well-differentiated adenocarcinoma, lower in differentiated or hormone-insensitive tumors (fibrosarcomas). A correlation was made between histologic type and receptor concentration (51).

Sometimes, especially when both HDT and HIT contain cytoplasmic AR, more sensitive biochemical methods should be used. Thus, using the effect of sodium molybdate and the photoaffinity labeling patterns of protein kinases with 8-azido-cAMP, a major difference between HDT and HIT was found, namely, that HDT contains a higher ratio of the type II/I regulatory subunits of protein kinase and a far greater level of proteolytic fragment (43K) than that of HIT. Thus, the estimation of protein kinases and their proteolytic fragments is a very sensitive method that can be used to distinguish between HDT and HIT containing the same amount of cytoplasmic ARs (14). R 3327 rat prostatic adenocarcinoma is devoid of progesterone receptors.

In addition to ER and AR, prolactin receptors (PLRs), insulin receptors (INRs) and an epidermal growth factor, urogastrone, were found in rat prostatic carcinoma cells derived from both Dunning R 3327 and R 3327 AT. However, there are great differences between the ratio of hormone receptor sites and histologic pattern. These data suggest a role of prolactin, insulin, and the epidermal growth factor urogastrone in the growth of prostatic carcinoma (33).

Renal Cell Carcinoma

Experimentally induced renal carcinoma (RCC) in laboratory animals has been extensively studied and can serve as an ideal model for renal tumor hormone dependency.

RCC induced by chemical carcinogens is influenced by sex hormones in mice and rats (65). In NZO mice dimethylnitrosamine (DMN) induced kidney tumors only in males; orchiectomy abolished tumor response. However, significant evidence for hormone-dependency of kidney tumors was found in male Syrian hamsters (*Mesocricetus auratus*). Both male and castrated female Syrian hamsters developed renal cell carcinomas after prolonged estrogen administration. These tumors are bilateral, extensive with metastases in lymph nodes and lungs, and histologically malignant. Their histologic pattern resembles that of human adenocarcinomas.

Estrogen-induced RCC in the hamster is mitigated or inhibited by estrogen antagonists, such as progesterone, testosterone propionate, and deoxycorticosterone (DOC). These tumors are transplantable in other hamsters, provided that they have been pretreated with estrogens or androgens. Although during serial transplantation these tumors can acquire some degree of autonomy or hormone independence, essentially their growth and evolution remains hormone dependent; thus they still respond to progesterone or androgens (43,44).

Recently, it has been shown that DES-induced and -dependent renal carcinoma of the Syrian hamster has a higher concentration of glucose 6-phosphate dehydrogenase (G 6-Pd) as compared with that observed in DES-induced but independent or autonomous renal carcinomas. Cytologic observations revealed irregular-shaped neoplastic cells in both dependent and independent renal tumor cells; however, in the DES-independent tumors,

C-type viruslike particles, more group-specific antigen, and reverse transcriptase activity were found (22).

Since the presence of possible oncogenic viruses has been reported in frog renal adenocarcinoma, fowl, and mouse (15), and also in Syrian hamster (22), it is possible that hormones act through the activation of a latent oncogenic virus preexistent in the normal kidney. Studies regarding the steroid receptors in estrogen-induced RCC demonstrated the presence of ER, PR, and AR. Although ERs and PRs were found in large concentrations, ARs were found only in low amounts and are not affected by estrogen administration (47). Renal cell carcinoma can be induced with estrogens also in male mice and in female guinea pigs. Thus, estrogen-induced RCC provides an excellent model for the study of hormone dependency of tumorigenesis and the data obtained from ablative or additive endocrine therapy can be extrapolated to human cancers and thus improve our understanding of the role of sex hormones on tumor growth. Both androgens and estrogens are essential for renal carcinogenesis in mice and hamsters.

Thyroid Carcinoma

Experimental thyroid tumors can be reproduced in laboratory animals, such as rats, hamsters, mice, and fish, by a chronic iodine deficiency, partial thyroidectomy, long-term administration of synthetic antithyroid compounds, chemical carcinogens (2-AAP), naturally occurring goitrogens, and irradiation of thyroid gland with radioactive iodine (^{131}I) and x-rays (50,52,77). These tumors, which grow extensively with lung metastases, are transplantable tumors similar to human thyroid carcinomas. The induction, development, and transplantability of thyroid tumors are largely dependent on the presence of thyroid-stimulating hormone (TSH). These are hormone-dependent, namely, TSH-dependent, tumors.

Their reproducibility, transplantability, morphology, and hormone dependency were extensively studied and correlated with thyroid hormone disorders, radioiodine uptake, and autoradiographic distribution by several laboratories, including ours (50,52). Combination of these factors, such as iodine deficiency and irradiation, or iodine deficiency and antithyroid compounds (methyl or propylthiouracil, MTU and PTU), markedly enhances the formation and invasiveness of thyroid tumors.

Cytologically, it was shown with the aid of light and electron microscopy that these are mainly benign tumors; only in few instances do anaplastic tumors occur. These benign tumors can incorporate radioiodine and manufacture thyroid hormones, although disorders in thyroid hormone synthesis and the occurrence of abnormal iodoproteins have been reported (50,77).

Inasmuch as the experimental thyroid hormones can grow and be transplanted only in the presence of TSH (animals should be made hypothyroid with a subsequent TSH secretion), these tumors can serve as a good animal model for the study of hormone dependency of human thyroid cancers.

If the thyroid tumors are transplanted in the absence of high TSH secretion, such as control hosts, these tumors fail to grow or lose their hormone dependency and acquire an advanced degree of autonomy, becoming anaplastic tumors. These anaplastic tumors are poorly differentiated, do not metabolize iodine, and have lost their hormone or drug sensitivity. There is a dose–response relationship with regard to hormone or drug administration.

It is interesting that the experimental thyroid tumors induced by chronic administration of thiouracil in rats can be successfully transplanted in neonatally thymectomized rats with intact thyroid. These findings raise questions regarding the role of immune host-defense systems and cell-mediated immunity in hormone-dependent thyroid tumors. Also, the hormone dependency can be facilitated by other hormones or physical agents. Thus, administration of thyroid extracts or thyroxine retards the growth and transplantability of these tumors, whereas estradiol and testosterone can facilitate it. Also, concomitant administration of radioiodine increases the formation and transplantability, whereas total-body irradiation by x-ray or cortisone administration has no effects (77). During serial transplantation, some thyroid tumors acquire a certain degree of autonomy, become hormone insensitive, and lose their differentiation and their ability to incorporate iodine and synthesize thyroid hormones. These findings indicate that thyroid hormones are composed of heterogeneous cell lines, some hormone sensitive, others hormone insensitive. Most retain their hormone dependency; however, after several passages the hormone-insensitive cell lines may regain control, explaining this propensity to autonomy and anaplastic pattern.

Paradoxically, a marked thyroid hyperplasia, adenomas, and papillary cystadenocarcinoma have been reported in rats after a prolonged administration of spirolactone (an aldosterone antagonist), probably by creating a hormonal environment with hyperthyroidism (49).

Lymphosarcoma and Leukemia

About 40 years ago, Lacassagne reported that prolonged administration of estrogens can induce lymphoid tumors of thymus in mice (46). More recently, it was also found that subcutaneous implantation of 20 percent DES–cholesterol pellets induced tumors of the thymus in BALB/c mouse (54). Lymphosarcoma occurred at the site of injection of DMBA in adult female mice of the noninbred CF-1 strain. Same mice developed lymphatic leukemia when feeding with DMBA (38). Murine transplantable lymphosarcomas are now available and can be maintained as a solid or an ascites tumor in homozygous DBA/2 mice. In addition to lymphoid tumors, several lines of transplantable lymphocytic leukemia were obtained in mice by chemical carcinogens or x-irradiation. Since 1944, intense investigations regarding the effects of glucocorticoid hormones on the development and regression of both lymphoid tumors and leukemias were carried out. Thus, Heilman and Kendall (30) showed the dramatic effects of corticoid hormones on lymphoid tumors. These workers demonstrated that large doses of cortisone caused regression of a solid transplantable lymphosarcoma in mice. However, these results proved only temporary in most animals; lymphoid tumors of adult male mice failed to regress after cortisone alone, and only a combination of cortisone and 17β-estradiol produced a rapid regression of these tumors. Cortisone administration can also prevent the development of spontaneous lymphatic leukemia and of lymphoid tumors after total-body irradiation in mice, whereas adrenalectomy enhances both spontaneous and radiation-induced carcinogenesis. Thus, administration of large amounts of hydrocortisone can produce a marked regression of thymic lymphosarcoma induced by x-irradiation in C57B1 mice (40). Most leukemic and lymphoid tumor transplantable lines are glucocorticoid sensitive and respond dramatically with regression to large amounts of corticoid hormones. However, there are differences regarding hormone sensitivity between these lines; some variants are hormone insensitive. Thus, in some neoplastic cell lines, glucocorticoids produce only inhibition of growth but not cytolysis, whereas other variants of lymphomas undergo lymphocytolysis when exposed to corticosteroids. There are also differences between mineralocorticosteroids and glucocorticosteroids. Aldosterone, for instance, was twice more effective as cortisol in the S49-1 line, but only one-twentieth as potent as cortisol against the ML388 line (29). Thus, many leukemic and lymphoid corticosteroid-sensitive cell lines are now available. Changes in chemical configuration of corticosteroids can enhance the tumor growth inhibitory effects. Ultrastructural studies showed that corticosteroids act first on nuclear chromatin, by inducing pyknosis and alterations of nuclear chromatin, and second on the cytoplasm (18). However, the corticosteroid effects are not cell cycle dependent.

Recent studies also demonstrated that hormone sensitive lines contain twice more glucocorticoid receptors than that found in hormone resistant lines. There are also significant differences with regard to glucocorticoid-sensitive and glucocorticoid-resistant cell lines (31,71).

Carcinoma of Scent Glands

The scent glands (flank organs) are ovoid and heavily pigmented, bilaterally situated in the costovertebral area of adult golden hamsters. Although these structures are present at birth, they do not reach full size until sexual maturity, being related to androgen secretion; they are androgen-sensitive organs and therefore more conspicuous in adult males than in female hamsters. Histologically, they are composed of large sebaceous glands and hair follicles and can play a role in the mating prelude, although they are not essential to this phenomenon.

Administration of androgens (testosterone propionate) alone induces a significant hyperplasia, whereas administration of androgens and estrogens (DES) together induces a malignant basal cell epithelioma in both male and female golden hamsters. Tumors of scent glands are also called chaetoepitheliomas, indicating that these tumors originate from the hair follicles present in these glands. Thus chaetoepitheliomas are hormone-dependent (i.e., androgen–estrogen-induced) tumors that metastasize and are transplantable as HDCs. The incidence of these tumors is lower in gonadectomized or hypophysectomized hamsters. Also, their propensity to autonomy is very low; even after 21 serial passages, the transplanted chaetoepithelioma does not become autonomous (42).

Similar hormone-dependent neoplasms were described in the perianal glands of dogs. These canine perianal tumors were found mostly in males; they are hormone dependent, since their growth is stimulated by androgens and inhibited by estrogens. Also, a reduction in tumor size or arrest of its growth occurred in castrated male dogs or after treatment with estrogens. Histologically, these are mainly benign tumors (adenomas); only few malignant (carcinomas) or mixed tumors are observed. Metastases are extremely rare. There is also a definite breed susceptibility for these tumors (a high incidence was observed in Cocker Spaniels and a low tumor incidence in Boxers). Treatment with DES produced a significant regression of these neoplasms (61).

Other estrogen-induced or spontaneous neoplasms, in Nb rats, such as tumors of adrenal cortex, pituitary, ovary (thecomas), uterus (leiomyomas), Leydig cells of the testis, thymus, pancreas, and salivary gland, can exhibit some hormone dependency during their transplantation. Estradiol receptors were recently found in a transplantable pancreatic carcinoma of the rat (57).

HUMAN HORMONE-DEPENDENT CANCERS

There is ample clinical and experimental evidence that ovarian hormones, particularly estrogens, play a key role in mammary carcinogenesis and in human breast cancer risks. Recently, it was demonstrated that other steroid hormones (progesterone, androgens, glucocorticoids) or polypeptidic hormones (prolactin, insulin, thyroid hormones) and prostaglandins can be implicated in the development or regression of experimental mammary carcinoma or human breast cancer (39,53). Hormone dependency of human breast cancer was first demonstrated by the end of the last century, when Beatson (1896) showed that a proportion of women with breast cancer benefited from combined treatment ovariectomy with administration of thyroid extract (4). During that time the only criterion for hormone dependency was the presence of particularly hormones for their growth and development; if the particular hormone is removed, the growth will stop or slow down, and in some patients the cancer will be extinguished.

At present, using more accurate methods, such as estimation of hormone receptors and autoradiographic and ultrastructural studies, it was revealed that a large proportion (about 35 percent) of human breast cancers are HDCs. It was also found that some breast cancers contain more than one hormone-receptor and can thus be dependent on one or more hormones or independent of all hormones. Yet one-third of breast cancers do not contain any kind of hormone receptors and are evaluated as HICs. Thus, a new and fascinating field was opened using the hormone receptor estimation, which provides more accurate knowledge in regard to hormone dependency, evaluation of cancer risks, and therapeutical decisions.

Breast Cancer

Human breast cancer recently became one of the most investigated of HCDs. However, the hormone involvement in the etiology and pathogenesis of human breast cancer is much wider than that delineated by receptor studies. As far as human breast cancer is concerned, there is no direct evidence that steroid hormones are carcinogenic per se; however, there is ample evidence that steroid hormones exert an important permissive role, by facilitating the primary action of other carcinogens (chemical, physical, viruses) or other hormones (prolactin, thyroid hormones) or by promoting cell proliferation, which allows carcinogens to initiate neoplastic changes; thus they act as cocarcinogens.

In an attempt to predict hormone dependency with greater accuracy, Bulbrook and associates carried out extensive studies of the pattern of steroid hormone metabolites excreted in the urine of breast cancer patients and compared the concentration of adrenal steroids with that of sex steroids (gonadal origin). Although some relationship with clinical response was established, this degree of correlation was not valid enough to influence therapeutic and prognostic decisions (3). This also indicates that hormonal control of breast neoplasms depends not only on plasma or urine concentrations of hormones, but also on the presence of hormone receptors. Recently several hormone receptors (estrogen receptors, progesterone, glucocorticoid, androgens, prolactin, insulin, and thyroid hormone) were detected on resected tumor specimens by mastectomy or in different cell lines (39,53,56). Quantitative determination of ER (estrophilin) content in excised tumor specimens revealed that most but not all patients with high content of ER respond to endocrine therapy, whereas women whose tumors contain low or negligible amounts of ER rarely respond to hormone therapy or endocrine ablation. ER (estrophilin) assays can predict hormone dependency correctly in 85 to 90 percent of cases. This can also predict the propensity for metastases and the probability of recurrence (39). It is generally accepted that ER are found in 50 to 80 percent of human breast cancer and that 55 to 60 percent of ER + tumors are likely to regress and respond to endocrine therapy, whereas those that do not contain ER (ER—) fail to respond (56). Similar ER were found also in male breast cancer. An interesting comparison between Japanese women (with a lower incidence of breast cancer) and those from Western countries (with a higher incidence) reveals some remarkable similarities and only few differences. Thus, the overall incidence of ER+ breast cancers is slightly higher in Western patients than in Japanese patients. There is a similar response to endocrine therapy, and 55 to 60 percent of ER+ patients respond to hormone therapy. The response rate in male cancers is similar to that in female breast cancers with positive ER (53). There is no correlation among tumor histopathology, clinical stage, lymph node metastases, and the presence of ER.

It is interesting to study why 40 percent of human breast cancer with ER+ fail to respond to endocrine therapy. It was believed that progesterone and androgen receptors might be the answer. However, it was found that most (nearly 57 percent) PgRs were present in ER+ breast cancers and only 11 percent of PgR were found in cancers with negative ER—. In these cases, with ER+ and PgR—, the response rate to endocrine therapy was very low. In contrast, when both receptors are present, the response rate was higher than in ER+ alone. In cases with ER— and PgR+, response rate was also low. PgRs were found also in a high proportion of male breast cancers.

A search for AR was also conducted to explain why this 40 percent of ER+ human breast cancers fail to respond to endocrine therapy. Thus, it was found that 38 percent of ER+ human breast cancers also contain AR, whereas only 23 percent of ER— cancers contain AR. Most patients with ER+ and AR— respond to endocrine therapy similarly to that of ER+ alone, yet the response is completely different from that of ER+ and PgR—, who fail to respond. The response rates in both ER+ and AR+ were found to be 66 to 75 percent, only slightly higher than those of ER+ alone (81). Recent studies also demonstrated the presence of extractable triiodothyronine receptors in excised biopsy specimens from primary and metastatic human breast cancer. Triiodothyronine receptor concentration was highly variable and showed no correlation among receptor concentration, endocrine status, histologic grading of the tumor, or concentrations of estradiol and progesterone receptors. Triiodothyronine receptors are nuclear receptors (13).

It is interesting to note that human breast tumors contain a mixture of cell sublines; some contain hormone receptors and are thus hormone-dependent, hormone-responsive cells, whereas other cell lines do not contain hormone receptors, and are hormone-independent or hormone-resistant clones. Sometimes, more hormone resistant or hormone-insensitive clones can be more predominant, taking over on the hormone-sensitive clones, which might explain the failure or escape of hormone therapy associated with a propensity to metastases and high malignancy. This concept of heterogeneous neoplastic cell lines—some positive hormone receptors, other negative hormone receptors—can explain the tumor evolution, its tendency to hormone independence or autonomy, and prediction as to prognosis and hormone therapy. Similar hormone receptors (ER, PgR) were also found in different cell sublines of human breast cancer transplanted to nude mouse (84). In addition to human breast cancers, cytosolic and nuclear estradiol receptors (ER and ER_o) and cytosolic and nuclear progesterone (PR and PR_o) receptors were found in human breast fibroadenomas. Their levels changed during the menstrual cycle or under hormonal treatment (estrogen–progestagen therapy) and provide valuable information regarding the hormone dependency of breast fibroadenomas (45).

Prostate Cancer

Spontaneous and hormonally induced prostate neoplasms in dogs, their regression after orchidectomy, and enhanced growth in the presence of androgens are relevant to human prostate cancer and furnish the proof that human prostate cancer is hormone responsive or hormone dependent. Thus, orchiectomy or administration of estrogens results in regression of human cancer of the prostate gland, whereas testosterone administration enhances the rate of growth of the neoplasm (36). Human prostate gland is a target organ for androgens. The gland atrophies after castration but regains its normal size and histologic characteristics after androgen supply. The prostate gland is also influenced by other hormones, such as estrogens and prolactin (26). Prostatic carcinoma is common in elderly men, reaching an incidence of 50 percent in men over 80 years of age. Still, little is known about the intrinsic mechanism of hormones in tumor development.

Studies of steroid receptors in normal and neoplastic prostatic tissue have improved our knowledge concerning the etiology and pathogenesis of prostatic carcinoma.

Studies of steroid receptors in normal human prostate are very few, because it is difficult to obtain normal prostatic tissue. The very high incidence of benign prostatic hypertrophy (BPH) in men over the age of 60 precludes the classification of prostatic tissue as normal in men over 50 years of age. Few observations on so-called normal prostatic tissue reveal the presence of ARs and ERs. Most receptor studies have been carried out on benign hypertrophic tissue and prostatic carcinoma. Thus, the presence of ARs, ERs, PRs, and glucocorticoid receptors was detected in patients with BPH, prostatic carcinoma, and metastases of prostatic carcinoma (23). Preliminary studies indicate that the estimation of hormone receptors in prostatic carcinoma may become of value for selection and individualization of therapy. However, at present receptor assays require large amounts of tissue and are not sensitive enough. If it becomes possible to obtain monoclonal antibodies against the hormone receptors, more sensitive immunoassays will be introduced that will also require far less tissue.

It seems likely that prostatic carcinoma, as mammary carcinoma, contains a heterogeneous cell population, some cell sublines being hormone-receptor positive, others receptor negative. Thus, a tissue from prostatic carcinoma estimated as receptor positive may also contain receptor negative cells.

Immunofluorescent techniques will make it possible to detect the receptor positive cells and thus to predict the value of endocrine therapy, as well as determine the most effective endocrine therapy. Recent findings indicate that in prostatic cells, zinc metabolism may influence androgen metabolism and the action of androgen receptors. One interesting biochemical feature of prostate carcinoma is the low zinc concentration as compared with hyperplastic or normal gland. Certain steroid hormones (dihydrotestosterone, dexamethasone, and hydrocortisone) as well as PGE_2 resulted in an increase of radioactive zinc (^{65}Zn) in the cytosol fraction, while estradiol and cortisone had no effect (24). These investigations, using PC-3 cells from human prostatic adenocarcinoma, have demonstrated that zinc metabolism is hormonally controlled. The mechanism by which zinc modulates specific functions is still unknown.

Renal Cell Carcinoma

Experimental observations strongly suggest that RCC is an HDT. Thus RCC has been induced with estrogens in male mice, female guinea pigs, as well as in male Syrian hamsters or in ovariectomized female or in female before reproductive maturity (when progesterone secretion is low). A delay in the occurrence of tumors in different organs, including kidney, was observed after ovariectomy in transplanted estrogen-induced renal carcinoma of the Syrian hamster (56).

Clinical observations such as the predominance of RCC in males, decrease after cessation of gonadal activity, racial differences (frequently in whites, seldom in blacks, and almost never in orientals), and a more frequent regression in males, led to the conclusion that human cell carcinoma is also a hormone-dependent neoplasm. The growth of this HDC is inhibited by certain estrogen antagonists, such as testosterone propionate, progesterone, deoxycorticosterone, and tamoxifen (67). It has also been found that corticosteroids may have an inhibitory effect on the growth rate of RCC, since adrenal cortex tumor has been found during the regression of RCC. Thus, corticosterods have been used either alone or in combination with progestigens to decrease the incidence of metastases and increase the tumor-free interval. Progesterone decreases the number of metastases in nephrectomized patients. Only 8 percent of nephrectomized and progesterone-treated patients developed metastases, as compared with 25 percent in nephrectomized-only patients (11).

Recently, steroid receptors were found in estrogen-induced RCC of Syrian hamsters, in normal human kidney, as well as in human RCC (8). Estrogen, progesterone, and aldosterone receptors were found in normal renal tissue surrounding the tumor area. Studies regarding the steroid receptors in renal cell carcinoma revealed ERs in approximately 61 percent and PRs also in 61 percent of patients with RCC; 39 percent of the tumors were positive for both ER and PR, and 17 percent were negative for both ER and PR. In addition to cytosol steroid receptor, nuclear estradiol receptors and progesterone nuclear receptors were found. Most patients with both ERs and PRs respond favorably to hormone therapy, while patients with both negative ERs and PRs failed to respond (17). All these data strongly suggest the hormone dependence of human RCC. When the tumor loses its steroid receptors (ER−, PR−), patients do not respond to hormonotherapy and should be treated with chemotherapy in association with radiation and immunotherapy.

Lymphoid Tumors and Leukemia

About 40 years ago it was shown that treatment with adrenocorticotropic hormone (ACTH) and cortisone resulted in temporary regression of human lymphatic leukemia and Hodgkin's disease (68). Since then, glucocorticoids (cortisone, hydrocortisone, prednisone, dexamethasone) are commonly used alone or in combination with other chemotherapeutic agents and produce a complete remission rate of 45 to 65 percent. The remission rate may rise to 88 percent or even 100 percent when more active chemotherapeutic drugs (methotrexate, mercaptopurine) are used (25). Although the use of corticosteroids in human leukemias and lymphomas produces a high rate of remission, suggesting the hormone sensitivity of these tumors, their precise mechanism on the lymphocytes remains unclear.

Recent work on the mechanism of action of corticosteroid strongly suggests that corticosteroids exert their biologic effects through the intracellular receptors located in the cytoplasm of sensitive target cells. Thus their hormone dependence is mediated through the receptor complexes. Several investigations in vitro demonstrated the presence of glucocorticoid receptors in normal and neoplastic human lymphoid cells. It was found in a large series of patients that almost all cases of malignant lymphoma have measurable titers of glucocorticoid receptors. A positive correlation between remission rate and favorable response to corticosteroid therapy of patients with lymphomas and acute lymphocytic leukemia (ALL) and the glucocorticoid receptors levels can be made; thus a useful selection of patients for hormonotherapy can be made by estimating the glucocorticoid receptors in these patients.

Although a parallelism exists between the glucocorticoid receptor content and response to hormone therapy, there is great variability as regards their distribution, since there are hormone-sensitive cell sublines and hormone-insensitive lines. For instance, thymocytes, which contain fewer receptors than peripheral lymphocytes, are more sensitive to the inhibitory effects of dexamethasone on RNA and DNA synthesis, than is found with circulating lymphocytes. This finding implies that the effects of glucocorticoids on lymphoid cells are mediated through other mechanisms in addition to receptor complexes. The lack of receptor complexes is not sufficient enough to preclude hormone sensitivity and hormone dependence of leukemic and neoplastic lymphoid cells (35). However, glucocorticoid both directly and indirectly controls the lymphoid cell population; by inducing cell death (hormone-induced cell death) by apoptosis, the lymphoid cells are mainly hormone-sensitive and hormone-dependent cells.

Endometrial Carcinoma

Clinical and pharmacologic evidence strongly suggests that uterine adenocarcinoma is hormone dependent. Thus, a high incidence of endometrial carcinoma after prolonged estrogen administration and increased incidence of endometrial hyperplasia and carcinoma in both postmenopausal women and in young women after long-term exposure to oral contraceptives, as well as the regression of this tumor after treatment with progestrogens and antiestrogens, demonstrate that endometrial adenocarcinoma is a hormone-dependent, hormone-sensitive tumor (27). Thus, endometrial adenocarcinomas are dependent on estrogens and sensitive to progestogens and antiestrogens. Treatment with progestogens can cure endometrial adenocarcinoma in situ in 60 percent of patients. In vitro studies reveal that estrogens act directly on their target cells, inducing mitosis, and the synthesis of a specific uterine protein. By contrast, progesterone adminstration induces cytotoxic effects on human endometrial carcinoma tissue in an organ culture system (66).

Recent investigations revealed the presence of ERs and PRs in endometrial carcinoma. Thus, ERs were detected in approximately 32 percent of tissue from patients with endometrial carcinoma. There is a high incidence of ER in well-differentiated tumors and a low content of ER in poorly differentiated tumors. Progesterone receptors were also detected sometimes in 15 to 20 percent of patients. It seems that estrogens stimulate progesterone receptor system; progesterone neutralizes the ER system and antiestrogens block it and induce PR synthesis (9). Analysis of steroid receptors in the heterogeneous cell population of endometrial carcinoma revealed ER-sensitive and ER-insensitive cell lines, as well as PR-sensitive and PR-insensitive lines. Thus, well-differentiated endometrial carcinoma retains much of the ability of the corresponding normal uterine tissue to respond to hormonal regulation.

Estrogen receptor concentrations decline after progestin administration

(Provera). Although there is no general agreement regarding a relationship between ER concentrations and the degree of cellular differentiation of uterine tumors, there is general agreement that PR concentrations are higher in well-differentiated than in poorly differentiated carcinoma. The number of cytoplasmic (cytosol) ER receptors is quite similar to that found at nuclear ER sites (69).

Thyroid Carcinoma

Experimental investigations demonstrate that the incidence, development, and regression of thyroid carcinoma are under the control of the hypothalamic–pituitary–thyroid axis. Thus, thyroid stimulating hormone (TSH) or thyrotropin markedly increase the incidence and growth of thyroid tumors in laboratory animals (mice, rats, and hamsters), whereas hypophysectomy and thyroxine administration decrease it (50,52,77). Regardless of its origin (chemical, chronic iodine deficiency, or radiation), thyroid carcinoma is a hormone-responsive tumor. There is a strong relationship between the degree of its cellular differentiation and hormone responsiveness. Well-differentiated thyroid tumors have a high iodine uptake, can synthesize active thyroid hormones, are stimulated by TSH administration, and regress after hypophysectomy or thyroxine treatment, whereas poorly differentiated or undifferentiated carcinomas exhibit a low iodine uptake and thyroid hormone synthesis and their hormone responsiveness to TSH and thyroxine is also low. Hence, well-differentiated thyroid carcinomas are mainly HDCs, while poorly or undifferentiated tumors are HITs. Thyroid cancers are mostly TSH-dependent tumors, as proved by the existence of TSH-receptors on thyroid tumors in experimental animals as well as in humans. This TSH-dependent cancer is regulated by the exogenous or endogenous TSH and thyroid hormones, according to the classic feedback mechanism: TSH stimulates the development and growth of thyroid tumors, whereas thyroxine administration and hypophysectomy inhibit it.

Although there is solid evidence that thyroid carcinoma cannot grow and develop in the absence of TSH in laboratory animals, this has not been shown for human thyroid cancer. Common thyroid carcinomas, which represent more than 80 percent of thyroid cancers, are papillary carcinomas and follicular carcinomas. Both types are partially TSH-dependent tumors, can pick up and metabolize iodine, and are able to synthesize thyroid hormones; they are also hormone responsive to thyroid suppressive therapy. Their metastases exhibit some degree of hormone dependency by incorporating radioiodine and manufacturing active thyroid hormone, as well as regressing after thyroxine administration. Histologic and ultrastructural studies show that these tumors are well-differentiated thyroid carcinomas. Recently thyrotropin-stimulating hormone (TSH) receptors were found in plasma membrane fractions of well-differentiated human thyroid tumors only. Since the number of receptor sites is similar to that found in normal human thyroid tissue, presumably these tumors retain their hormone dependency, and their growth and metabolic activity is affected by TSH (1). Thyroglobulin markers are also helpful in distinguishing between well-differentiated, hormone-dependent thyroid carcinomas and undifferentiated or poorly differentiated, hormone-independent thyroid tumors. The latter type includes medullary thyroid carcinoma (MTC) and anaplastic thyroid carcinoma. Light and electron microscopy as well as autoradiography and receptor studies demonstrate loss of follicular pattern and the presence of irregular and bizarre cells. Medullary thyroid carcinomas are predominantly composed of C cells that synthesize excess amounts of calcitonin, as well as other polypeptides or ectopic hormone (ACTH, serotonin, and possibly MSH). In addition, they can secrete endorphins, kallikrein, prostaglandins, CEA, CRF, somatostatin, substance P, nerve growth factor and melanin. Recently, an immunoreactive thyroglobulin-like protein or "C-thyroglobulin" was found in these tumors which is identical to that found in canine C-cells and is a 27S protein. Medullary carcinomas neither incorporate iodine nor are they hormone-responsive tumors. They are familiar and often associated with pheochromocytomas (multiple endocrine neopasia, MEN type III).

The anaplastic carcinoma is a rare, invasive tumor, an undifferentiated, hormone-unresponsive tumor that carries a poor prognosis. Neither TSH receptor nor adenylate cyclase activity was detected in this tumor, suggesting that its growth and metabolic activity are independent of TSH (i.e., it is a hormone-independent tumor).

Thus, cellular differentiation and receptor estimation determine to a large extent the type of hormone dependency, therapy required, as well as the prognosis for survival of patients with thyroid cancer.

Other Suspected Human Hormone-Dependent Cancers

The assay of hormone receptors demonstrates the presence of steroid hormone receptors in different solid tumors, namely ovarian carcinoma, colon cancers, melanoma, and liver malignant tumors. Both ERs and PRs have been found in patients with ovarian carcinoma at levels correlated with antiestrogen therapy. Most patients with well-differentiated tumors exhibit both ER and PR and respond favorably to estrogen antagonists (tamoxifen). However, there is a great variability as regards the titer of hormone receptor proteins (HRPs), which reflects the dependence of the tumor cells; it is likely that this is due to heterogeneous cell populations that compose the tumor, with only some cell lines being hormone dependent (58). Steroid hormone receptors have also been found in a significant number of patients (male and female) with colon cancers. Estrogen receptors, PRs, androgens (dihydrotestosterone-DHT), and glucocorticoid receptors (GRs) have been detected among patients with colon cancers. Approximately 70 percent of colon tumors contain one or more hormone receptors, and approximately 26 percent contain all three receptors, 22 percent of which are receptor negative.

Thus, the presence of steroid hormone receptors in primary colon malignancies suggests that some colon cancers may be hormone dependent; therefore, hormonal manipulation should be undertaken on an experimental basis in those patients with primary and metastatic colon cancer whose tumors contain hormone receptors (2).

The possible hormone dependence of human melanoma has been speculated on for many years. Clinical observations suggest that women have a better prognosis than men, that women respond more favorably to therapy than do men, and that an exacerbation of preexisting melanomas occurs during pregnancy, followed by regression with cessation of pregnancy. A search for steroid hormone receptors has shown the presence of ERs in 45 percent, of PRs in 22 percent, of ARs in 17 percent, and of GRs in 19 percent. In studies on human melanoma transplanted into nude mice, it was shown that one cell line, which is ER+, grows slower in females than do ER− cell lines; also, ER+ lines exhibit an increased latency as compared with the ER− line. Thus, the data from several cancers indicate that only a small percentage of patients have tumors that contain specific high hormone receptors as compared with breast cancers, and there is not strong correlation between the presence (or absence) of steroid hormone receptors and the response to endocrine manipulation in melanoma (59).

Some testicular tumors (interstitial cell or Leydig cell tumors, Sertoli cell tumors, seminomas) exhibit a partial or incomplete hormone dependency during their evolution. Primary tumors and their metastases retain their steroid-synthesizing capacity, and there is an excellent correlation between the level of human chorionic gonadotropin (hCG), especially beta units (hCG-β) and response to therapy. Radioimmunoassay for hCG-β is the test of choice for diagnosis and follow-up assessments in these patients.

It is well demonstrated that the hypothalamic–pituitary–testicular axis plays an important role in the growth and function of testis, and gonadotropins act on testosterone secretion, possibly by regulation of the number of LH receptors on the plasma membrane of the Leydig cells.

Basic Mechanism(s) of Hormone Dependency

Hormone-dependent tumors provide convincing evidence that hormones are directly involved in tumor growth regulation, invasiveness, and regression. These tumors are totally or even partially dependent on the presence of one particular hormone. This hormone is required for the development of normal target tissues in which the tumor originate (mammary gland, prostate gland, thyroid gland). These target cells normally develop only in the presence of hormones that govern their growth and maintenance. In the absence of these hormone(s), these tissue cannot grow, their cells will die. Thus, the neoplastic cells that arise in these target tissues retain their hormone dependency either totally or partially. A target tissue can be dependent on the presence of one or more hormones (mammary gland, prostate gland), as reflected in the hormone dependency of their tumors.

Neoplasms that arise in target tissues or hormone-dependent tissues cannot be transplanted in the absence of certain hormones, which should be supplemented to hosts in which tumor is grafted—otherwise, the neoplastic cells will shrink and finally die. Thus, these tumors grow only in hormone-conditioned hosts. Also, the parent or original tumor cannot develop if the hormone is surgically removed or counteracted by administration of synthetic hormone antagonists, in which case the neoplastic cells would regress and die. During successive transplantations, some neoplastic cells will gradually lose their hormone dependency and move toward a partial or total autonomy or hormone independence.

It is of great importance to recognize the HDTs for prognosis and treatment of patients. These cancers usually respond favorably to endocrine therapy (additive hormone therapy or ablative endocrine therapy). All tumors that arise in target tissues—either spontaneously or chemically, virally or radiation induced—retain their hormone dependency.

The precise mechanism(s) of hormone dependency are more complex and still not clearly understood. Significant progress in this field was made during the last decade with the introduction of more sensitive and accurate methods, such as electron microscopic autoradiography, enzyme determination, and particularly the estimation of tumor receptor status. It was demonstrated in animal tumors, as well as in human cancers, that all hormone-dependent neoplasms exhibit high concentrations of hormone receptors (receptor-rich tumors), whereas the amount of hormone receptors in HITs is very low or practically negligible (receptor-poor tumors). An increasing number of hormone receptors can now be accurately estimated in different types of tumors. Hence, steroid hormone receptors (ERs, PRs, ARs, GRs) or polypeptide hormone receptors [prolactin receptors (PLRs), insulin receptors (INRs), thyrotropin receptors (TSH-Rs), prostaglandins (PGs), or other epidermal growth factor receptors] are frequently found in experimental and human cancers. In most cases a correlation between the titer of hormone receptors and the number of their site(s) has been established.

The same tumor can possess one or more hormone receptor sites. The hormone receptors bind either to cytoplasm (or cytosol receptors) or to nuclear chromatin (nuclear receptors). Numerous laboratories are accumulating data on the correlation of cytoplasmic and nuclear hormone receptors with hormone responsiveness or dependency. Cytoplasmic or cytosol estrogen receptors are chiefly identified with ^{3}H-estradiol and analysis by the sucrose-gradient technique as 8S and 4S estrogen receptors. There is a strong correlation between the concentration of hormone receptors and hormone dependency. Although hormonal autonomy or hormone independence is associated with a lack of hormone receptors, not all positive HRTs are hormone responsive. Furthermore, few negative hormone receptor neoplasms are still hormone responsive. This suggests that hormone receptors are in a nonfunctional state in some tumors, while other tumors may contain functional hormone receptors. Also, hormone dependency can be in a silent or dormant stage. The dormant neoplastic cells can retain their hormone dependency for several years. This hormone dependency can be elicited by hormone supplementation. This diversity of tumor receptor status can also be explained by the heterogeneity of the cell population. Electron microscopic and SEM studies show that tumors are composed of several cell sublines. Each cell line exhibits characteristic organelle distribution and cell surface features. Also, some cell lines contain hormone receptors and are hormone responsive, whereas others are hormone insensitive. Thus, cell kinetic studies indicate that only 70 to 90 percent of the total tumor cell population are hormone sensitive, whereas 8 to 30 percent do not contain receptors and are hormone sensitive in a transplantable rat prostatic adenocarcinoma.

The precise mechanism by which the hormone interacts with its receptors is still unclear. It is postulated that the steroid hormone interacts with the cytoplasm (or cytosol receptor) or form a complex. This complex appears to be translocated into the nucleus and to bind to a nuclear acceptor site (nuclear receptor) that may be DNA or DNA modified by chromatin proteins; the result of this nuclear translocation is the initiation of messenger RNA (mRNA) synthesis, and consequently the synthesis of new proteins, usually enzymes, which bring about the response of the cell to the steroid (41). Thus, the union of hormone with the receptor sets into motion a series of events that culminate in the tissue response to the hormone (48). This hormone–receptor complex is manifested in inactive and active forms. The presence of a hormone antagonist (e.g., estrogen antagonist, or nafoxidine) competing for the same receptor site binds to the receptor proteins and forms a new antagonist receptor–protein complex that fails to initiate the mRNA synthesis and shuts down the entire system. Thus, tumor growth will be stopped or even regressed.

Thus, when the complex receptor steroid (or polypeptide) hormones enter the nucleus and bind to the chromosomes, they stimulate the synthesis of new mRNA and consequently synthesis of new proteins, acting in the expression of new genetic material in the target cells. Hence, the intracellular concentration of hormones will greatly increase in hormone-dependent cells, while it is low in hormone-independent or nontarget cells in which the hormone enters and goes through the cell membrane (Figs. 5–1a, b).

The phenomenon of positive receptor, yet hormone-unresponsive cells, can be explained by an inhibition in the translocation of cytoplasmic receptor into the nuclear receptor site or by the presence of a modulator, a cytoplasmic molecule associated with the receptor and functions as a modulator receptor activation. Hence, not only is the presence of hormone receptors important,

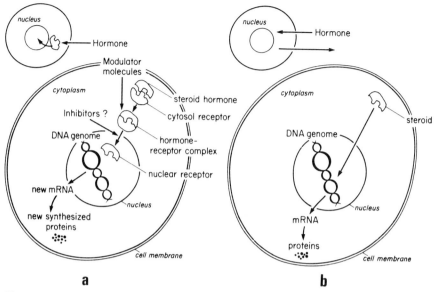

Figure 5-1 Mechanism of hormone receptors and intracellular concentrations of hormones in (a) hormone-dependent cancer and (b) hormone-independent cancer.

but other mechanisms, such as receptor activation and the existence of inhibitory factors of this activation, are decisive for hormone dependency. Some hormone-resistant or hormone-independent cell lines contain a high concentration of receptor translocation inhibitors. It should be pointed out that not all steroid-resistant cells are associated with high concentrations of receptor translocation inhibitor nor can the presence of a modulator molecule, which is also associated with the receptor, explain the hormone insensitivity of these neoplastic cells. Thus, in some cell lines of Morris hepatoma (9633, 9618A) the unresponsiveness or resistance to glucocorticoids was not attributable either to low receptor levels or to inhibition of translocation of the receptor complex to the nucleus, but rather to other factors that intervene at the nuclear level that cannot be analyzed as yet (41). Thus, the mechanism(s) by which hormones control hormone sensitivity and hormone dependency of neoplastic cells are more complex, and the role of receptors in carcinogenesis is unclear. It is possible that change in hormonal metabolism may induce loss of sensitivity to hormonal control, which subsequently predisposes the tissue to tumor development. However, no correlation was found between the ER content of the mammary glands of some strains of mice and the susceptibility of these strains to develop spontaneous tumors. Also, hyperplastic alveolar nodules in rat mammary glands containing low ER concentrations do not develop into mammary tumors (20).

It appears that receptors are not directly involved in tumor induction;

however, they are involved in the progression of tumors toward autonomy and, to some degree, in the cellular differentiation of a tumor.

A correlation between the content of hormone receptors and hormone ability to modify thymidine uptake in vitro as well as in vivo has also been recently reported. Estradiol administration stimulated thymidine incorporation, and a chronically deficient supply of estradiol to a cell line (CAMA-IN) derived from human breast cancer induced a loss of thymidine uptake, whereas glucocorticoid administration inhibits the ^{3}H-thymidine uptake. Cell lines from patients with acute myelocitic leukemia containing significant receptor concentrations exhibit a low thymidine uptake after glucocorticoid administration; by contrast, cell lines from patients that lacked receptors showed no progression of their disease and low levels of thymidine uptake. Hence, a correlation among receptor concentrations, thymidine incorporation, and the ability of hormones to control responsiveness and hormone dependency is also critical to prognosis and to therapy (79).

There are also differences regarding the electrophoretic pattern of some enzymes between HDTs and HITs. Thus the faster the G 6-Pd isoenzyme binding pattern, the more concentrated is the DES-induced and DES-dependent RCC of the Syrian hamster, as compared with that of DES-induced but DES-independent tumor. Independent or autonomous tumors are also associated with C-type RNA viruslike particles and reverse transcriptase activity (22). After the steroid hormone binds to its cytosol receptors and forms a steroid–hormone complex, it enters the nucleus, where it binds to the genome, forming a new species of mRNA and subsequently newly synthesized proteins (Fig. 5–1).

During neoplastic transformation, or by serial transplantation, some neoplastic cells lose their morphologic and electrophoretic patterns and their ability to synthesize new mRNA species required for hormone dependency; they also become more independent or autonomous. Therefore, the transitional stages from hormone dependency to hormone independence or autonomy are accompanied by a series of morphologic, electrophoretic, and possible electron microscopic autoradiographic changes in DNA synthesis. Newly synthesized species of mRNA and proteins are clearly different in hormone-dependent cells as compared with independent or autonomous neoplastic cells.

COMMENTS AND CONCLUSIONS

Although the terms HDCs and HICs are not new, our understanding of how hormones control neoplastic growth and its responsiveness stems directly from advances in pertinent methods, and hence has undergone enormous changes over the past several years. Refinements in methodology have been numerous, and new technical approaches have been developed in recent years, such as estimation and possible visualization of hormone receptors, autoradiographic distribution of ^{3}H-thymidine uptake, and DNA synthesis, and ultrastructural and kinetic studies of neoplastic cells. All these procedures demonstrate most neoplasms to be composed of several cell lines that differ both in cytology and in behavior. Some of these cell sublines contain hormone receptors and are hormone dependent and hormone responsive; others do not contain hormone receptors and are hormone insensitive, hormone independent, or autonomous.

The degree of hormone dependency can be directly correlated with the number of responsive neoplastic cells containing hormone receptors; when the number of cellular receptors declines, the tumor loses its hormone dependency and moves toward autonomy. Since there are transitional stages between hormone dependency and autonomy, tumors contain a mixture of heterogeneous cell populations and receptor status.

These findings have improved our knowledge regarding the neoplastic growth regulatory mechanism and its hormone dependency or autonomy and have also enabled us to select patients for endocrine therapy—a tremendous boon to clinical research, since earlier attempts at endocrine therapy were both disappointing and inconclusive.

Although the terms hormone dependent and hormone responsive tend to be used synonymously, not all HRTs are hormone-dependent neoplasms, and vice versa. The term HDT should be reserved to describe those tumors that develop in the hormone-dependent or target tissues (mammary gland, prostate, thyroid, uterine, ovary, and kidney) and that grow and propagate only in the presence of respective hormone. If this hormone is removed (by ablation or antagonists), the tumor will regress and eventually die. Almost all HDTs (65 to 85 percent) contain one or more specific receptors (monoclonal or multiclonal tumors) demonstrating that their neoplastic cells are responsive to one or more hormone. In most instances these tumors and their metastases respond favorably to endocrine therapy. There are only eight recognized HDTs in humans and laboratory animals.

A larger series of HRTs that occur and develop in different organs (lymph nodes, thymus, skin, colon, liver, and lung) exhibit hormone receptors (15 to 60 percent) of varying degrees and respond particularly well to endocrine therapy. Although the presence of hormone(s) can facilitate their development and propagation, these tumors can grow and propagate in the absence of hormones. They also contain receptors for one or several hormones. Their response to hormone therapy ranges from inconclusive to dramatic. It seems likely that these neoplasms contain hormone-sensitive cell lines in their heterogeneous population. Despite the fact that approximately two-thirds of HDTs are hormone responsive, one-third of HDTs (breast cancers) that contain receptors still do not respond to endocrine therapy. Thus, it is clear that the presence of hormone receptors does not guarantee the responsiveness to that particular hormone. Also, a maximal cellular response can occur without maximal receptor binding, possibly because of the presence of spare receptors. Such spare receptors are found for insulin and for other polypeptide hormones.

The growing interest in hormone receptors in recent years has improved our knowledge on hormone action in tumor development and progression. Many receptor defects and mutations in neoplastic cells have been discovered, hence the complexity of the receptor model and its interactions with other cellular systems becomes more apparent. Tumor progression from preneoplastic to neoplastic stages was also correlated with hormone-receptor concentrations. Hyperplastic alveolar nodules with low ER concentrations do not develop into mammary tumors in rats (20). It is possible that circulating hormones regulate the level of their own intracellular receptors or those of other hormones; for instance, increased prolactin levels results in increased ER concentrations, and high progesterone concentrations suppress the replenishment of ER in the uterus and in DMBA-induced mammary tumors (72).

Clearly, the role of hormone receptors in controlling the growth and function of target tissues and their dependent tumors is extremely complex. In spite of these drawbacks and some lack of specificity, the value of hormone receptors for endocrine therapy is well established and should be part of routine evaluation. Determination of hormone responsiveness of a tumor and its receptor status should always complement the histopathologic diagnostic of a tumor (60).

From the clinician's standpoint, the most valuable information to be gained from ER (estrophilin) determinations is the presence or absence of ERs, which permit good estimations regarding prognosis and hormonal therapy. Ninety-five percent of ER− tumors do not respond to any type of hormonal therapy (ablative or additive), while ER+ tumors tend to respond (33 to 66 percent to sequential endocrine therapies. There is no correlation between ER content and either the histopathologic pattern of primary tumor or axillary lymph node histology. In addition to hormone receptors, which are good tumor markers providing immense help in selecting hormone therapy, the estimation of calcitonin (CT) is also an accurate marker for medullary thyroid carcinoma (MTC). In hormone-dependent thyroid cancers, thyroglobulin (TG) is a valuable tumor marker for diagnostic purposes and for determining prognosis of their hormone responsiveness, while CT is worthwhile for diagnosis of medullary thyroid tumors. It has recently been shown that prostatic acid phosphatase (PAP) is a valuable marker for the detection of intracapsular prostatic cancer. Thus, 90 percent of prostatic carcinoma can be detected before metastasis, with the result that the survival rate is significantly improved.

Hormonal dependency is also preserved during the dormant or quiescent status, when the tumor does not proliferate and grow and can be evoked by administration of the hormone. Thus, experimental estrogen-induced tumors in rats can be evoked by estrogen administration from the dormant stage. In some HDTs (breast cancers) the receptor assay can predict correctly the hormone responsiveness in almost 85 to 90 percent of cases (39). Estimation of hormone receptors is also important in predicting the occurrence of metastases and their response to endocrine therapy. Cutaneous and lymph node metastases are more likely to regress and respond favorably to endocrine therapy than are bone metastases; brain metastases have a poor prognosis. When hormone receptor concentrations are high in either the primary tumor or its metastases, the patient should be placed on endocrine therapy; low concentrations call for placing the patient on chemotherapy. Some benefits of chemotherapy—especially in premenopausal patients over the age of 40— could be due to a drug-induced ovarian failure. Potent nonsteroidal antiestrogens, such as tamoxifen and nafoxidine, apparently act by competitive binding to estrogen receptors. Clinical trials of these agents show that they can induce remissions in patients with metastatic breast cancer.

Recent findings support the hypothesis that antiestrogens control the growth of breast cancer by acting directly on the ER located on cancer cells (16). It has been also proposed that antiestrogens could be acting via a receptor specific for antiestrogens, but not for estrogens. However, there is no correlation between the estrogen receptor values and histologic grade in human breast cancer (79). It has also been suggested that estrogens may control the tumor growth and its hormone dependency by induction of specific growth factors that stimulate the growth of hormone-responsive cells in mammary, pituitary, and kidney tumors. Extracts of rodent uterus, kidney, or liver contain specific growth factors for these three tumor cell lines (75). Thus, in addition to hormone receptors, hormones can modulate hormone responsiveness by other mechanism(s), such as the induction of specific growth factors, enzyme formation, and synthesis of specific proteins.

Studies of hormone receptors also provide useful information in establishing the prognosis and treatment of other human hormone-dependent cancers, such as prostate carcinoma, RCC, thyroid carcinoma, lymphoid tumors, and leukemia. When the tumor loses its receptors and hormone dependency (receptor-negative tumor), patients should be placed on chemotherapy associated with radiotherapy and immunotherapy.

From a general physiologic point of view, hormone receptors are components of target cells that specifically bind the hormones and convey the hormonal message to the intracellular machinery. There are nuclear receptors (thyroid hormones), nuclear and cytoplasmic receptors (steroid hormones), and plasma membrane receptors (polypeptide hormones and neurotransmitters). The action of many hormones on their receptors is controlled by a self-regulating mechanism. Thus, insulin, growth hormone, LH-hCG, TRH, glucagon, vasopressin, catecholamines, and calcitonin are able to induce a decrease in the number of their own receptors. However, ACTH and TSH receptors cannot be regulated by their hormone concentrations, and the regulation is independent of hormone concentration. The hormone resistance

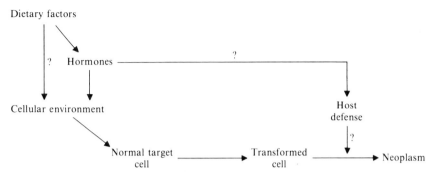

Figure 5-2 Possible mechanism by which hormones and dietary factors control cellular evolution and neoplastic transformation.

or hormone insensitivity of target cells is due mainly to a loss of receptors as well as to the preexposure of the cell to the hormone. The loss of receptors is an active phenomenon induced by variation in hormone concentration and required protein synthesis. Thus, the hormonal regulation of cell responsiveness is a very complex process, depending on both cell and hormones (78).

Furthermore, recent data regarding international epidemiology of HDCs suggests that the distribution of the endocrine-dependent cancers (breast cancer, prostate cancer, thyroid cancer, and colon cancer) is related to dietary factors. For example, a predominantly high-protein high-fat diet imposed in early life can make persons susceptible to the development of these cancers (5). Clinical evidence shows associations among breast cancer, colon cancer, and endemic goiter. Experimental evidence provides some support for this hypothesis (12). Thus, caloric restriction has a general inhibitory influence on tumorigenesis, while dietary fat tends to promote tumorigenesis, but only of mammary tumors. The incidence of DMBA-induced mammary tumors in rats increased from about 70 percent to 95 percent when the level of dietary fat was raised from 0.5 percent to 20 percent by weight. It is possible that dietary factors act on target cells by modifying the level of hormones. It is known that change in diet can significantly influence growth hormone, thyroid hormones, and steroid hormones. Thus, a correlation among hormones, nutrition, and carcinogenesis should also be made (Fig. 5-2). Although the development, propagation, and regression of HDTs are mainly regulated by hormones and cellular receptors, other factors can influence their evolution as well; hormone dependency is a more complex phenomenon that is not yet fully understood.

REFERENCES

1. Abe, Y., Ichikawa, Y., Muraki, T., Ito, K., and Homma, J.: Thyrotropin (TSH) receptors and adenylate cyclase activity in human thyroid tumors: Absence of high affinity receptor and loss of TSH responsiveness in undifferentiated thyroid carcinoma. *J. Clin. Endocrinol. Metab.* 52:23–28 (1981).

2. Alford, T., Do, H., Geelhoed, G., Tsangaris, N., and Lippman, M.: Steroid hormone receptors in human colon cancers. *Cancer 43*:980–984 (1979).

3. Atkins, H., Bulbrook, R., Falconer, A., Hayward, J., MacLean, K., and Schurr, P.: Ten years experience of steroid assays in the management of breast cancer. *Lancet 2*:1255–1260 (1968).

4. Beatson, B.: On treatment of inoperable carcinoma of the mammal: Suggestions for a new method of treatment, with illustrative cases. *Lancet 2*:104–107; 162–165 (1896).

5. Berg. J.: Can nutrition explain the pattern of international epidemiology of hormone dependent cancers? *Cancer Res. 35*:3345–3350 (1975).

6. Bloom, H., Baker, J., Dukes, W., and Mitchley, B.: Hormone dependent tumours of the kidney. II. Effect of endocrine ablation procedures on the transplanted oestrogen induced renal tumor of the Syrian hamster. *Br. J. Cancer 17*:646–656 (1963).

7. Bodwin, J., Clain, T., and Cho-Chung, J.: Inverse relation between estrogen receptors and cyclic adenosine 3',5'-monophosphate binding proteins in hormone dependent mammary tumor regression due to dibutyryl cyclic adenosine 3',5'-monophosphate treatment or ovariectomy. *Cancer Res. 38*:3410–3413 (1978).

8. Bojar, H., Wittliff, J., Balzer, K., Dreyfurst, R., Boeninghaus, F. and Staib, W.: Properties of specific estrogen binding components in human kidney and renal carcinoma. *Acta Endocrinol.* [Kbh] (suppl.) *193*:51, (1975), abstr.

9. Bonte, J.: Hormonal dependence of endometrial adenocarcinoma and its hormonal sensitivity to progestogens and antiestrogens. In Iacobelli, S., King, R., Lindner, H., and Lippman, M. (eds.) *Hormones and Cancer.* New York, Raven Press, 1980, pp. 443–455.

10. Boyland, E.: Human hormone dependent tumors. *Prog. Exp. Tumor Res. 2*:145–157 (1961).

11. Bracci, U., and DiSilverio, F.: Attuali orientamenti nella diagnosi e terapia dei carcinomi del rene. L'ormonodipendenza. *Atti Soc. Ital. Urol. 1*:167–189 (1976).

12. Carroll, K.: Experimental evidence of dietary factors and hormone dependent cancers. *Cancer Res. 35*:3374–3383 (1975).

13. Cerbon, M., Pichon, M., and Milgrom, E.: Thyroid hormone receptors in human breast cancer. *Cancer Res. 41*:4167–4173 (1981).

14. Chung, L., Thompson, T., and Breitweiser, K.: Sensitive biochemical methods to distinguish hormone dependent and independent Dunning tumors of prostatic origin. *Proc. West Pharmacol. Soc. 24*:305–310 (1981).

15. Claude, A.: A spontaneous, transplantable renal carcinoma of the mouse. Electron microscopic study of the cells and of an associated virus-like particle. *J. Ultrastr. Res. 6*:1–18 (1962).

16. Coezy, E., Borgna, J., and Rochefort, H.: Tamoxifen and metabolites in MCF$_7$ cells: Correlation between binding to estrogen receptor and inhibition of cell growth. *Cancer Res. 42*:317–323 (1982).

17. Concolino, G., Marocchi, A., Conti, C., Tenaglia, R., DiSilverio, F., and Bracci, U.: Human renal cell carcinoma as a hormone dependent tumor. *Cancer Res. 38*:4340–4344 (1978).

18. Cowan, W., and Sorenson, G.: Electron microscopic observations of acute thymic involution produced by hydrocortisone. *Lab Invest. 13*:353–370 (1964).

19. Cronkite, E., Shellabarger, C., Bond, A., and Lippincott, S.: Studies on radiation-induced mammary gland neoplasia in the rat. I. The role of the ovary in the neoplastic response of the breast tissue to total or partial body x-irradiation. *Radiat. Res. 12*:81–93 (1960).

20. Dao, T., Sinha, D., Christakos, S., and Varela, R.: Biochemical characterization of carcinogen induced mammary hyperplastic alveolar nodule and tumor in the rat. *Cancer Res. 35*:1128–1134 (1975).

21. De Sombre, E., Kledzik, G., Marshall, S., and Meites, J.: Estrogen and prolactin receptors concentrations in rat mammary tumors and response to endocrine ablation. *Cancer Res. 36*:354–360 (1976).

22. Dodge, A.: Fine structural, HaLv gs antigen and reverse transcriptase study of the Syrian hamster stilbestrol induced renal carcinoma. *Lab. Invest. 31*:250–257 (1974).

23. Ekman, P., Dahlberg, E., Gustafsson, J., Hogberg, B., Pousette, A., and Snochowski, M.: Present and future clinical value of steroid receptor assays in human prostatic carcinoma. In: Iacobelli, S., King, R., Lindner, H., and Lippman, M. (eds.): *Hormones and Cancer.* (New York, Raven Press, 1980), pp. 361–370.

24. Giles, P., and Cousins, R.: Hormonal regulation of zinc metabolism in a human prostatic carcinoma cell line (PC-3). *Cancer Res. 42*:2–7 (1982).

25. Goldin, A., Sandberg, J., Henderson, E., Newman, J., Frei, E., and Holland, J.: The chemotherapy of human and animal acute leukemia. *Cancer Chemotherap. Rep. 55*:309–507 (1971).

26. Griffiths, K., Peeling, W., Groom, G., Sibley, P., and Harper M.: Protein hormones and prostatic cancer. In Iacobelli, S., King, R., Lindner, H., and Lippman, M. (eds.): *Hormones and Cancer.* New York, Raven Press, 1980, pp. 185–192.

27. Gusberg, S.: Hormone dependence of endometrial cancer. *Obstet. Gynecol. 30*:287–293 (1967).

28. Harmon, J., and Hilf, R.: Insulin and mammary cancer. In Kellen, J., and Hilf, R. (eds.): *Influences of Hormones in Tumor Development,* vol. II. (Boca Raton, Fl., CRC Press, 1979), pp. 111–178.

29. Harris, A.: Differentiated functions expressed by cultured mouse lymphoma cells. *Exp. Cell. Res. 60*:341–353 (1970).

30. Heilman, F., and Kendall E.: The influence of 11-dehydro-17-hydroxy-corticosterone (compound E) on the growth of a malignant tumor in the mouse. *Endocrinology 34*:416–420 (1944).

31. Hollander, N., and Chiu, J.: In vitro binding of cortisol-1, 2-^{3}H by a substance in the supernatant fraction of P1798 mouse lymphosarcoma. *Biochem. Biophys. Res. Commun. 25*:291–297 (1966).

32. Hollander, V., and Diamond, E.: Hormonal control in animal breast cancer. In Sharma, R., and Criss, W. (eds.): *Endocrine Control in Neoplasia.* (New York, Raven Press, 1978,) pp. 93–119.

33. Hollenberg, M., and Inon, M.: Binding of insulin and epidermal growth factor urogastrone to normal and tumorigenic rat prostatic tissue. *Fed. Proc. 37*:897 (1978), abstr.

34. Holtzman, S., Stone, J., and Shellaberger, C.: Synergism of estrogens and x-rays in mammary carcinogenesis in female ACI rats. *J. Natl. Cancer Inst. 67*:455–459 (1981).

35. Homo, F., Duval, D., Harousseau, J., and Thierry, C.: Glucocorticoid receptors in normal and neoplastic human lymphoid cells. In Iacobelli, S., King, R., Lindner, H., and Lippman, M. (eds.): *Hormones and Cancer,* (New York, Raven Press, 1980), pp. 387–401.

36. Huggins, C.: Endocrine induced regression of cancers. *Science 156*:1050–1054 (1967).

37. Huggins, C., Grand, L., and Brillantes, F.: Critical significance of breast

structure in the induction of the mammary cancer in the rat. *Proc. Natl. Acad. Sci USA 45*:1294–1300 (1959).

38. Huggins, C., and Uematsu, K.: Induction of lymphatic leukemia in non inbred mice and its control with glucocorticoids. *Cancer 37*:177–180 (1976).

39. Hensen, E.: Hormone dependency of breast cancer. *Cancer 47*:2319–2326 (1981).

40. Kaplan, H., and Nagareda, C.: On the possibility of cure of malignant lymphoid tumors. I. Treatment of autochthonous lymphoid tumors in $C_{57}Bl$ mice with massive doses of lymphocytolytic agents. *Blood 18*:166–175 (1961).

41. Kenney, F., Lane, S., Lee, K., and Ihle, J.: Glucocorticoid control of gene expression. In Criss, W., Onto, T., and Sabine, R. (eds.): *Control Mechanisms in Cancer.* (New York, Raven Press, 1976), pp. 25–35.

42. Kirkman, H., and Algard, T.: Androgen-estrogen-induced tumors. I. The flank organ (scent gland) chaetoepithelioma of the Syrian hamster. *Cancer Res. 24*:1569–1580 (1964).

43. Kirkman, H., and Bacon, R.: Estrogen induced tumors of the kidney. I. Incidence of renal tumors in intact and gonadectomized male golden hamsters treated with diethyl stilbestrol. *J. Natl. Cancer Inst. 13*:745–755 (1952).

44. Kirkman, H., and Bacon, R.: Estrogen induced tumors of the kidney. II. Effect of dose, administration, type of estrogen and age on the induction of renal tumors in intact male golden hamsters. *J. Natl. Cancer Inst. 13*:711 (1952).

45. Kultenn, F., Fournier, S., Durand, J., and Mauvais-Jarvis, P.: Estradiol and progesterone receptors in human breast fibroadenomas. *J. Clin. Endocrinol. Metab. 52*:1225–1229 (1981).

46. Lacassagne, A.: Sarcomes lymphoïdes apparus chez des souris longuement traitées par des hormones oestrogènes. *Conpt. Rendu Soc. Biol. (Paris) 126*:193–195 (1937).

47. Li, S., Li, J., and Villee, C.: Significance of the progesterone receptor in the estrogen induced and dependent renal tumor of the Syrian golden hamster. *Ann. NY Acad. Sci. 286*:369–383 (1977).

48. Litwack, G., and Singer, S.: Subcellular actions of glucocorticoids. In Litwack, G. (ed.): *Biochemical Actions of Hormones*, vol. 2. (New York, Academic Press, 1972), pp. 113–163.

49. Lumb, A., Newvorne, P., Rust, R., and Wagner, B.: Effects in animals of chronic administration of spironolactone. A review. *J. Environ. Pathol. Toxicol. 1*:641–660 (1978).

50. Lupulescu, A., and Petrovici, A.: *Ultrastructure of the Thyroid Gland.* (Baltimore, Williams & Wilkins, 1968), pp. 44–46.

51. Marklan, F., Chopp, R., Cosgrove, M., and Howard, E.: Characterization of steroid hormone receptors in the Dunning R-3327 rat prostatic adenocarcinoma. *Cancer Res. 38*:2818–2825 (1978).

52. Matovinovic, J., Hilbert, R., Armstrong, W., and Helgensen, R.: Thyroid tumor and thyroid transplant tumor in iodine deficient rat. In Cassano, C., and Andreoli, M. (eds.): *Current Topics in Thyroid Research.* (New York, Academic Press, 1965), pp. 920–932.

53. Matsumoto, K., and Sugamo, H.: Human breast cancer and hormone receptors. In Sharma, R., and Criss, W. (eds.): *Endocrine Control of Neoplasia.* (New York, Raven Press, 1978), pp. 191–208.

54. McCain-Lampkin, J., and Potter, M.: Response to cortisone and development of cortisone resistance in a cortisone-sensitive lymphosarcoma of the mouse. *J. Natl. Cancer Inst. 20*:1091–1109 (1958).

55. McGuire, W., Huff, K., Jennings, A., and Chamness, G.: Mammary carcinoma: A specific biochemical defect in autonomous tumors. *Science 175*:335–336 (1972).

56. McGuire, W., Pearson, O., and Segaloff, A.: Predicting hormone responsiveness in human breast cancer. In McGuire, W., Carbone, P., and Vollmer E. (eds.): *Estrogen Receptors in Human Breast Cancer.* (New York, Raven Press, 1975), pp. 17–30.

57. Molteni, A., Rao, M., and Reddy, J.: Estradiol receptors in transplantable pancreatic carcinoma of the rat. *Fed. Proc. 37*:897 (1978), abstr.

58. Myers, A., Moore, G., and Major, F.: Advanced ovarian carcinoma: Response to antiestrogen therapy. *Cancer 48*:2368–2370 (1981).

59. Neifeld, J., and Lippman, M.: Steroid hormone receptors in melanoma. *J. Invest. Dermatol. 74*:379–381 (1980).

60. Nenci, I.: Estrogen receptor cytochemistry in human breast cancer. Status and prospects. *Cancer 48*:2674–2686 (1981).

61. Nielsen, S., and Aftosmis, J.: Canine perianal gland tumors. *J. Am. Vet. Med. Assoc. 144*:127–135 (1964).

62. Noble, R.: Hormonal control of growth and progression in tumors in Nb rats and a theory of action. *Cancer Res. 37*:82–94 (1977).

63. Noble, R.: The development of prostatic adenocarcinoma in Nb rats following prolonged sex hormone administration. *Cancer Res. 37*:1929–1933 (1977).

64. Nomura, Y., Abe, Y., and Inokuchi, K.: Specific estrogen receptor and its relation to response to oophorectomy in rat mammary cancer induced by 7,12-dimethylbenz(a)antracene. *Gann 65*:523–528 (1974).

65. Noronha, R.: The inhibition of dimethylnitrosamine-induced renal tumorigenesis in NZO/B_1 mice by orchiectomy. *Invest. Urol. 13*:136–141 (1975).

66. Nordquist, R.: Hormone effects on carcinoma of the uterine body studied in organ culture. A preliminary report. *Acta Obstet. Gynecol. 30*:287–293 (1967).

67. Patterson, J., and Battersby, L.: Tamoxifen: An overview of recent studies in the field of oncology. *Cancer Treatm. Rep. 64*:775–779 (1980).

68. Pearson, O., Li, M., Rawson, R., Dobriner, K., and Rhoads, C.: ACTH- and cortisone-induced regression of lymphoid tumors in man. *Cancer 2*:943–945 (1949).

69. Pollow, K., Boquoi, E., Schmidt-Gollwitzer, M., and Pollow, B.: The nuclear estradiol and progesterone receptors of human endometrium and endometrial carcinoma. *J. Mol. Med. 1*:325–342 (1976).

70. Rose, D., and Noonan, J.: Influence of prolactin and growth hormone on rat mammary tumors induced by N-nitrosomethyl urea. *Cancer Res. 42*:35–38 (1982).

71. Rosen, J., Rosen, F., Milholand, R., and Nichol, C.: Effects of cortisol on DNA metabolism in the sensitive and resistant lines of mouse lymphoma P1798. *Cancer Res. 30*:1129–1136 (1970).

72. Sasaki, G., and Leung, B.: On the mechanism of hormone action in 7,12-dimethylbenz(a)anthracene-induced mammary tumors. I. Prolactin and progesterone effects on estrogen receptor in vitro. *Cancer 35*:645–651 (1975).

73. Sellitti, D., Tseng, Y., and Latham, K.: Effect of 3,5,3'-triiodo-L-thyronine on the incidence and growth kinetics of spontaneous mammary tumors in C_3H/HeN mice. *Cancer Res. 41*:5015–5019 (1981).

74. Shafie, S., Cho-Chung, Y., and Gullino, P.: Cyclic adenosine 3',5'-monophosphate and protein kinase activity in insulin-dependent and insulin-independent mammary tumors. *Cancer Res. 39*:2501–2504 (1979).

75. Sirbasku, D.: Estrogen induction of growth factors specific for hormone-responsive mammary, pituitary, and kidney tumor cells. *Proc. Natl. Acad. Sci. USA 75*:3786–3790 (1978).

76. Smolev, J., Coffey, D., and Scott, W.: Experimental models for the study of prostatic adenocarcinoma. *J. Urol. 118*:216–220 (1977).

77. Taylor, S.: Induction of thyroid cancer in rats on low-iodine diet. In Cassano, C., and Andreoli, M. (eds.): *Current Topics in Thyroid Research.* (New York, Academic Press, 1965), pp. 976–981.

78. Tell, G., Haour, F., and Saez, J.: Hormonal regulation of membrane receptors and cell responsiveness: A review. *Metabolism 27*:1566–1592 (1978).

79. Terenius, L., Simonsson, B., and Nilsson, K.: Glucocorticoid receptors, DNA synthesis, membrane antigens and their relation to disease activity in chronic lymphatic leukemia. *J. Steroid Biochem. 7*:905–909 (1976).

80. Thoresen, S., Tangen, M., Stoa, K., and Hartveit, F.: Oestrogen receptor values and histological grade in human breast cancer. *Histopathology 5*:257–262 (1981).

81. Trams, G., and Maas, H.: Specific binding of estradiol and dihydrotestosterone in human mammary cancers. *Cancer Res. 37*:258–261 (1977).

82. Walsh, P., and Wilson, H.: The induction of prostatic hypertrophy in the dog with androstanediol. *J. Clin. Invest. 57*:1093–1097 (1976).

83. Young, S., Cowan D., and Sutherland, L.: The histology of induced mammary tumors in rat. *J. Pathol. Bacteriol. 85*:331–340 (1963).

84. Yu, W., Leung, B., and Gao, Y.: Effects of 17β-estradiol on progesterone receptors and the uptake of thymidine in human breast cancer cell line CAMA. *Cancer Res. 41*:5004–5009 (1981).

Chapter 6

HORMONES AND CHEMICAL CARCINOGENS: THEIR MECHANISM OF ACTION (DNA, RNA, PROTEIN SYNTHESIS)

GENERAL CONSIDERATIONS

The idea that cancer evolves as a series of sequential heritable cellular changes is quite old. It began with the discovery of chromosomes and has had its ups and downs.

With the use of modern methods in cancer research, a tremendous bulk of material has accumulated during the past two to three decades indicating that conversion of a normal population of cells to one showing malignant neoplastic behavior requires a series of molecular events. These events are intimately related, and the ultimate focal point of such sequences is the cell—the smallest integrating unit in the biologic systems.

To understand how cancer develops with chemicals or hormones, it is necessary to integrate the molecular and biochemical changes with the cellular

182

and tissue biologic responses or to collaborate between micromolecular and macromolecular levels, which is in fact the pathogenesis and nature of cancer.

The neoplastic transformation, the process by which a normal cell is transformed into a precancerous and later into a potential cancer cell, involves a plurisequential stage of which not necessarily all steps are mutational (14,52,55). There is increasing evidence that a great number of tumors are dependent on the presence of an appropriate hormonal milieu, immune surveillance, and tissue factors (chalones, growth factors). Still, the fundamental problem in the field of cancer biology, that is, the primary event leading to the occurrence of abnormal proliferative or malignant transformed cells, remains unsolved.

In recent years, a heated debate started between proponents of somatic mutation, which advocates biochemical lesions in the structure of DNA as the major or single cause of neoplastic transformation (genetic theory) (9,11,12, 40,57) and the proponents of epigenetic theory or developmental changes (alterations in gene expression without changes in the DNA sequences) (13,52,55,60). However, considerable evidence supporting somatic mutation as a model of cancer causation has accumulated in the recent years.

Hence, to date, efforts have been concentrated on DNA synthesis, with some interest in RNA and proteins. Because of the relative ease with which the interactions between a labeled carcinogen and nucleic acids can be visualized in a target organ in vivo by autoradiography with tritiated ^{3}H-hydrocarbons, DNA was assumed to be the significant cellular target for carcinogens (11,12,40). However, because of the long DNA molecules, it is possible that the interaction between carcinogen and DNA is taking place in more than one site and no single region of high affinity has been found (38,40). Thus, miscoding in DNA is often considered most relevant. In addition to miscoding, other alterations in DNA, such as recombinations, translocations, and gaps may be important in the incipient stages of cancer development. In fact, some investigators (14,57) have suggested that mutagenesis may be of only minor importance in the early stages of carcinogenesis and the genetic transposition of large segments in the genome might be more relevant to the process. Also, a possible role of histones and nonhistones in chromosomal proteins should be foreseen. However, the limited evidence available suggests that most human cancers are not caused by conventional mutagens, but can be the result of genetic transposition. Despite the fact that the molecular biology of transposition is only beginning to be understood, it remains promising (14). New techniques and approaches should be developed in order to fully understand the environmental factors that influence its frequency.

Although many chemical carcinogens exhibit a mutagenic action, none of the hormones (including DES), nor any of their metabolic products, has so far been shown to be convincingly mutagenic; however, an interaction between DNA and DES, especially a covalent binding of DES metabolites to DNA in short tests, has been reported (19).

Although there is ample evidence suggesting interactions between chemical carcinogens and DNA, this evidence is scarce in regard to interactions between hormones and DNA.

This review emphasizes the mechanisms, and not the phenomena, regarding carcinogens and hormones. Thus, we will briefly describe the interactions of chemical carcinogens and hormones with the macromolecules of DNA, RNA, and proteins.

CHEMICAL CARCINOGENS AND DNA SYNTHESIS

DNA Synthesis

Although the initial cellular target of chemical carcinogens has not yet been unequivocally identified, the existing evidence strongly suggest DNA damages (DNA synthesis, DNA repair) as an important step in neoplastic transformation. Previous experiments by Brookes and Lawley indicated a correlation between the binding of polycyclic aromatic hydrocarbons to DNA of mouse skin and their carcinogenic potential (11).

DNA Synthesis

Further evidence for an association between carcinogenesis and perturbation in DNA synthesis was provided by the higher rate of development of cancers in patients with hereditary diseases (e.g., xeroderma pigmentosum, Bloom's syndrome, and ataxia telangiectasia). Thus, patients with xeroderma pigmentosum (XP), who lack the ability to repair DNA damages induced by ultraviolet irradiation and certain chemicals, have a marked tendency to develop malignant neoplasms. Like mutations induced in bacteria (*Escherichia coli* and *Salmonella typhimurium*) by ultraviolet light, the cells of XP patients have a defect in DNA excision that makes them 10 times more sensitive to the lethal (16,37) and mutagenic effects of most mutagens (26,42). Also, patients with ataxia telangiectasia (AT), who are unable to repair DNA damage caused by ionizing radiation, have a marked susceptibility to malignant neoplasms (59).

Bloom's syndrome and Fanconi's anemia, two other inherited diseases associated with chromosomal abnormalities, show a high incidence of leukemia and malignant diseases (25). All these data suggest that cancer is mainly due to somatic mutations (12,14,57). In addition, a good correlation exists between carcinogenic and mutagenic effects of many chemical carcinogens; most carcinogens are also mutagens. However, not all mutagens are carcinogenic. This mutagenic activity is now widely used for the early detection of chemical carcinogens, by the so-called Ames test, which is rapid and less expensive as compared with classic tests using laboratory animals (2). However, not all data obtained from these simple tests using microbial systems can be extrapolated to animal models and humans, which are more complex.

The essence of the interactions between chemical carcinogens and DNA can be summarized as follows. Most carcinogens are mutagens, whether intact or after modification by microsomal enzymes. Most known carcinogens are mutagenic in at least one test system (53). Although some noncarcinogenic chemicals have been found to be mutagenic, only a few chemical carcinogens are not mutagens (54). There is also a qualitative correlation between the conversion of procarcinogens to ultimate carcinogens with increased chemical reactivity for DNA and their ability to act as mutagens in microbial systems. Also, there is good evidence to indicate that the sensitivity of some inbred strains of animals to carcinogenesis induced by polycyclic aromatic hydrocarbons is largely dependent of the capacity of these animals to convert the inactive form (procarcinogen) into the active form (or ultimate carcinogen) (47). Some evidence also suggests that organ specificity (lung, liver, skin) of some carcinogens is at least partially related to the ability of these tissues to excise the damaged bases from DNA, as well as to the dynamics of formation of the alkylating derivatives of carcinogens (50). Thus the somatic mutation theory is also supported by the pharmacogenetics and dynamics of carcinogen metabolism.

Further evidence supporting a relationship between carcinogenesis and DNA damages has come also from studies of cellular transformation by the base analog Brd Urd (5-bromodeoxyuridine). Brd Urd transforms cells in culture only if the cells are irradiated with UV light subsequent to incorporation of Brd Urd into DNA. Thus, treatment of Syrian hamster embryo cells with Brd Urd followed by near-UV irradiation in the S period of the cell cycle, but not those treated in the G_1 period or in late S/G_2 phase, underwent neoplastic transformation. These findings demonstrate that a direct lesion of DNA is sufficient to initiate neoplastic transformation, in strong support of the important role of DNA damages in carcinogenesis (5). Most chemical carcinogens exhibit the highest carcinogenic activity during the S phase (DNA synthesis) of the cell cycle (they are cell-cycle dependent). Furthermore, not all carcinogens (chemical, viral, or physical) can induce neoplastic cells in which DNA synthesis was inhibited (40).

Other workers believe that chemical carcinogens act on the cells containing genes capable of inducing neoplastic transformation if expressed at abnormal levels (17).

It seems that neoplastic transformation may result from a single alteration in the genome (one hit response) and subsequently chemical carcinogens act by inducing somatic mutations. Chemical carcinogens can act at different loci of the long molecule of DNA. To date, no single region of high affinity has been found (20).

Most tumors are of monoclonal nature. This was demonstrated in animal tumors (epidermal tumors induced by DMBA or MCA) as well as in human cancers by using A and B types of the enzyme G 6-PD (glucose 6-phosphate dehydrogenase). More than one somatic mutation can be expressed in a given cell, and many, perhaps all, cancers require a sequence of two or more genetic errors in order that malignancy can be expressed. However, neoplastic transformation requires more than one stage, of which not necessarily all are mutational and not every mutant cell gives rise to a cancer cell.

DNA Repair

The indirect support that DNA repair may be a critical factor in chemical carcinogenesis comes from the well-known high incidence of skin cancer (melanoma) in patients with XP. All these XP patients have lost their ability to repair DNA after exposure to UV and also to some chemical carcinogens and mutagens (25).

Other human diseases (ataxia telangiectasia, Fanconi's anemia, Bloom's syndrome) also show deficiency in DNA repair as well as increased risk for neoplasia. Fibroblasts in culture from these patients (mainly XP patients) show a defect in DNA repair (26). Thus, it was often postulated that our major protection against cancer resides in our efficiency to repair the DNA damaged by the many carcinogens and mutagens in our environment. Although a chemical lesion in DNA is by no means synonymous with the development of cancer, the DNA damage is involved in cancer initiation in most instances. Drugs, chemicals, diet and hormones modulate this phenomenon. Recent cytogenetic studies add further support to the existence of specific human "cancer genes". Some tumors, such as retinoblastoma, Wilm's tumor and renal cell carcinoma are frequently associated with a chromosomal deletion occurring in tumor cells.

DNA damage can be in a structural (structural DNA) segment or in regulatory segment (control DNA) or it can involve more complex rearrangements or larger segments of DNA, such as in transpositions.

All these data strongly suggest that neoplastic transformation can be the direct result of a perturbation in nuclear DNA. For most known chemical carcinogens, nuclear DNA is a direct target for their action (11,40,62). However, there are carcinogens that act directly on mitochondrial DNA (4,48).

Thus, administration of aflatoxin B_1 (hepatic carcinogen) to experimental animals preferentially attacks the mitochondrial DNA and consequently results in covalent binding to liver mitochondrial DNA in concentrations three to four times higher than in nuclear DNA. Also, mitchondrial transcription and translation remain inhibited up to 24 hr, suggesting a long-term effect of aflatoxin B_1 on the mitochondrial genetic system during hepatic carcinogenesis (48). The chemical modification of mitochondrial DNA is accompanied by a pronounced inhibition of mitochondrial RNA and protein synthesis. Using labeled aflatoxin B_1 (^3H AFB_1), it was found to be located primarily in mitochondrial DNA of hepatocytes. It is also known that most neoplastic cells exhibit an impaired structure and function of mitochondria. Similarly, some activated metabolites of benzo(a)pyrene and other polycyclic aromatic hydrocarbons incubated with tissue culture cause substantially greater damage to mitochondrial DNA than to nuclear DNA (4). The persistent high level of AFB_1 in circular mitochondrial DNA can be due to a lack of excision system in these organelles (45). Thus, these observations show that AFB_1 as well as other chemical carcinogens, including N-nitrosodimethylamine to mitochondrial DNA in vivo and of polycyclic aromatic hydrocarbons in vitro, indicate that mitochondrial DNA is a critical target for chemical carcinogens.

It is possible that modifications of mitochondrial DNA by carcinogens lead in the long run to mitochondrial mutations and may contribute to neoplastic transformation. However, a great discrepancy still remains in the biochemical advances regarding DNA synthesis, DNA repair, and chemical carcinogens; the expressions of this modifications at cellular level are poorly understood. Most studies regarding the intrinsic mechanism of DNA repair, starting with a simple one, such as base excision, to a more complex form of damage, such as removal of interstrand crosslinks in postreplication repair, are done mainly in vitro systems and to a much lesser extent in vivo.

The discovery of some enzymes in bacteria that can intervene in transmethylation process by removing the methyl group ($-CH_3$) from the O^6-positive of guanine in DNA and later its transfer to a S-containing moiety of protein, raise the question of action of these enzymes in methylating carcinogens.

At present, however, we cannot detect these discrete and incipient modifications in DNA molecule in the first steps of carcinogenic process, namely, their expression at cellular level. We have to use more sensitive methods, such as electron microscopy, high-resolution autoradiography, and SEM and develop new approaches for the detection of these incipient (initial) cellular transformation and the primary target of carcinogens in the cell machinery.

To determine the preferential target of carcinogens, namely, at which stage of DNA metabolism, DNA synthesis, or DNA replication our knowledge of chemical oncogenesis will be improved. Some differences in response to chemical carcinogens might be explained in terms of differences in binding of carcinogen to replicating or nonreplicating DNA.

Thus, several experiments demonstrate that effects of chemical oncogen are much increased in DNA synthesis (S phase) and are highly cell cycle dependent. Most chemical carcinogens exert their maximum effect in S phase or in the boundary of G_1-S period. Using mouse fibroblast cells synchronized by arginine deprivation it was found that a chemical carcinogen (N-methyl-N'-nitro-N-nitrosoquanidine, MNNG) exerts its maximal oncogenic transformation in the late G_1 and beginning of S phase (G_1-S and S periods) (8).

However, little is understood of the molecular events that occur during the DNA synthesis and DNA replication. It is likely that the onset of DNA synthesis is related to the synthesis of some regulatory proteins. These regulatory proteins were already identified in late G_1 and are required for the initiation, but not for the progression, of DNA synthesis; others believe that membrane changes are responsible for triggering the S phase (22).

Since most chemical carcinogens are also mutagens, this supported the somatic mutation theory of cancer, originally proposed by Boveri (9). It is also possible that some chemical carcinogens, including MNNG induced selective mutation in bacteria containing replicating forks (dividing) than in bacteria in which DNA synthesis was complete (nondividing) (15). Whereas most chemical oncogens exert their potential malignant transformation in late G_1 and S phase, some viral carcinogens (polyomavirus) have been reported to be twice as efficient in transforming G_2 phase than in other phases of the cell cycle (6). This hypothesis, which postulates that DNA is a major target of chemical carcinogens, led to the use of several short-term tests for detection of carcinogenic activity of many suspected environmental carcinogens. These tests are accurate in almost 80 percent of cases, since most carcinogens are mutagens. However, in several cases, only the ultimate carcinogen is the active product; most of carcinogens should be enzymatically converted from procarcinogens to ultimate carcinogen, a process called "activation" (Figs. 6–1 and 6–2). If DNA repair is the crucial factor in carcinogenesis, our protection against cancer consists in the cell's capacity to repair DNA after exposure to different carcinogens. Thus, there is a very good correlation in a

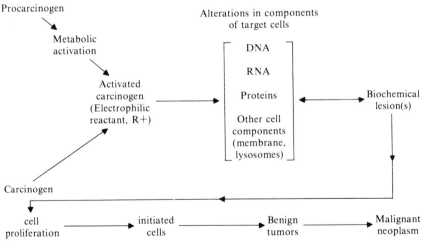

Figure 6-1 Diagrammatic representation of the metabolic activation of chemical carcinogens and their interactions with cellular components, cell proliferation, initiation, and neoplastic transformation.

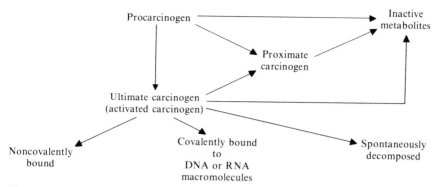

Figure 6–2 Different pathways by which the ultimate carcinogen may operate.

series of more than 300 compounds between the mutagenesis (back mutations to histidine auxotrophy in various strains of *Salmonella*) and carcinogenic activity, with approximately 10 percent false positives and 10 percent false negatives (30).

Transfection

Transfection is another interesting phenomenon that arises from the induction of transformation by the transfer of DNA or chromatin to susceptible cell lines. Thus, DNA from cells transformed in vitro or in vivo with chemical or viral carcinogens was shown to induce transformation. High-molecular-weight DNA of cells transformed by DNA fragments induces transformation with high efficiencies in secondary transfection assays. Interestingly, DNA from normal cells was equally effective, suggesting that normal cells contain genes capable of inducing transformation. Hence, these findings indicate that DNA of both chemically transformed and normal cells is capable of inducing transformation or transfection. It is possible that potential transforming genes are encoded in the genome of normal cells (17). Thus, DNA from chemically transformed cells can act by disorganizing the host genome as a result of mutational alteration of cis-acting regulatory sequences that controls expression of endogenous transforming genes. It seems that a variety of spontaneous or chemically induced tumors contain transforming genes that are transmissible with high efficiency by transfection. This opens a new, promising, and intriguing field for cancer research. Thus, chemical carcinogens can act by covalent binding to a normal or modified nuclear (or mitochondrial) DNA or its associated proteins.

The carcinogenic process can be the result of long-term exposure to chemical carcinogens and requires more than one necessary event, so-called multiple-hit theory of carcinogenesis (3). Thus, latent cancer can be due to a smaller number of hits. Also, increasing incidence of cancer with age might be due to continued or increased exposure to a carcinogen (multiple hits) or to an indirect but unknown effect of aging, such as reduced capacity to repair the damaged DNA. This defective DNA repair mechanism is apparently the result of a deficient exonuclease enzyme. Although most chemical carcinogens exert their initial effects by inducing DNA damage, certain known carcinogens (several pesticides, herbicides, and xenobiotics) do not exhibit or generate mutagenic or DNA damaging effects. This can be due to technology which is deficient in detecting this early lesion or may suggest other pathways in carcinogenesis that do not involve DNA damage.

Nevertheless, proponents of the theory that DNA is the main target of carcinogens (oncogens) argue that most aspects of the total cancer origin revolve around the DNA behavior. Thus an abundance of evidence supports the assertion that the interference of different chemical, viral, drugs, or physical agents to DNA, in almost any conceivable way, is likely to be the prelude of cancer induction. Or, put in another way, it is difficult to believe that there are recognizable carcinogenic events that have not involved DNA modification. Since DNA is the biochemical repository of the genetic inheritance of cells, it exerts a dominant influence over cell growth, division, and differentiation, and DNA replication is a necessary precondition for cell division, thus DNA constitutes the key vulnerable target for the action of carcinogens. Hence, the biochemical basis for many agents to act as potential carcinogens is plausibly related to their capacity to interact with DNA. It is clear that one of the most common and widespread responses to assaults on DNA is the strand breakage.

Recently, various types of spontaneous lesions in DNA, of which the commonest is depurination, followed by depyrimidation and deamination of cytosine, were reported. These all appear to be recognized and repaired without mutagenesis. Other spontaneous lesions involving internal changes in the bases themselves are also important in either giving rise to informational errors or, in postmitotic cells, damage manifested as an increase in single-stranded DNA molecules (38).

The result of any physical or chemical assault on DNA in vivo is the occurrence of mutations. Due to the ease and extreme sensitivity of mutagenicity, it has been established that the great majority of known carcinogens are mutagens, so that mutagenic assays have been adopted as indispensable short-term tests in screening programs for the detection of potential carcinogens. However, the relationship between mutagenic activity (mutagenicity) and the potential for carcinogenesis is still a hotly debated issue (62).

Apparently most interactions between chemical carcinogens and DNA are irreversible. However, new and more sensitive methods should be developed in order to detect the precise site(s) of chemical carcinogens and DNA interactions. The pursuit of these findings and the role of DNA repair mechanisms in normal and damaged cells will increasingly attract the attention of cytologists and biochemists over the coming decades.

CHEMICAL CARCINOGENS AND RNA SYNTHESIS

Despite the fact that by far most of the effort has been focused on DNA synthesis and replication, there are other molecular targets for chemical carcinogens, including RNA and protein synthesis. However, RNA and proteins have received only some interest in chemical oncogenesis.

It is now clear that many chemical carcinogens and irradiation produce alterations of all the major macromolecules of the target cells including RNA, proteins and DNA. Some of the RNA tumor viruses, such as Rous sarcoma virus, have all the information to convert a susceptible target cell to a malignant neoplastic cell by an essentially one-step process in RNA synthesis (60).

There are differences among carcinogens; thus a virus or irradiation induced in mice always induces leukemia of T lymphocyte origin, whereas a chemical carcinogen (7,12-dimethyl-benz(a)anthracene, DMBA) induced a leukemia of B-lymphocyte origin (29).

Thus, in contrast to proponents of somatic mutation theories who advocate that DNA is the critical cellular target in chemical carcinogenesis, a neoplasm may originate from a number of essential aberrations from the normal which can affect DNA, RNA, proteins or other cell components (membrane, lysosomes) (Fig. 6-1). First, a procarcinogen or carcinogen should be converted by metabolic activation to an activated carcinogen (electrophilic reactant (R^+)) that can attack one preferential cellular target or more, inducing alterations in DNA, RNA, proteins, or other cell components, and consequently biochemical lesions of target cells with cell proliferation and initiated (neoplastic) cells.

However, not all activated or ultimate carcinogen is critically bound to the macromolecules of DNA or RNA; other portions are converted to inactive metabolites, noncritically bound or spontaneously decomposed (Fig. 6-2).

Thus, chemical carcinogens act on the target cells by a sequence of complex events, many of which are controlled and modified by numerous endogenous and exogenous factors. In addition to species, strain, sex, and age differences, hormonal, nutritional and immunologic factors are involved heavily and may enhance or decrease the extent and rate of the carcinogenic process by modifying macromolecular synthesis, control of differentiation, and gene action systems (Figs. 6-3a,b).

At present there is no definite evidence that somatic mutation due to damages or alterations in DNA synthesis or DNA repair mechanism is the solely responsible mechanism for carcinogenesis. There is not a quantitative correlation between carcinogenic and mutagenic potentials of many chemicals. Thus, a substantial number of noncarcinogenic chemicals have also produced mutations in the Ames test; some of the most powerful carcinogens are only weakly mutagenic or nonmutagenic. Also, we have to recognize that carcinogenic potential of individual chemicals varies widely when administered in different strains or species of mammals. Also, tumor induction

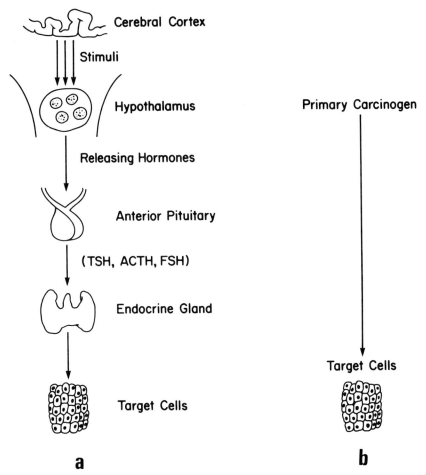

Figure 6-3 Mechanism of primary carcinogen on target cells in hormone dependent tumor (*a*) and hormone independent tumor (*b*).

depends on the physical state of carcinogenic material. Thus, tumors can be induced by simply inserting a solid sheet of chemically inert material into rat tissue (1). If the material is made porous or is inserted in fibrous form, tumors do not occur. The neoplastic transformation results in this instance from the physical state of the material. There is no sign that carcinogenic material enters into the cell and the main effect seems to be due to disruption of the organized cells. Also, steroid hormones, which are normal body constituents, when applied in large amounts are carcinogenic and these tumors transplanted into the spleen of the original host causes them to become neoplastic (24).

Thus, for several types of carcinogenesis, the somatic mutation seems a dubious explanation at best (55).

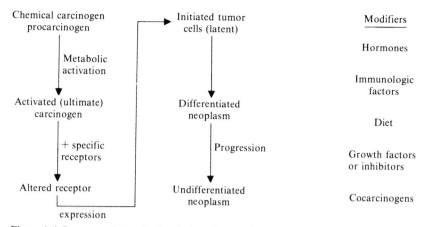

Figure 6-4 Sequence of steps in chemical carcinogenesis controlled and modified by numerous factors.

Epigenetic Changes Induced in Animal and Plant Cells

It has been established that nuclei could be transplanted from cells of differentiated frog tissues into eggs containing inactivated nuclei and that the transplanted nuclei would direct the development of all tissues of a mature frog (27). This finding showed that inheritable changes of differentiated tissues can be brought about without a change in the primary structure of DNA. Also, the nuclei from a frog kidney carcinoma transplanted into the egg preside over the development of the full range of tissues of a tadpole, showing no evidence of tumor formation (43). All these findings in tumor-free tadpoles indicate a more direct implication of an epigenetic mechanism in cancer induction; and nonmutational changes in cells can bring about neoplastic transformation. Also, the transdetermination experiments suggest a relationship between the type of epigenetic control involved in the development and loss of control in cancer. It has been shown that imaginal disks of *Drosophila* larvae capable of forming structures as legs or wings could be transplanted into the adult for many generations, yet retain the ability to form these structures (28). However, due to transdetermination, another structure appeared. If the transplantations in adults were continued for many generations, the imaginal disk grew at an increasingly rapid rate and eventually became tumorous. The relationship between transdetermination and the onset of cancer suggests that cancer occurs because of a disruption in the highly integrated organizational controls that permit expression of the normal intact structures, and is not due to changes in the primary structure of the genome.

Also, the occurrence of teratocarcinoma is widely regarded as a truly epigenetic mechanism. Teratocarcinomas arise from parthenogenetically activated germ cells or from germ cells transplanted into ectopic sites, which frees them of normal controls over cellular division (41). When cells from diploid mouse teratocarcinomas or tumor cell lines are injected into normal blastocytes, tumor-free chimeric animals can develop. This relocation of teratocarcinoma cells into an embryonic environment containing normal development signals can convert the teratocarcinoma cells back into normal embryonic cells. Hence, the totipotency of teratocarcinoma cells suggests that teratocarcinoma is a tumor induced by an epigenetic switching event (44).

Several reports also indicate that neoplastic transformed cells retain the capacity to form normal tissues. Thus, the exposure of several different rat tumors to embryonic inductors in the primitive streak of chick embryos causes the tumors to differentiate and lose their carcinogenic properties (18). Also, the cultivation at low density of cells transformed with polyomavirus can induce the formation of variants with a reversion of certain properties characteristic of neoplastic transformation.

Plant cells are particularly useful in distinguishing between genetic and epigenetic changes because complete plants can be regenerated from individual somatic cells with different phenotypes. Thus, crown gall teratomas of tobacco are a good example of a tumor in which transplantation (grafting) to the proper environment can lead to differentiation of the tumor cells into morphologically normal cells, including seeds which give rise to tumor free plants (10). A similar event occurs during progression to autonomous growth of crown gall tumors under the stimulation of an infected agent; these findings with uninfected cells indicate that a key event in carcinogenesis can be an epigenetic one.

Epigenetic Changes Induced by Chemical Carcinogens

If malignant transformation generally occurs via an epigenetic rather than a mutational mechanism, one might predict the existence of chemical carcinogens without mutagenic effects. However, most chemical carcinogens or their metabolic intermediates are mutagens. There are approximately 10 to 23 percent of known chemical carcinogens which are not mutagens; these are inactive in the *Salmonella* reverse mutation test. Several of the chemicals that are negative in the *Salmonella* assay are also negative in most other short-term tests (34). Other chemicals which are inactive in all short term tests could be acting via epigenetic or nonmutational mechanisms. One of these nonmutational mechanisms might be promotion, which could be possibly the mechanism of action of some carcinogenic steroid hormones, such as 17β-estradiol.

There is no requirement that the carcinogen interact directly with the DNA of the cell. The initial events might just as well occur in the cell membranes as in the genome. A known chemical carcinogen, such as

3-methylcholanthrene, is soluble in the lipids found in membranes. It could destabilize the cellular membranes and thereby possibly initiate a set of changes that lead to irreversible loss of the capacity of the cell to interact with other cells. Indeed, the malignant transformation can occur in cell culture with a fairly high incidence in the absence of any known carcinogen (49). Thus, the carcinogenic event appears to be more a deprivation of normal cell interactions than the result of any positive influence of a chemical carcinogen on the cellular genome.

Therefore, it seems likely that the carcinogenic potential of chemicals can best be tested in animal cell systems that express the full social behavior of cells. To use bacteria as a test for carcinogens is to eliminate totally the factors involved in cell association so crucial to the expression of malignancy; it can also be the initial target in the origin of neoplastic transformation.

The use of bacteria as test models (e.g., Ames test) is based on the assumption that a somatic mutation is the cause of cancer, when in fact we do not know the cause with any certainty. Genetic and epigenetic changes can operate in a mutual manner, and not in an exclusive one. Another interesting epigenetic phenomenon is the suppression of malignant phenotype by cellular differentiation and the cellular differentiation can "cure" the malignant potential of cells in a number of neoplasms. A good example of this phenomenon occurs in keratinizing squamous cell carcinoma. These tumors contain a population of dividing and invasive stem cells, some of which may differentiate into squamous cells and form the pearls in the core of the tumor. Differentiation of the malignant stem cells is accompanied by a cessation of cell division and disappearance of malignant cells (51). Also, differentiation of metastatic neuroblastomas and ganglioneuroblastomas into mature ganglion cells has been reported in several patients. Differentiation of some clones of myeloid leukemia cells in the presence of macrophages and granulocyte inducers is accompanied by a cessation of proliferation (21). The macrophages are important effector cells in tumorigenesis. They can produce collagenase, elastase, numerous complement components, kallikrein, and prostaglandins. They interact with lymphocytes, granulocytes, and platelets. These observations led to the assumption that the fundamental lesion in cancer is a lack in the ability of stem cells to differentiate normally (51).

There is also evidence for epigenetic control of expression of 40 early gene products of Simian virus in teratocarcinoma cells, which suggests that host cell differentiation controls viral function (39).

CHEMICAL CARCINOGENS AND PROTEIN SYNTHESIS

The hypothesis that focuses on protein or RNA requires a complex network of indirect interlocking effects as compared with the hypothesis that focuses directly on DNA, the simplest hypothesis. For this reason, the hypothesis accepting proteins or RNA as preferential or critical targets for carcinogens is more difficult to be accepted or proved. Also, it is difficult to explain how the macromolecules of proteins or RNA that are apparently not self-duplicating and that show continual or intermittent turnover are capable of storing information for relatively long periods of time (latent period or latency).

Until now, many important theories regarding the mechanism of cell response to a variety of hormonal and chemical carcinogens accept as explanation that a variety of mutation events may occur that involve either specific genes of the host cell or the integration of viral genes into host genomes.

However, after consideration of these theories, a major critique emerges, namely, that in some instances cells exposed to carcinogenic agents do not exhibit either structural aberration of chromosomes or their numbers, and accordingly it seems possible that, at least in the early stages, other factors are involved in carcinogenesis.

Recently, many fetal proteins, including fetal enzymes and particularly isozymes, have been found in tumor cells; that is, fetal proteins (α-fetoprotein) are present in the chromatin of some animal tumors (13). The rise in serum of α-fetoproteins in animals exposed to carcinogens coincides with the early appearance of nodular hyperplasia. It seems likely that the fetal mechanisms that would normally block the continued growth and development of fetal cells are not expressed in neoplastic cells because of the lack of systems that operate during fetal growth. Thus, again, fetal proteins, a propriety of malignant neoplasms, appear well before cancer can be recognized. Control of cell growth and differentiation is very complex and still not well understood; this includes positive and negative extracellular factors, cytoplasmic elements, including repressors and derepressors, receptors, and specific gene sets in the nucleus. These gene sets or batteries include genes operating in normal adult cells, genes operating in fetal tissue cells, and ribosomal protein genes for the synthesis of ribosomes. Mechanisms and gene expression and protein synthesis control are similar in fetal cells to that of normal adult cells. However, the genes involved in normal phenotypic cell functions are different from those required for cell growth, invasiveness and metastasis (Fig. 6–4).

According to the operon model (Chapter 2), an adult cell responds to extracellular stimulus (S_1) by forming intracellular stimulus receptor complexes (S_1R_1) that activate genes G_1–GR_n and such responses for hormonal stimuli have been already demonstrated (O'Malley and Means, quoted in Chapter 2). Interactions of S_1R_1 complexes with nucleolar genes increases ribosomal RNA (rRNA) and subsequently ribosome synthesis. Activation of genes G_1–GR_n also produces the messenger RNA (mRNA) and rRNA that form polysomes. Reduction or termination of stimulus results in a decrease of ribosome and polysome formation (Fig. 6–5a).

In fetal tissues, the intracellular stimulus receptor complexes (S_1R_1) act and activate the fetal genes, which control the synthesis and release of fetal

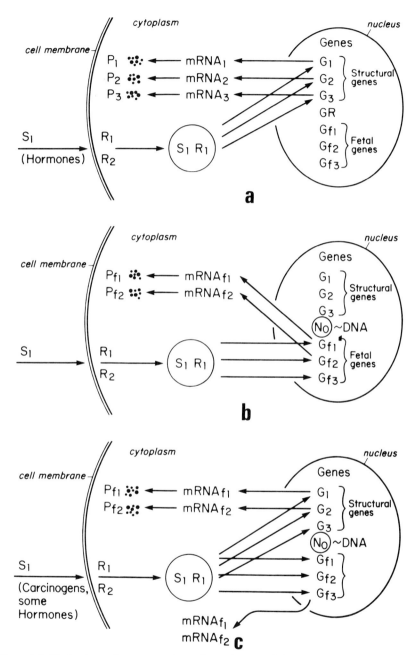

Figure 6-5 Mechanisms of gene expression and protein synthesis in (a) adult tissue, (b) fetal tissue, and (c) carcinogenesis.

proteins (α-fetoprotein). Most neoplastic cells express fetal structural genes for specific enzymes and antigenically active fetal proteins, called oncofetal proteins, such as carcinoembryonic antigen and α-fetoproteins, found in patient serum (56) (Fig. 6–5b). In *carcinogenesis*, the intracellular stimulus receptor complexes (S_1R_1) act on both structural and fetal genes by derepressing certain fetal genes which are related to control of cell growth and division, invasiveness, and metastasis, and consequently lead to expression of the phenomena of abnormal growth, invasiveness, and metastasis, the characteristic properties of carcinogenic process. Cancer cells no longer produce the suppressors or blockers which inhibit the gene expression and synthesis of new phenotypically cell proteins. Thus the cancer cells that emerge from the exposure to different chemical and hormonal carcinogens have a fundamental fixed mechanism that includes operation of both fetal and specialized genes (Fig. 6–5c). Electron microscopic observations show an increase in ribosomal and polysomal synthesis in the early steps of carcinogenesis, whereas a decrease and disorganization of ribosomal and polysomal populations predominate in the later stages. Electron microscopic autoradiography using ^{3}H-leucine clearly demonstrates that the free ribosomes and polysomes are the specific sites for the synthesis of sedentary or growth protein synthesis required for the growth of cancer cells. We do not know whether carcinogens (oncogens) preferentially attack the rRNA and directly attack protein synthesis, or whether they attack first the mRNA and consequently the rRNA and protein synthesis. In later stages, some cells are destroyed by carcinogens, causing a disarray in gene expression and protein synthesis, with cell death. Also, the occurrence of several structural and antigenically abnormal proteins in several types of tumors has been reported (thyroid cancers, colon, lung and liver). Therefore the shut-off or "turn-off" specific mechanisms are missing in cancer cells, whereas they are operating normally in fetal tissues.

It seems likely that most of tumor promoters (PMA-phorbol myristate acetate, isolated from croton oil and anthralin) which play an important role in skin tumorigenesis, act mainly on protein synthesis, microtubule polymerization, enzyme synthesis and release of prostaglandins (61).

HORMONES: MECHANISM(S) OF ACTION IN CARCINOGENESIS

The mechanism(s) by which hormones result in cancer development is not yet understood. Approximately 20 years ago, a comparison between carcinogens and hormones stressed that carcinogens are agents that bring about an apparently irreversible modification of the cell's hereditary nuclei acid (DNA) with loss of ability to respond properly to homeostatic regulators, whereas hormones are promoters or inhibitors of cell homeostasis. They regulate growth and function of cells but do not produce cancers. The general belief was that if cancer arises in a hormone-stimulated organ, we had better search for another force (23). Although there is ample evidence that hormones exert a powerful role in initiation and development of tumors induced by either of the three categories of carcinogens—chemical, viral, or physical (radiation)—and offer many possibilities for controlling certain tumors, there is still no direct evidence that hormones are carcinogenic per se. Thus, there is no hard evidence that hormones are able to initiate the malignant transformation by pushing normal cells into uncontrolled proliferation; however, prolonged exposure to large doses of hormones markedly increases the incidence of some cancers. Hence, the main question—Are hormones carcinogens, cocarcinogens, or only tumor promoters?—still remains unsolved. A comparison between carcinogens and hormones shows some similarities, but mostly dissimilarities as regards their mechanism of action at the macromolecular level. Thus, most chemical carcinogens need to be activated by microsomal enzymes before they are active or true carcinogens; carcinogens induce neoplastic transformation both in vivo and in vitro; short exposure to carcinogens produces irreversible changes in cells; cell division and proliferation are necessary before true neoplasia occurs; and most chemical carcinogens appear to be mutagens and subsequently somatic mutations may be involved in neoplastic transformation.

It has been known for some time that tumors of endocrine glands appear primarily as a result of imbalance or hormonal disequilibrium, with subsequent overproduction or underproduction of specific hormones. It is well demonstrated that most hormonal homeostasis is governed by a feedback mechanism. These so-called thermostats maintain a constant level or equilibrium between the specific hormones secreted by endocrine organs and the pituitary and hypothalamic hormones, thus a hypothalamic–pituitary–endocrine gland axis is very important in pathogenesis of endocrine cancers (Chapter 4). A hormonal imbalance can result in tumorigenesis in endocrine organs and their target tissues. Thus, the chief questions regarding the mechanism of hormones need to be resolved: Are hormones acting as true carcinogens or mainly as tumor promoters where other carcinogens (chemicals, viral, radiation) may be the true carcinogen? Hormones thereby provide only a proliferating tissue on which other carcinogens can act directly. There is still no definite answer to this question; however, in some circumstances, at least some steroid hormones might act as carcinogens (46). Also, hormones may be essential to carcinogenesis by preparing the background against which tumors ultimately arise. For instance, hormones (estrogens, corticosteroids, and prolactin) are essential factors in the development of mammary cancer, although this does not mean that they exert direct carcinogenic action. In mice, both estrogens and prolactin increase the incidence of mammary neoplasms by directly stimulating the development of mammary gland. Estrogens and prolactin, and probably progesterone, all contribute to the development of mammary tumors in rats exposed to carcinogens. But the role of estrogens is even more complex, since estrogens can stimulate prolactin secretion.

However, in studying the mechanism(s) of hormones in carcinogenesis, we have to take into account some essential differences regarding the metabolism of hormones in different species, animal strains, and their status of reproductive physiology, such as animals with spontaneous estrus cycles, with functional corpora lutea (dog) and without (mice and rats), or with reflex ovulation (rabbit), which may respond differently to exogenous hormones. Also, pregnancy alters the response to hormones by conferring a relative protection against mammary cancer in humans and in rats, while increasing the risk of breast cancer in mice. Hence, in vivo studies of hormonal effects are almost impossible to interpret. It is difficult to define a target cell, since cell populations—benign or malignant—are heterogeneous, and consequently exhibit various responses to hormones. Only a fraction of the cell population will respond synchronously and homogeneously to any hormone, and in the same manner (36). After malignant transformation, the cells still retain some characteristics of their tissue of origin; thus the cell and its progeny require the same cell environment in order to survive and grow and hormones are part of this environment. Also, hormones play an important role in tumor transplantation; some transplantable tumors are definitely dependent on the hormonal milieu of the host. In the presence of hormones, these dependent tumors can be transplanted and maintained for several generations, while in their absence, the tumors cannot take in, grow, or develop, hence they will shrink and eventually die (Chapter 8).

In recent years, more accurate epidemiologic studies regarding the use of hormones as therapeutic agents and cancer incidence in humans indicate a higher frequency of cancer of the vagina and cervix after DES treatment; anabolic steroids may produce hepatocellular carcinomas in patients with aplastic anemia, and oral contraceptives are suspected in the increased incidence of hepatomas.

It is possible that steroid hormones might only contribute to enhancing the carcinogenic activity of unknown compounds by competing for the same biotransformation systems in liver. Hormones may act in the initiation phase of carcinogenesis by providing either a normal background (permissive role) or abnormal conditions (teratogenic role) for subsequent action of chemical, viral, or physical agents, or they may act in the promotion phase by enhancing or facilitating the growth and metastatic process of tumors after they have been initiated. There are several possible mechanisms by which hormones can act or intervene in carcinogenesis. Some of these mechanisms have not yet been demonstrated and remain speculative:

1. Hormones may stimulate the DNA synthesis and mitosis essential for fixation of the transformed state.
2. Hormones may act by binding to and modification of nuclear DNA and its associated proteins.

3. Hormones may act in the transcriptional, namely posttranscriptional stage, by enhancing the gene expression and thus the synthesis of new proteins (i.e., increase the synthesis of mRNA and rRNA).
4. Hormones may increase the covalent binding of chemical carcinogens to macromolecules (or other cellular components) by influencing metabolic activation systems.
5. Hormones may compete with chemical carcinogens for the same biotransformation systems (in liver and skin).
6. Hormones may compete with chemical carcinogens for the same cellular receptors.
7. Hormones may activate the production of oncogenic viruses (e.g., mammary tumor virus, MTV, in mice).
8. Hormones may produce preneoplastic lesions which provide an environment for the survival of cells with an abnormal potential.
9. Hormones may enhance the rate of transformation or progression of neoplastic cells to neoplastic cells.
10. Hormones may preferentially stimulate the proliferation of abnormal cell populations, from a heterogeneous cell population.
11. Hormones may exert an immunosuppressive role and subsequently could accelerate tumor induction and development.
12. Hormones, by stimulating the proliferation of normal cells, may exhaust the normal cell population and consequently eliminate their inhibitory influence over the abnormal cell proliferation.
13. Hormones may act by an imbalance of cell homeostasis in a target organ, by increasing cell proliferation over functional differentiation.
14. Hormones may act on cell environment, by creating a hormonal milieu that can enhance or reduce some specific synthetic and secretory activities and thus enhance or reduce the tumorigenic potential.
15. Some hormones may exhibit a weak mutagenic activity.
16. Hormones may act on the operon system by stimulating derepression genes, thereby bringing about abnormal cell proliferation.
17. Hormones may act indirectly through growth factors (GF): first, hormones increase the formation of growth factors, in turn increasing the development of cancer by chronic overstimulation of the target cells.
18. Hormones may act by conversion to another substance with more carcinogenic potential (e.g., androgens to estrogens).

Although many chemical carcinogens are mutagens and show a parallelism between their covalent binding to DNA and mutagenic action, only few steroid hormones, including DES metabolites, exhibit a covalent binding to DNA and a weak mutagenic activity in short-term tests that indicate interactions with DNA.

However, most studies regarding the mutagenic action (or mutagenicity) of sex steroid hormones were carried out before a statistical model for mutagenic tests was developed and are therefore inconclusive. Also, mutagenic studies regarding sex steroids using mammalian germ cells, such as cytogenetic studies on oocytes, and spermatocytes are scarce. Only two dominant lethal tests—one a combination of mestranol and lynoestranol and the other on norethisterone acetate—have been considered positive (19).

Therefore, additional studies are required before a definite statement regarding mutagenic action of sex steroids can be made.

Many sex steroid hormones cause embryotoxic and fetotoxic effects in several species when administered during pregnancy; these effects are usually dose related. Some estrogens also produce teratogenic effects in exposed offspring. Furthermore, a brief exposure of newborn mice to estrogens leads to a high incidence of different cancers in later life (58).

Neonatal mice provide a useful model for studying the long-term effects of prenatal exposure of humans to DES and other sex steroids (7). Both mice and rats are born with incompletely developed genital tracts. In mice the injection of sex steroids or DES during the first few days after birth may induce irreversible changes in the genital tract. Despite the fact that hormones injected into neonatal mice are not metabolized by the placenta (as are those occurring in humans exposed prenatally), the responses are similar to those that occur in mice exposed prenatally. Some of these responses, such as vaginal adenosis and cysts, resemble those seen in humans after transplacental exposure to DES (32).

Nonneoplastic changes in the genital tract are commonly found in girls born to women who received DES during pregnancy. Also, some clinical observations suggest a high incidence of vaginal cancer in the daughters of women who received brief DES therapy during the first trimester of their pregnancy; effects are detected at 15 to 22 years of age (31,32). These observations suggest that even brief exposure to steroid hormones can induce cancers, and some steroid hormones may act as carcinogens. Some hormones and hormonelike substances (prostaglandins, growth factors, chalones) may act on DNA synthesis of preneoplastic and neoplastic cells. They act mostly during S phase (DNA synthesis), and possibly during DNA replication.

Light and electron microscopic autoradiography using ^{3}H-thymidine shows marked enhancement of ^{3}H-thymidine incorporation and also of DNA content in preneoplastic and neoplastic nuclei of epidermal and thyroid tumors. There is an increase of many folds of DNA synthesis after various types of hormone administration, including thyroxine, glucagon, estradiol, calcitonin, and prostaglandins, as well as a sharp decrease in neoplastic nuclei after corticosteroid (hydrocortisone, cortisone) administration, hypophysectomy, and castration.

These findings suggest that hormones may act on carcinogenesis by interfering with DNA synthesis. With the aid of high-resolution autoradiography it is possible to detect the early damages in DNA repair mechanism(s) after exposure to chemical carcinogens.

A certain hormonal environment may facilitate or inhibit the DNA repair mechanism(s), subsequently enhancing or mitigating tumor growth and development.

COMPARISON BETWEEN HORMONES AND CHEMICAL CARCINOGENS IN REGARD TO THEIR MECHANISM OF ACTION IN CARCINOGENESIS

Despite the many efforts focused upon regarding the mechanism(s) of action of diverse chemical carcinogens, only a few were made regarding the intrinsic mechanism(s) of hormone action in the process of carcinogenesis. Recent findings suggest some similarities and dissimilarities between these two classes:

1. Both chemical carcinogens and hormones require a certain latent period (latency). This period is shorter in the case of chemical carcinogens and much longer for hormones. Most chemical carcinogens need to be metabolized, chiefly by microsomal enzymes in order to be active carcinogens; thus many chemical carcinogens must first be activated before they become active (or ultimate) carcinogens (Fig. 6–3). However, there is no need for hormones to be metabolized before they become active.

2. Both chemical carcinogens and hormones exhibit tissue selectivity or responsiveness. Thus, 3-methylcholanthrene and benzopyrene generally cause skin tumors, whereas DMBA generally induces skin tumors, mammary carcinomas, and leukemia; urethane primarily causes lung tumors, and zinc causes testis tumors. Hormones cause tumors mainly in the target tissues (mammary gland, thyroid, ovary, prostate gland). However, hormones may accelerate or inhibit tumor induction by chemical, viral, or physical agents in several organs (liver, lung, lymphoid tissue, skin).

3. Dose dependence: Hormones always require prolonged, continuous administration, namely large doses, whereas most chemical carcinogens can induce cancers after a single dose administration. However, administration of small and repeated doses can increase the incidence of tumors by shortening the latent period. Both chemical and hormone effects appear to be dose dependent.

4. Most carcinogens are tumorigenic both in vitro and in vivo, while most hormones are tumorigenic only in vivo.

5. Most chemical carcinogens are mutagenic and act preferentially on DNA by covalent binding and secondarily on RNA and protein synthesis, whereas hormones act primarily on mRNA (by inducing gene expression) and rRNA and secondarily on DNA synthesis and repair mechanism(s). Most hormones are not mutagens or are only weak mutagens.

6. Most tumors produced by chemical carcinogens are of a malignant nature with high tendency to local invasiveness and metastasis, whereas most tumors induced by hormones are benign in nature, exhibiting a local invasiveness and, in very rare instances, metastases.

7. Most hormone-induced tumors regress or disappear after treatment is discontinued or stopped, whereas tumors induced by chemical carcinogens continue to grow and develop after being initiated by even a single dose.

8. Tumors caused by hormones can be transplanted only in the presence of a particular hormone, whereas those induced by chemical carcinogens do not require the presence of hormones for transplantation; however, hormones can facilitate their transplantation.

9. There is a great variability among hormone-induced tumors in regard to species, sex, and age of the animals involved, although this variability also exists for chemical carcinogens, but to a much lesser degree.

10. Most cellular changes are irreversible after chemical carcinogens, while they are reversible after hormonal treatment.

11. Cellular proliferation is a fundamental requirement in both systems (chemicals or hormones), before neoplastic transformation occurs.

Table 6-1. COMPARISON BETWEEN MECHANISM(S) OF ACTION OF HORMONES AND CHEMICAL CARCINOGENS

HORMONES	CHEMICAL CARCINOGENS
Not mutagenic; weakly mutagenic only in some instances	Most are mutagens
Act preferentially on mRNA and proteins	Act preferentially on DNA
Tumorigenic only in vivo	Tumorigenic both in vivo and in vitro
Not necessary to be metabolized, before becoming active	Metabolic activation essential in most cases
Prolonged and continuous administration required	A single dose can be sufficient
Hormonal tumorigenesis is highly species and sex dependent	Chemical cancers are sex and species dependent to a much lesser degree
Initially reversible cellular changes	Initially irreversible cellular changes
Most tumors are of benign nature; locally invasive tumors	Most tumors are of malignant nature with metastasis
Latent period (latency) is much longer	Latency is shorter after chemicals
Tumor regression after discontinuation or cessation of treatment	No tumor regression occurs when treatment is discontinued
Cellular proliferation is necessary	Cellular proliferation is also required

COMMENTS AND CONCLUSIONS

Looking at the diverse list of chemical carcinogens and hormones currently thought to be carcinogenic or cocarcinogenic, the chief question before the oncologist is: How do these diverse chemicals and hormones act in the process of carcinogenesis?

Although the involvement of hormones in carcinogenesis was suspected long ago, only a few efforts were made at clarifying their mechanism(s) of action at macromolecular levels.

Further research should be developed in the area of hormonal and chemical carcinogenesis in vitro. Even though most evidence suggests that many chemical carcinogens are working by acting on DNA synthesis and the DNA repair mechanism, a good correlation can be made between mutagenic action (mutagenicity) and carcinogenic potential (carcinogenicity); there is less evidence regarding the intrinsic mechanism of hormones at the cellular level.

For this reason, their basic mechanism(s) is not yet understood and sometimes speculative. Since most experimental cancers are caused only after repeated or prolonged exposure to a carcinogen or hormone and similarly most human cancers appear in old age, it is logical to believe that several steps are required to convert normal cells into an invasive and malignant cell. Some steps from this long chain of events, which finally result in malignant or neoplastic transformation of a cell, are still not clearly understood.

By using modern methods, which are more accurate and sensitive as compared with classic ones, we are in a better position to detect the initial events that occur in a transformed cell and are still a long way from fully clarifying these intrinsic mechanism(s) at macromolecular levels. Are carcinogens real inducers of the abnormal cell proliferation, or do they just stimulate the already existing abnormal cells from a so-called normal cell population? Thus, a carcinogen (chemical, viral, hormonal) is merely a selector of already transformed cells present in the population before application of the chemical. Thus, application of a carcinogen would provide neoplastic cells with a great competitive advantage and perhaps liberate them from the inhibition of surrounding normal cells. This fact can explain why only a small portion of an exposed cell population is converted into malignant and neoplastic cells; not all cells undergo malignant transformation when exposed to the same carcinogen. This suggests that cells capable of responding to carcinogenic agents are those that have already undergone the first steps in tumor progression and they become the prime target (52).

Transfection experiments support the hypothesis that even normal cells contain latent transforming genes that may be exposed when their usual environment is disrupted (17). Hence a gene does not have to be abnormal in the sense of directing the synthesis of a faulty product, to cause cancer. Neoplastic transformation may be caused by the activation of dormant cellular genes, possibly as a result of gene arrangement. This suggests that there is more than one pathway to transformation.

Thus, many carcinogens are only activating these dormant genes already existing in normal cells. The activation of dormant genes can be due to a derepression process. Abundant evidence has been accumulated in recent years which supports the assertion that interference of an oncogen with DNA is very likely to be the prelude to the cancer induction. As a result of any physical or chemical assault on DNA in vivo is the production of mutations. The hypothesis that cancer begins with a somatic mutation was first proposed by Boveri (1912). Although the somatic mutation theory has been challenged primarily because not all chemical carcinogens are mutagens and not all mutagenic substances are potential carcinogens, the close correlation between mutagenicity and carcinogenicity recently revived many tests using bacterial systems and mammalian somatic cells in culture for screening of several environmental carcinogens. One of these, the Ames test using *Salmonella typhimurium* with its three mutations and its ability to grow in a histidine-free medium, found almost 85 percent of known carcinogens to be mutagenic. However, this test does not explain how mutation causes cancer. Despite the acceptance of the Ames test for the general screening of environmental and industrial carcinogens, the main problem still remains: Can results obtained from bacterial systems or cell culture models be extrapolated to human cancers?

In the opinion of this author, these simple tests cannot explain how carcinogens act on human cells, which require a more complex cell environment than bacteria or even animal cells. Thus, there is a need to develop more ideal systems close to human oncology, since most intermediate steps in carcinogenesis are largely dependent on their cellular environment.

Another important problem widely debated among oncologists and endocrinologists is whether hormones are true carcinogens. Due to widespread use of hormones as therapeutic agents in several endocrine and nonendocrine diseases, this raises many questions regarding the cancer incidence after a long period (15 to 20 years) following hormonal treatment or in the daughters of pregnant women.

Studies using neonatal mice and rats for the long-term effects of prenatal exposure to DES and sex steroids showed that both mice and rats were born with incompletely developed genital tracts in a stage similar to that in the first trimester in humans. Also, vaginal adenosis and other preneoplastic lesions resemble those seen in humans after transplacental exposure to DES have been reported (32). However, it should be remembered that placenta of different species can metabolize the DES and sex steroids in a different way from that seen in human placenta.

Although there is ample evidence that hormones are crucial factors in controlling the growth, development, and propagation of several neoplasms, there is no direct evidence, except in a few instances (sex steroids, estrogens), that hormones are carcinogenic per se. Since cancer is considered primarily a disease of cellular differentiation, rather than a direct result of a somatic mutation, the study of hormones in controlling cell differentiation will be of increasing significance.

Because most investigations recently focused on the molecular genetics of carcinogenesis and because of the concept that initial cellular changes are always irreversible, the control of neoplastic transformation was conceived as almost impossible. Inasmuch as recent evidence suggests that an abnormal cell differentiation in the primordial lesions and some cells from some tumors (teratocarcinoma in mice, squamous cell carcinoma in rats) can be restored to normal cells, few tumors, such as keratinizing squamous cell carcinoma, retain a high capacity of self-cure by cell differentiation (51). Additional studies should be directed on the effects of hormones on cell differentiation to control this process by hormonal manipulations.

Thus hormones may lead to neoplastic changes, not by mutations in the sense of aberrations in DNA structure, but through epigenetic changes. Hence, carcinogens and some hormones may act by modifying the gene function and not the gene structure. Steroid hormones might directly or indirectly induce epigenetic changes leading to an abnormal cellular differentiation or cell autonomy, without modifying nuclear DNA (Fig. 6–6). The cellular mechanisms controlling normal differentiation are similar to those involved in cancer, with the exception that in carcinogenesis, expression of cell developmental pattern is abnormal.

Recent evidence suggests a relationship between hepatocarcinogenesis (development of hepatocellular cancers) and an androgen environment both in humans and in experimental animals. Thus, an increased number of hepatocellular carcinomas (HCC) were reported in patients with or without anemia (Fanconi's anemia), and taking long-term androgens (metiltestosterone) for different reasons (cryptorchidism, impotence). Also, idiopathic hepatocellular carcinomas in North America occur more frequently in males than in females; this difference is even higher in the black population (36). However, it is not certain whether the hormonal milieu may contribute to the differences of cancer incidence in males and females. Additional studies are needed to explain the role of hormones in the occurrence and development of spontaneous tumors and also in sex differences of some cancers (lung, breast, bone, brain, lymphomas, digestive organs, melanomas, leukemia, endocrine glands, and urinary tract). Since 1964, when Brookes and Lawley first demonstrated that polynuclear aromatic hydrocarbons strongly bind to nuclear DNA in mouse skin, thus making DNA the significant cellular receptor of carcinogenic hydrocarbons, evidence mounted to indicate the genotoxic effects of chemical carcinogens, such as chromosomal aberrations, mutagenesis, inhibition of DNA synthesis, and DNA repair. It was also demonstrated that all

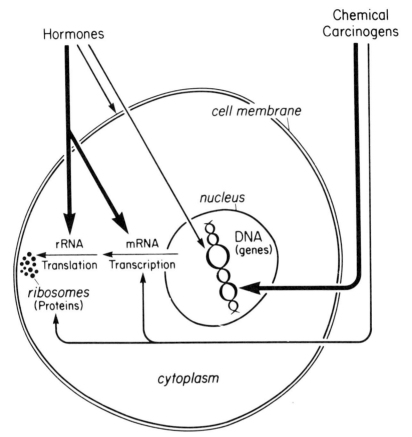

Figure 6-6 Basic mechanism(s) of action of hormones and chemical carcinogens on DNA, RNA, and protein synthesis. Major or principal mechanisms are indicated by thick arrows, secondary mechanism by thin arrows.

three major types of DNA damages—base damage, strand breakage, and crosslinkage—elicit DNA repair. Thus, several tests for the study of nuclear DNA damage and repair in a variety of ways were developed in recent years.

Although it is generally believed that most chemical carcinogens act in their initial steps by a covalent binding to DNA and that these short tests, using bacterial systems or mammalian cells in culture, are accurate enough to permit early detection of chemical environmental carcinogens, we must keep in mind that some carcinogens may operate by other molecular mechanisms without inducing DNA damages and repair. Also, not entirely activated or ultimate carcinogen is critically bound to nuclear DNA macromolecules, some noncritically bound or degraded to inactive metabolites or spontaneously decomposed.

Although hormonal carcinogenesis was demonstrated long ago, the initial events of so-called carcinogenic hormones at the macromolecular level are not yet clarified. There are certain differences between the intrinsic or basic mechanism of chemical carcinogens and hormones at the cellular level. Thus, most chemical carcinogens critically bind to DNA macromolecules, whereas hormonal carcinogens act primarily on mRNA and proteins. Chemicals may operate predominantly by inducing chromosome and gene abnormalities, whereas hormones operate principally by expressing new gene formation and acting through cellular differentiation. Most initial interactions of chemical carcinogens are irreversible, while those of hormones are reversible.

All hormones are of endogenous origin; chemical carcinogens are exogenous (mainly) and endogenous in nature. A single dose of a chemical carcinogen is sufficient to elicit tumors in various organs; only a repeated administration of large doses of hormones can induce tumors. Most hormone-induced neoplasms are benign, developing first in the target tissues. Most hormones act on DNA and RNA, not by a critical covalent binding, but through their nuclear or cytoplasmic receptors. Only after formation of these hormone-receptor complexes can hormones elicit their carcinogenic effects. However, in spite of the above-mentioned differences, there are many similarities regarding the cellular mechanisms of hormones and chemical carcinogens; many chemical carcinogens have significant side effects on the endocrine glands and indirectly increase hormone secretion (hypersecretion) → cellular over-stimulation → carcinogenesis. Also, several natural and synthetic hormones possess (especially in large doses) different pharmacologic and toxic effects similar to carcinogens, and consequently should be treated like other chemical with intrinsic carcinogenic potential. Accordingly, more sensitive tests should be developed in order to assess the carcinogenic potential of natural and synthetic hormones as well as to evaluate the carcinogenic risks of hormones to humans. Inasmuch as most hormones are not mutagenic, as many chemical carcinogens are, it is difficult, if not impossible, to develop short-term tests as are used with bacterial systems (Ames test); we have to rely for the most part on animal models. These models are slower, more costly, and time consuming, but they provide data that can be extrapolated to humans.

Also, data obtained from short-term tests are insufficient in declaring chemicals as potential carcinogens. For assessment of the carcinogenic potential of hormones or chemical carcinogens in humans, further investigations using animal models must be performed.

Several hormones undergo a complicated intermediate metabolism before they can become active; some of their intermediate metabolites may act as carcinogens. These metabolic differences may explain the species differences fundamental to hormonal carcinogenesis. Steroid hormones (glucocorticoids, estrogens, and androgens) exert differential effects regarding mRNA species and their ability to synthesize new proteins (33).

Although DES exhibits only a weak mutagenic activity in bacterial systems and mammalian cells (by slightly increasing the sister chromatid exchanges in a pseudodiploid Chinese hamster cell line), it exerts important embryolethal and teratogenic effects in experimental animals as well as in humans. DES taken during pregnancy significantly increases the frequency of vaginal and cervical clear cell adenocarcinomas in daughters. There is also an increased risk of endometrial carcinoma in young women with Turner's syndrome and treated with DES (19). Thus, there is strong evidence that estrogens, including diethylstilbestrol are casually related to the occurrence of cancers in experimental animals and humans. These hormones should be cautiously used in women, especially during pregnancy. In recent years, an increasing number of hormonelike substances of hormonomimetic agents have been discovered. These agents cause hyperactivity and hormonal imbalance in many instances and may act as carcinogens or cocarcinogens.

Further investigations are required in order to assess their carcinogenic potential and to clarify their intrinsic mechanism(s). Since hormones and chemical carcinogens may use more than one means to express their carcinogenic potential, a rigid distinction between these two classes seems inappropriate.

The major concern is still related to a direct carcinogenic effect of hormones. In my opinion, hormones act mainly as cocarcinogens or weak carcinogens, by inducing epigenetic changes through mRNA, critical in controlling cellular differentiation, whereas most chemicals act as strong carcinogens, through DNA, by inducing genetic and mutational changes. Thus, due to the use of more accurate and sensitive methods for the study of DNA, RNA, and protein synthesis, an improved understanding of intrinsic mechanisms of hormones and chemical carcinogens at cellular and macromolecular levels has emerged in recent years (Fig. 6–6).

REFERENCES

1. Alexander, P., and Horning, E.: Observations on the Oppenheimer method of inducing tumors by subcutaneous implantation of plastic films. In Wolsterholme, G., and O'Connor, M. (eds.): *Carcinogenesis, Mechanism of Action.* (Boston, Little, Brown, 1958), pp. 12–22.
2. Ames, B.: Carcinogenicity test. *Science 191*:241–243 (1976).
3. Ashley, D.: The two "hit" and multiple "hit" theories of carcinogenesis. *Br. J. Cancer 23*:313–328 (1969).
4. Backer, J., and Weinstein, J.: Mitochondrial DNA is a major cellular target for dihydrodiolepoxide derivative of benzo(a)pyrene. *Science 209*:297–299 (1980).
5. Barrett, J., Tsutsui, T., and Tsio, P.: Neoplastic transformation induced by a direct perturbation of DNA. *Nature 274*:229–232 (1978).
6. Basilico, C., and Marin, G.: Susceptibility of cells in different stages of the mitotic cycle of transformation by polyoma virus. *Virology 28*:429–437 (1966).
7. Bern, J., Jones, L., Mori, T., and Young, P.: Exposure of neonatal mice to steroids: long term effects on the mammary gland and other reproductive structures. *J. Steroid Biochem. 6*:673–676 (1975).

8. Bertram, J., and Heidelberger, C.: Cell cycle dependency of oncogenic transformation induced by N-methyl-N'-nitro-N-nitrosoguanidine in culture. *Cancer Res. 34*:526–536 (1974).
9. Boveri, T.: *The Origin of Malignant Tumors.* (Baltimore, Williams & Wilkins, 1929).
10. Braun, A., and Wood, H.: Suppression of the neoplastic state with the acquisition of specialized functions in cells, tissues and organs of crown gall teratomas of tobacco. *Proc. Natl. Acad. Sci. USA 73*:496–500 (1976).
11. Brookes, P., and Lawley, P.: Evidence for the binding of polynuclear aromatic hydrocarbons to the nucleic acids of mouse skin: relation between carcinogenic power of hydrocarbons and their binding to deoxyribonucleic acid. *Nature 202*:781–784 (1964).
12. Burnet, F.: Cancer: somatic genetic considerations. *Adv. Cancer Res. 28*:1–79 (1978).
13. Busch, H.: A general concept for molecular biology of cancer. *Cancer Res. 36*: 4291–4294 (1976).
14. Cairns, J.: The origin of human cancers. *Nature 289*:353–357 (1981).
15. Cerda-Olmedo, E., Hanawalt, P. and Guerola, N.: Mutagenesis of the replication point by nitrosoguanidine map and pattern of replication of the Escherichia coli chromosome. *J. Mol. Biol. 33*:705–719 (1968).
16. Clever, J.: Repair of alkylation damage in ultraviolet sensitive (xeroderma pigmentosum) human cells. *Mutat. Res. 12*:453–462 (1971).
17. Cooper, C., Okenquist, S., and Silverman, L.: Transforming activity of DNA of chemically transformed and normal cells. *Nature 284*:418–421 (1980).
18. DeLustig, E., and Lustig, L.: Accion de inductores embryionaires sobre tejidos tumorales. *Rev. Soc. Argent. Biol. 40*:207–216 (1964).
19. Diethylstilbestrol and diethylstilbestrol propionate. In *Evaluation of the Carcinogenic Risk of Chemicals to Humans, IARC Monograph*, vol. 21. (Lyons, International Agency for Research on Cancer, 1979), pp. 173–231.
20. Farber, E.: Chemical carcinogenesis: A biologic perspective. *Am. J. Pathol. 106*: 271–296 (1982).
21. Fibach, E., Landau, T., and Sachs, L.: Normal differentiation of myeloid leukemia cells induced by a differentiation inducing protein. *Nature (New Biol) 237*:276–278 (1972).
22. Fujiwara, Y.: Effect of cyclohexamide on regulatory protein for initiating mammalian DNA replication at the nuclear membrane. *Cancer Res. 32*:2089–2093 (1972).
23. Furth, J.: Vistas in the etiology and pathogenesis of tumors. *Fed. Proc. 20*:865–873 (1961).
24. Gardner, W., Pfeiffer, C., and Trentin, J.: Hormonal factors in experimental carcinogenesis. In Homburger, F. (ed.): *Physiopathology of Cancer.* (New York, Harper & Row, 1959), pp. 152–237.
25. German, J.: Bloom syndrome II. The prototype of human genetic disorders predisposing to chromosome instability and cancer. In German, J. (ed.): *Chromosomes and Cancer.* (New York, Wiley, 1974), pp. 601–617.
26. Glover, T., Chang, C., Trosko, J., and Li, S.: Ultraviolet light induction of diptheria toxin resistant mutants in normal and xeroderma pigmentosum human fibroblasts. *Proc. Natl. Acad. Sci. USA 76*:3982–3986 (1979).
27. Gurdon, J.: Adult frogs derived from the nuclei of single somatic cells. *Dev. Biol. 4*:256–273 (1972).
28. Hadorn, E.: Proliferation and dynamics of cell heredity in blastema cultures of Drosophila. *Natl. Cancer Inst. Monogr. 31*:365–397 (1969).
29. Haran-Ghera, N., and Peled, A.: Thymus and bone marrow derived lymphatic

leukemia in mice. *Nature 241*:396–398 (1973).

30. Heidelberger, C.: Mammalian cell transformation and mammalian cell mutagenesis in vitro. *J. Environ. Pathol. Toxicol. 3*:69–87 (1980).

31. Herbst, A., Kurman, R., Scully, R., and Postkanzen, D.: Clear cell adenocarcinoma of the genital tract in young females: Registry Rep. *N. Engl. J. Med. 287*:1259 (1972).

32. Herbst, A., Scully, R., and Robbey, S.: Vaginal adenosis and other diethylstilbestrol related abnormalities. *Clin. Obstet. Gynecol. 18*:185–194 (1975).

33. Higgins, S., and Gehring, U.: Molecular mechanisms of steroid hormone action. *Adv. Cancer Res. 28*:313–397 (1978).

34. Hollstein, M., McCann, J., Angelosanto, F., and Nichols, W.: Short term tests for carcinogens and mutagens. *Mutat. Res. 65*:133–226 (1979).

35. Johnson, F.: Androgenic anabolic steroids and hepatocellular carcinoma. In Okude, K., and Peters, R. (eds.): *Hepatocellular Carcinoma*. (New York, Wiley, 1976), pp. 95–110.

36. Kellen, J.: Animal models for cancer research. In Kellen, J., and Hilf, R. (eds.): *Influences of Hormones in Tumor Development*, vol. I. (Boca Raton, Fl., CRC Press, 1979), pp. 1–9.

37. Kleijer, W., Lohman, P., Mulder, M., and Bootsma, D.: Repair of x-ray damage in DNA of cultivated cells from patients with xeroderma pigmentosum. *Mutat. Res. 9*:517–523 (1970).

38. Lindahl, T.: In "DNA repair processes and cellular senescence" Preprint 1977, quoted in Burnett, p. 28.

39. Linnenbach, A., Huebner, K., and Croce, C.: DNA transformed murine teratocarcinoma cells: Regulation of expression of simian virus 40 tumor antigen in stem versus differentiated cells. *Proc. Natl. Acad. Sci USA 77*:4875–4879 (1980).

40. Marquardt, H.: DNA—the critical cellular target in chemical carcinogenesis? In Grover, P. (ed.): *Chemical Carcinogens and DNA*, vol. II (Boca Ratan, Fl., CRC Press, 1978), pp. 159–179.

41. Martin, G.: Teratocarcinomas and mammalian embryogenesis. *Science 209*:768–776 (1980).

42. Mayhr, B., Turnbull, D., and DiPaolo, J.: Ultraviolet mutagenesis of normal and xeroderma pigmentosum variant human fibroblasts. *Mutat. Res. 62*:341–353 (1979).

43. McKinnell, R., Deggins, B., and Larat, D.: Transplantation of pluripotential nuclei from triploid frog tumors. *Science 165*:394–396 (1969).

44. Mintz, B.: Gene expression in neoplasia. *Harvey Lect. 71*:193–246 (1976).

45. Miyaki, M., Yatagai, K., and Ono, T.: Strand breaks of mammalian mitochondrial DNA induced by carcinogens. *Chem. Biol. Interact. 17*:321–329 (1977).

46. Nandi, S.: Comparison of the tumorigenic effects of chemical carcinogens and hormones. *J. Anim. Sci. 40*:1263–1266 (1975).

47. Nebert, D.: Pharmacogenetics: An approach to understanding chemical and biological aspects of cancer. *J. Natl. Cancer Inst. 64*:1279–1290 (1980).

48. Niranjan, B., Bhat, N., and Avadhani, N.: Preferential attack of mitochondrial DNA by aflatoxin B_1 during hepatocarcinogenesis. *Science 215*:73–75 (1982).

49. Parshad, R., and Snafor, K.: Effect of horse serum, fetal calf serum, bovine serum and fetuin on neoplastic conversion and chromosomes of mouse embryo cells in vitro. *J. Natl. Cancer Inst. 41*:767–779 (1968).

50. Pegg, A.: Metabolism of N-nitrosodimethylamine. *IARC Sci. Publ. 27*:3–22 (1980).

51. Pierce, G.: Differentiation of normal and malignant cells. *Fed. Proc. 29*:1248–1254 (1970).
52. Prehn, R.: Tumor progression and homeostasis. *Adv. Cancer Res. 23*:203–236 (1976).
53. Rinkus, S., and Ligator, M.: Chemical characterization of 465 known or suspected carcinogens and their correlation with mutagenic activity in the Salmonella typhimurium system. *Cancer Res. 39*:3289–3318 (1979).
54. Rosenkrantz, H., and Poirer, L.: Evaluation of the mutagenicity and DNA modifying activity of carcinogens and noncarcinogens in microbial systems. *J. Natl. Cancer Inst. 62*:841–871 (1979).
55. Rubin, H.: Is somatic mutation the major mechanism of malignant transformation? *J. Natl. Cancer Inst. 64*:995–1000 (1980).
56. Sarcione, E.: Alpha fetoprotein: Detection, isolation and characterization. In Busch, H. (ed.): *Methods in Cancer Research*, vol. 10. (New York, Academic Press, 1973), pp. 85–104.
57. Straus, D.: Somatic mutation, cellular differentiation and cancer causation. *J Natl. Cancer Inst. 67*:233–241 (1981).
58. Takasugi, N., Kimura, T., and Mori, T.: Irreversible changes in mouse vaginal epithelium induced by early post-natal treatment with steroid hormones. In Kazda, S., and Denenberg, V. (eds.): *The Post-Natal Development of Phenotype*. (London, Butterworths, 1970), pp. 229–251.
59. Taylor, A., Harden, D., Arlett, C., Harcourt, S., Lehmann, A., Stevens, S., and Bridges, B.: Ataxia telangiectasia: A human mutation with abnormal radiation sensitivity. *Nature 258*:427–429 (1975).
60. Temin, H.: Mechanism of cell transformation by RNA tumor viruses. *Annu. Rev. Microbiol. 25*:609–648 (1971).
61. Van Duuren, B.: Tumor promoting and cocarcinogenic agents in chemical carcinogenesis. In Searle, C. (ed.): *Chemical Carcinogens*. (Washington, D.C., American Chemical Society, 1976), *173*:24–51
62. Waring, M.: DNA modification and cancer. *Annu. Rev. Biochem. 50*:159–192 (1981).

Chapter 7

HORMONES AND THE METASTATIC PROCESS

GENERAL CONSIDERATIONS

Metastasis is defined as the transfer of neoplastic cells from the primary tumor of one organ, or part of it, to another not directly connected with it. Each metastase is a clone of the primary tumor; therefore, the growth of neoplastic cells in metastasis has a similar rate to that of primary tumor. However, in multiple metastases, the growth rate, receptor content, and hormone responsiveness will be different for each metastases. Distribution of metastases or the cell's capacity to metastasize is not directly related to the histology of primary tumor (stage at diagnosis) or immunocompetence, but can be related to presence or absence of hormone receptors and thus to endocrinologic responsiveness. The metastasizing capacity is also different for each anatomic type of tumor.

    We do not know the factors that govern progressive metastatic growth or those factors that can arrest it. It is amazing how some microscopic cancers can lie dormant as latent neoplastic foci for many years, as in prostate, thyroid, and breast. The capacity of primary tumor to metastasize and the spread of metastases are dependent on a particular endocrine milieu. Thus in about one-third (35 percent) of women with mammary cancers, the neoplastic metastases are dependent on this particular endocrine milieu. The hormonal

214

treatment can produce a rapid and total disappearance of large metastatic lesions in a substantial number of patients with breast, thyroid, and prostatic cancers.

This chapter focuses on the role of hormones in governing the metastic process and only briefly reviews the biologic mechanisms of cancer invasiveness and metastases (11,37,41,47).

BIOLOGIC MECHANISMS OF THE METASTATIC PROCESS

The mechanisms of the metastasizing process are complex. The metastatic potential of tumor cells is difficult to evaluate in many tumors. It is assumed that more than one factor enhances the metastatic process. Every day millions of neoplastic cells are shed from the primary tumor, but the number of overt clinical metastases that arise is far fewer. That means there are also inhibitory factors or rate-limiting steps in the development of the metastatic process. Hence, the dissemination, location, and proliferation of primary neoplastic cells outside the primary tumor are governed by several factors, some enhancing or stimulating the metastatic capacity of neoplastic cells, others inhibiting it. Thus the stimulatory and inhibitory factors or agents play a cardinal role in the metastatic process. Recently, several laboratories including ours, using such modern methods as electron microscopy, autoradiography, immunochemistry, and scanning electron microscopy revealed that many primary tumors are composed of heterogeneous cell populations. These subpopulations of neoplastic cells exhibit a different antigenicity, ultrastructural morphology, receptor(s) sites, growth rate, karyotypes, and cell surface characteristics. Also their susceptibility and responsiveness to different cytotoxic, hormonal, or physical agents are greatly variable. Although the histologic studies demonstrated that metastatic cells originate in the primary tumors and there are morphologic similarities between primary tumors and the metastasis, only some primary neoplastic cells exhibit the gamut of properties needed to accomplish the complex process of metastasis. The ability of neoplastic cells to metastasize requires several properties, somewhat similar to the case of athletes who compete in a decathlon, requiring several qualities for this event. Thus, cellular morphology (cell deformability), cell surface properties, cell interactions, increased vascular permeability, immune host–cell relationship, defects in basement membrane, and so on are important factors in the metastatic process and could be a selection process of the super cells for metastasis.

TUMOR AS A HETEROGENEOUS CELL POPULATION

By a repetitive selection process of B-16 melanoma cells from the primary tumor, it was possible to obtain metastatic cell strains differing from their parent somatic cells and exhibiting increased mobility and invasiveness. These super metastatic cells differ in several parameters from the primary tumor cells, having a greater electrophoretic mobility, lack of intercellular connections, increased lytic or degradative enzymes, surface glycoproteins, and also diminished or lack of hormone receptors. At present, it is not established as to whether this cell selection occurs in humans as well. Through the use of modern methods, investigators were able to identify cell subpopulations; hence the cellular population of a primary tumor is not homogeneous, as was previously thought. For instance, subpopulations of cells were found in a line of Chinese hamster ovary (CHO). SEM showed that UV-induced murine fibrosarcoma syngeneic to the C_3H mouse exhibit a heterogeneous cell population with different cell subpopulations. Thus colonies displaying a bizarre morphology always exhibit a high metastatic potential, whereas the small round colonies show a low metastatic potential. The number of pulmonary metastases was higher among cells obtained from bizarre colonies than in those obtained from round colonies (8,11). Electron microscopy and SEM also show that murine squamous cell carcinoma exhibits a heterogeneous cell population. Some neoplastic cells exhibit a bizarre ultrastructural morphology and cell surface changes suggest that these cells are more malignant than others that are close to normal, and display an increased tendency for invasion and metastases. Similar studies on basal cell carcinoma induced by chemical carcinogens in rats revealed a more homogeneous cell population; the basal neoplastic cells are more regular and their cell surface more flattened. The intercellular connections are well preserved in basal cell carcinoma. These ultrastructural and cell surface characteristics could explain the low invasiveness and tendency to metastasize of basal neoplastic cells as compared with that of squamous neoplastic cells, which exhibit a high metastatic potential. Thus the ultrastructural morphology and cell surface changes can be well correlated with the frequency of metastases and malignancy and can be used as a sensitive method for detection of metastatic potential (26,27). Therefore, the tumor is not a cellular entity, but is composed of many cell subpopulations, each having a different metastatic potential.

The biologic mechanisms for cancer invasion and metastasis remain unclear and are probably dependent on both host factors and intrinsic characteristics of neoplastic cells. Although spontaneous metastases seldom occur in experimental animal cancers, metastases are the most devastating aspect of neoplasia, failure of therapy, and cause of death in human cancers.

There are three main steps in the metastatic process: detachment of neoplastic cells from primary tumor, mobilization and migration by different routes (hematogenous, lymphatic, or direct extension), and implantation or seeding of neoplastic cells in another organ. It is well demonstrated by clinical and experimental observations that metastasizing cells have a selective preference in their location or implantation, preferring some organs over others, according to the so-called seed-and-soil hypothesis described by Paget long ago (32). He assumed that neoplastic cells find some organs more fertile ground than others for metastatic growth. There is an organ specificity for the metastatic process and migratory neoplastic cells are in need of a microenvironment for implantation and growth. From several thousands of detached neoplastic cells originating in primary tumors every day, only a few are able to locate and grow as metastases; the great majority die. Thus the metastatic process is one of the most devastating causes of death as well as a major obstacle in the therapy of cancers. The pathogenesis of metastatic process is an intricate and more complex process due to a series of events or cascade of events, since the neoplastic cells are released from the primary tumor, then disseminate into circulation and locate to distant sites (Fig. 7-1b.). It is well known that some tumors, such as oat cell carcinoma and malignant melanoma, exhibit a high metastatic potential, whereas other, such as basal cell carcinoma, have a very low metastatic ability. Recently, several investiga-

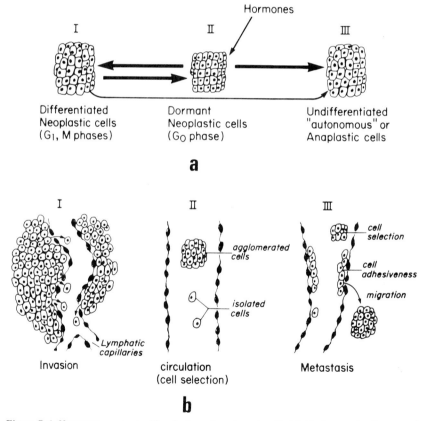

Figure 7-1 Hormones as controlling factors of metastatic cells (a). Pathogenesis of metastatic process (b).

tions were focused on the metastatic process in order to determine and clarify the pathogenesis of metastasis. Many questions arise:

Are metastatic cells cancerous cells or not?

Which are the controlling factors of the spread and fate of neoplastic cells, since they enter the circulatory system?

What factors control the large pool of dormant cells or dormancy state of neoplastic cells?

What factors control the ability of neoplastic cells to locate and grow in a selective site(s), and thus develop a new tumor, identical cellularly to primary neoplasm?

Are the metastases sensitive or responsive to the same therapeutic agents?

Can we detect the early metastases (micrometastases) before they develop into clinical or macrometastases?

The development of metastasis represents the end stage of this intricate process. It is well known that the great majority of disseminated cells from the primary tumor die before they reach their final destination. However, some of these circulating cells exhibit a peculiar ability and are able to locate and rapidly grow in the sites located far from and cytologically different from the primary tumor, thus exceeding its size, being the major cause of therapeutic failure and death. Recent investigations using electron microscopy, SEM, autoradiography, and biochemical and receptor studies show that the primary neoplasm is a mosaic of cells composed of different cell subpopulations, from which some exhibit a highly metastatic potential due to their adhesiveness, cell surface morphology, biochemical cell surface properties, absence of receptor site(s), and finally their ability to interact with the host cells. All these cellular and humoral parameters can modify the location, development, and extent of subsequent metastases. Therefore the metastatic cells are neoplastic cells that exhibit a characteristic cell surface morphology, biochemical and biophysical properties, diminished antigenicity, increased dividing capacity, increased anaploidy, detachability, and adhesiveness, which endow these cells with a special ability to survive, locate, and grow in a different site. The metastatic strain cells are one of the extreme malignant phenotypes. The metastatic process is influenced by a multitude of factors about which very little is known. The study of biogenesis and the mechanism(s) of the metastatic process are very important, since most cancer deaths are not caused by the primary tumor, but rather by the secondary growths or metastases.

ORGAN SPECIFICITY (ORGANOTROPISM) OF METASTASES

One curious aspect of metastasis is its distinctive distribution or tropism for different organs. Thus, patients with melanoma have a high risk of developing liver metastases, those with breast tumors bone metastases, those with testicular tumors lung metastases, and those with thyroid tumors lung and bone metastases. This organ preference or tropism suggests some sort of affinity between tumor cells and specific organs somewhat similar to seeds that can grow only in a specific soil (seed-and-soil hypothesis), as well as to certain hormonal factors. For instance, it was found that in rats with implanted fragments of lung, kidney, spleen, heart, skin, and thyroid tissue intravascular administration of S_{19} melanoma cells formed metastases only in transplanted lung tissue, suggesting that lung is the only suitable "soil" in which melanoma cells can grow (24,30). Hormonal factors can also play an important role in the development of metastases. For instance, the osteo-tropism of breast tumors can be explained by the fact that these neoplastic cells can synthesize large amounts of prostaglandins and other osteolytic factors. These patients develop bone metastases and hypercalcemia due to osteolytic activity. This osteolysis can be inhibited in vitro by prostaglandin synthesis inhibitors, such as aspirin and indomethacin, which inhibit the prostaglandin synthetase (4,35). Also, administration of aspirin and indo-methacin inhibits the development of metastases and hypercalcemia in rats with Walker tumor (36).

CHARACTERISTICS OF METASTATIC CELLS

Recently attention has been paid to the study of alterations in cell surface carbohydrates during the neoplastic transformation. Thus the role of sialic acid was recently investigated and the ability of murine tumor cells (B_{16} mouse melanoma) to metastasize spontaneously from subcutaneous sites was positively correlated with the total sialic acid content in cell culture and most strongly with the degree of sialylation of galactosyl and acetylgalactosaminyl residues in cell surface glycoconjugates. The increased syalylation of glycocon-jugates on cell surface may enhance the metastatic behavior of tumor cells by increasing their adhesiveness, by increasing the formation of large cell emboli, by increased capacity to aggregate blood platelets, or by a decreased cell susceptibility to destruction by host immune defense mechanisms (52).

Cell surface properties and adhesiveness of neoplastic cells were the subject of intensive investigations in the 1940s. It was assumed that neoplastic cells lose their adhesion due to a defective mechanism, causing cell detach-ment and consequently cell mobilization and tendency to metastasize to occur. It was suggested that this low adhesion of neoplastic cells can be due to a decrease in calcium bridges between adjacent cancer cells (9). Although this notion was found to be incorrect, it is generally true that neoplastic cells are more easily detached from each other than are normal cells; most probably, as a result of inherent defects in their peripheral regions, the intrinsic mechanism of cell detachment and active mobilization, one of the main characteristics of metastatic behavior, are still not fully understood (18,34,37,41,46). Current

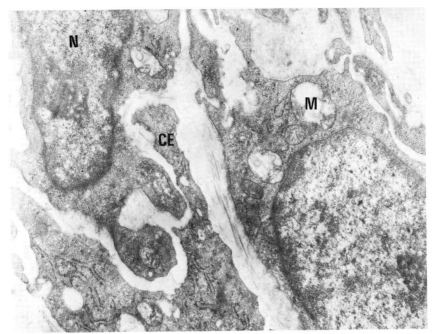

Figure 7-2 Electron micrograph showing metastatic epidermal cells (Squamous cell carcinoma). Complete lack of intercellular connections and poor differentiation. Long cell extensions can be seen (CE). N (nuclei) and abnormal mitochondria (M). Epon, uranyl acetate, and lead citrate, ×15,000.

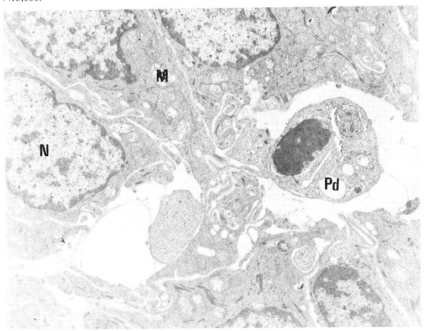

Figure 7-3 Electron micrograph showing metastatic cells (squamous cell carcinoma): They are poorly differentiated, tend to migrate by emitting extensive pseudopods (Pd). Nuclei (N) and mitochondria (M). Epon, uranyl acetate, and lead citrate, ×15,000.

ultrastructural studies show that in many instances cancer cells lose their intercellular connections, such as desmosomes and junctional complexes or terminal bars; they are separated by widened intercellular spaces with several microvilli and cell extensions, indicating an active cell mobilization. Hence, in addition to their defective physicochemical surface properties, metastatic cells exhibit some abnormalities in their intercellular connections (Fig. 7-2). It was also found by other investigators that cell and tissue interactions are disturbed in most tumors. Although a number of observations indicate that intercellular communications are abnormal in many neoplasms, the precise mechanism of these disturbances exhibited by neoplastic cells remains unknown (46). (Fig. 7-3).

FACTORS CONTROLLING THE METASTATIC PROCESS

It is possible that several humoral and cellular host factors can influence the cellular interactions between cancer cells and host tissues. For instance, stress can significantly affect the cellular detachment. Other factors can affect the metastatic process (or metastasibility) of experimentally induced neoplasms, as well. Thus, experiments with MCA-induced sarcoma in C57BL/6J mice show a decreased metastasibility when this tumor is transplanted or injected subcutaneously or intravenously in the nude mouse, which is an athymic or T cell-deficient animal. Concomitant administration of thymus cells to the nude mice bring the metastasibility and transplantability to the level of that observed in syngeneic mice. Also, spontaneous metastases from the same MCA-induced sarcoma did occur in the nude mice when specifically sensitized spleen cells were supplemented. These findings suggest that spontaneous metastases can be facilitated by weak immunoresponses. The occurrence of spontaneous metastasis is due mainly to the incapability of these mice to develop thymus-dependent immunoresponses (6). Also, the increased incidence of experimental metastases in nude mice is associated with a low level of natural killer (NK) cells. The metastatic incidence can be significantly decreased or inhibited by increasing NK-cell activity by a concomitant administration of bacterial adjuvants and interferon (19). Interferons are proteins derived from fibroblasts and leukocytes and possess antitumor activity. It is assumed that NK-cells are a subset of helper T-cells; they are cytotoxic cells. Hence, the metastatic potential is well correlated with the low levels of natural killer cell-mediated cytotoxicity.

The migration of metastatic cells is also under the influence of chemotactic factors. Thus injection of C_5-derived chemotactic factor into the peritoneal cavity of Sprague-Dawley rats induced diffuse mesenteric metastases after intravenous injection of Walker carcinosarcoma cells. Intraperitoneal injection of histamine or trypsin-treated albumin induced fewer metastases. Trauma, injury, and inflammation can also increase the incidence and location of metastases, possibly because of the generation of C_5-related chemotactic factors in that region. Thus mobilization and movement of neoplastic cells from the circulation may be under the influence of chemotactic factors somewhat similar to the responsiveness of neutrophils to leukotactic stimuli (25). There are also specific organ differences as regards the proliferation kinetics of tumor cells, which could explain the organ specificity of some metastases or seed-and-soil hypothesis. Thus there is a difference in labeling indexes by using tritiated thymidine (^{3}H-Tdr) autoradiography between tumor cells of rat ascites hepatoma (AH7974) arrested in the blood vessels of the brain to that of choroid plexus in both single and continuous tritiated thymidine administration (23). Also, specific aggregation occurs when tumor cells are suspended with purified organ cells. When pulmonophilic B-16 melanoma cells are suspended with different partially purified organ cells (liver, kidney, lungs, spleen, and red cells), the aggregation occurs mostly with lung cells. So, the affinity of these B-16 melanoma cells is much greater for lung cells as compared with liver, kidney, spleen, or red cells. These findings suggest that factors at the tumor cell–endothelial capillary cell interface are important for organ selection of metastases (30). Immunologic factors may also affect the pattern of metastasis; thus immunosuppression by high doses of cortisone or cyclophosphamide induces a wider distribution of labeled tumor cells after intravenous injection (17). Clinical and experimental observations show a predilection of certain neoplasms to implant and grow in specific organs; thus metastasis is a selective process. Recently selective cell lines that can metastasize preferentially in brain, lung, adrenal gland, or ovary were developed by repeated in vivo selections. Also, the reticuloendothelial system (RES) may play a role in clearance or retention of malignant cells, since this system is known to be responsible for the removal of foreign bodies from circulation; agents that stimulate or blockade the RES activity alter tumor growth. Thus, ^{125}I Urd-labeled cells from B-16 melanomas were injected into mice, and the lung retention of these malignant cells was determined. Experiments were performed in mice pretreated with endoxin or zymosan, modifying the RES activity. Thus, a retardation of arrested melanoma cells from the lung and a consequent increase of pulmonary metastases were observed in mice injected with endotoxin or zymosan. On the other hand, fewer metastatic nodules were observed in mice chronically treated with endotoxin. These experiments indicate that RES may play an important role in the control of dissemination of malignant cells and metastasis formation (16). The dissemination of neoplastic cells can also be influenced by some large glycoproteins such as *laminin* and *fibronectin*. Originally laminin is found in the basement membranes (namely in the lamina lucida) and is synthesized by a number of normal and neoplastic cells. However, recent studies indicate that laminin may either stimulate or inhibit the cell attachment, depending on the type of cells. *Fibronectin* due to its close contact to microfilaments, increases the contact and adhesion of neoplastic cells by interacting across the plasma membrane with actin microfilaments.

Hence both glycoproteins may play an important role in neoplastic cell dissemination.

DORMANT TUMOR CELLS

Clinical and experimental observations clearly suggest that a large population of neoplastic cells can be in a quiescent or dormant state. These poorly proliferating or nonproliferating cells can persist for several years, coexisting in some kind of symbiosis with the host cells (12,49). Thus, several histologic studies found, for example, in randomly examined thyroid at autopsy, that a large number of thyroids (49.5 percent) contained nodules from which 2 percent were histologically malignant. This 2 percent is a significant number, since the incidence of clinical thyroid cancer is only six in 1 million (29). Similar findings were made in studies regarding carcinoma of the prostate. Also, after the introduction of exfoliative cytology as a technique for cancer detection, it was found that a vast number of cervical carcinoma were carcinoma in situ. Altogether, these data demonstrate that a larger-than-expected number of cancers are in a clinically quiescent state or tumor dormancy (41). Autoradiographic studies show that most of these dormant cells are in a nonproliferating state or in the G_0 phase of the cell cycle (42). Probably several immunologic and hormonal factors must act to restrain these dormant or precancerous cells to proliferate into overt neoplasia. Recently several experimental models for the study of dormant cells were developed, showing that intravenously inoculated normal thyroid cells can survive for a long time, particularly in the lung. However, when these animals (mice) are rendered thyroxine deficient (hypothyroidism) by the administration of methylthiouracil (MTU), the thyroid cells proliferate and form typical follicles. Similar observations were made with thyroid cells obtained from hyperplastic or neoplastic glands; they remained in a dormant state for a long time until the animals were rendered thyroxine deficient. Hence, these neoplastic cells do not die, but remain in a dormant or quiescent state, yet are still responsive to hormonal stimuli, in this case, TSH (45). Also, trauma (such as repeated laparatomy and liver manipulation) markedly increased the liver metastases in rats following intraportal injection of Walker 256 carcinosarcoma cells. Tumor regrowth was possible even after a latency of 5 months (12). Also, dormant pulmonary metastases were described in rats. However, when these rats were immunologically suppressed by whole-body x-irradiation or thoracic duct drainage, these dormant or micrometastases develop into macrometastases (10). These experiments suggest an immunologically mediated restraint of dormant cells. Dormant neoplastic cells can be also hormonally stimulated. Thus in an estrogen-dependent experimental tumor, stimulation of dormant cells was achieved by estrogen administration after 10 months of dormancy (31).

The clinical importance of dormant cells is demonstrated by the late occurrence of metastases in patients with carcinoma of the breast, prostate carcinoma, malignant melanoma, thyroid carcinoma, and hypernephroma. These clinical and experimental observations demonstrate that the neoplastic cells can be kept quiescent or dormant for a long period of time; this latency or dormancy is an important state in therapy and prophylactic control of cancers.

ENDOCRINOLOGIC MODULATION OF DORMANT NEOPLASTIC CELLS AND MICROMETASTASES

Experimental observations suggest that dormant cells are mostly located extravascularly and are still under hormonal control. Since it has been demonstrated that hormones and hormonelike substances exert an important modulating effect on the onset, development, and regression of primary neoplasms (Chapter 4), it is logical to assume that hormones influence the metastatic process as well. However, investigations into the role of hormones on cancer invasion and metastasis formation are few and sporadically reported. Inasmuch as the metastatic cells are neoplastic cells similar to those of the parent tumor, they partially preserve the hormone responsiveness due to retention of receptor site(s) (Fig. 7–1a).

Thus, experimental and clinical investigations of mammary cancer, thyroid carcinoma, and prostrate neoplasms revealed that the presence of estrogen receptors, TSH receptors or androgen receptors indicate a poorly metastasizing process and a favorable response to hormonal manipulation, whereas the absence of hormone receptors indicate a high metastatic potential and tendency to invasiveness. These data provide some hopes of controlling the treatment and prophylaxis of metastases. Thus, in breast cancer with advanced metastases, the ablation of estrogen producing organs (ovariectomy, adrenalectomy) can favorably affect the evolution of metastases. Also, metastases from differentiated thyroid carcinoma (in lymph nodes, bones, or lung) are still dependent and responsive to TSH stimulation for growth. Suppression of TSH secretion by exogenous thyroxine shrinks, and in some cases, both in animal and human cancers, arrests the metastatic process. Ultrastructural studies show that thyroid metastatic cells in lymph nodes exhibit most of the ultrastructural characteristics of parent thyroid cells from primary tumor; these neoplastic cells also incorporate radioiodine and synthesize thyroglobulin, which can be used as a marker for these metastates.

Prostate cancer and its metastases provide a similar clinical and experimental model. Most of the earlier investigations focused on the effects of corticosteroid hormones on metastatic induction. Thus, cortisone administration induced a marked inhibition or arrest of local growth of transplantable mammary carcinoma in C_3H mice. Metastases of transplanted adenocarcinoma were never observed in nontreated animals. However, multiple metastases occurred at about 5 to 6 weeks after transplantation in cortisone-treated mice. The longer the animal survived, the greater was the incidence of cortisone-induced metastases. These cortisone-induced metastases are histologically similar to local growth of transplanted tumor; they can be also transplanted and produce local growth. However, the transplanted metastases did not grow unless cortisone was given to the new host. It is possible that the metastasizing action of cortisone is similar to that of hyaluronidase, which enhances the propagation of neoplastic cells. Estrogens and steroid hormones potentiate these hyaluronidase effects. Also, it is likely that cortisone acts on immune neoplastic–host cell relationships by inhibiting the immune host-defense mechanism (1,28). Cortisone administration also increases the incidence of lung metastases after intravenous injection of tumor cell suspension from Krebs II adenocarcinoma, but not with Sarcoma 37 in mice. This discrepancy is attributable to differences of local tissues or "soil," since the same marked discrepancy occurs in the distribution of both tumors after injection in the left ventricle of animals with or without cortisone treatment. Tissue reactivity around metastases develops concomitantly with recovery of reticulo-endothelial system (RES). Thus cortisone may act first on RES by decreasing the tissue-specific antibody production (33). The metastasizing effect of cortisone, and perhaps the role of other hormones on the metastatic process, can be explained by the effect on RES activity, and especially production of specific tissue antibodies. Supporting this hypothesis is our previous investigation regarding cortisone effects on RES activity, in which it was demonstrated that administration of cortisone acetate and hydrocortisone markedly decreases the phagocytic activity of Kupffer cells in rat liver (Lupulescu, 1958). Enhancement of metastatic process by cortisone administration has also been demonstrated in mice implanted with DMBA (dimethylbenzanthracene) tumors. Whereas the untreated animals develop no tumors, the cortisone-treated mice develop a large number of metastases. Also, original methylcholanthrene-tumors showed enhanced metastasis formation (3). Cortisone appears to affect the local milieu of the disseminated neoplastic cells. Thus, cortisone can induce metastases from tumors that ordinarily do not metastasize.

Another important observation is that cortisone not only enhances metastatic formation, but causes a shift in the organ distribution of metastases. Thus, pretreatment with cortisone shifts the predominant site of metastases from the lung in normal mice to the liver in cortisone-treated mice (28). A suspension of carcinosarcoma cells from Sarcoma 180, Krebs-2, and Ehrlich ascites was injected into pretreated-cortisone mice, producing primarily liver metastases, while as in normal mice, lung metastases predominate—clear evidence of the existence of a difference in "soil," which can be altered by hormones, namely cortisone. The Walker carcinosarcoma is another cortisone-sensitive tumor. Pretreatment with cortisone inhibits tumor growth by about 50 percent. Cortisone also significantly inhibits the growth rate of the Ehrlich ascites tumor in CGW mice. The inhibition is dose-related. However, the growth rate of the Ehrlich tumor is significantly increased in adrenalectomized mice (48).

In our series of experiments using squamous cell carcinomas and basal cell carcinomas induced with MCA in mice and rats concomitantly treated with cortisone or hydrocortisone, because the tumor development was markedly inhibited by cortisone, no metastasis formation was observed (see ref. 49a). Also, an increase in the frequency of spleen metastases was observed in the patients with advanced breast cancer and treated with cortisone and/or prednisone. Thus among 31 cortisone-treated patients with disseminated breast cancers, the autopsy showed spleen metastases in eight cases, whereas no spleen metastases were found in patients not treated with cortisone (21).

Possible mechanisms of cortisone metastasizing action were evoked, such as decreased adhesiveness of neoplastic cells, increased permeability of connective tissue and blood capillaries, decreased activity of the RES system, and consequently of antibody production, creating favorable conditions for the implantation of neoplastic cells by altering the local milieu. Body irradiation and pregnancy may increase metastatic frequency. Thus other hormones, such as estrogens, can increase metastatic process. Also pituitary growth hormones (GH) can increase the incidence of lung metastases after intravenous injection of Sarcoma T_{241} cells. Pretreatment with GH of the recipient mouse increases the number of lung metastases and also accelerates their growth. However, GH given after cell injection was ineffective (50). It was recently reported that 17β-estradiol and insulin are essential for MCF-7 human breast carcinoma and tumor metastasis. Thus, MCF-7 are able to metastasize to lungs, liver, and spleen. 17β-Estradiol treatment increases both the growth rate and frequency of metastases. Castration or diabetes prevents metastasis formation, but treatment with estrogens or insulin restores the metastatic capacity. High levels of collagenase were also found in chemically induced (by MCA) papillomas and carcinomas of dorsal mouse skin and in carcinomas of human urinary bladder. Carcinomas had higher enzyme levels as compared to papillomas. The infiltrative growth of the carcinoma may be directly related to high collagenase activity. An enhanced collagenase production by the fibroblasts was recently found in human basal carcinomas (3a). By using immunofluorescent staining it was found that collagenase activity was always higher in tumor tissue as compared to normal surrounding tissue. The collagenolytic activity can be correlated to tumor differentiation. The activity is higher in poorly differentiated adenocarcinomas; it was also higher in medullary than in scirrhous tumors and was weak in benign tumors. There is evidence that metastatic cells can produce a specific collagenase for basement membranes. These findings indicate that connective tissue and collagenase may play an important role in tumor invasion and poorly understood metastatic process. Hormones may change the collagenase activity. Since both estrogens and insulin enhanced the production of collagenases in culture media, it was postulated that these hormones exert their metastasizing effects by enhancing collagenase production (39).

Prostaglandins (PGs) E_2 and $F_{2\alpha}$ (PGE_2 and $PGF_{2\alpha}$) markedly enhance the growth of primary tumor and also slightly increase metastasis formation. In our investigations regarding the effects of PGE_2 and $PGF_{2\alpha}$ on tumor development and the metastatic process, it was found that they significantly increase the incidence and development of squamous cell carcinomas induced by topical application of MCA on mouse skin. However, only in a few instances were spontaneous metastases observed in the stomach, lung, and eye. These metastases are histologically similar to parent neoplasms. Human breast carcinomas contain and synthesize more PG-like material than is seen either in normal breast tissue from the same patients or in benign tumors. A higher PG activity was detected in the suspensions of neoplastic cells from patients with advanced breast carcinoma, bone metastases and osteolytic activity and it was postulated that prostaglandins may play an important role in the evolution of tumor metastases (4,35,36). Although most investigations demonstrate that PGE_2 and $PGF_{2\alpha}$ enhance the growth of primary neoplasm and only slightly the incidence of spontaneous formation, a few indicate that prostacyclin (PGI_2), one of the most potent antithrombogenic agents, and PGD_2, exert antimetastatic effects. Accordingly, the effect may result from the platelet antiaggregatory action of prostacyclin and can be potentiated by phosphodiesterase inhibitors (theophylline). Thus a concomitant administration of theophylline and prostacyclin markedly reduces lung metastasis formation in mice injected with cell suspension from a B-16 amelanotic melanoma. Inhibitors of prostacyclin synthesis increase metastasis formation. It is postulated that prostacyclin in vivo may play an important role in controlling the metastatic process (20).

THERAPEUTIC STRATEGIES REGARDING METASTASES

Significant progress in the treatment of metastases was recently made due to the studies regarding the cell kinetics, cell population growth, and cell cycle in the metastatic foci as compared with that of primary tumor. By using electron microscopy and SEM it was shown that the metastatic cells are qualitatively different from their parent somatic cells in primary tumors. Recent studies using ^{3}H-thymidine autoradiography demonstrate that metastatic cells are also quantitatively different from parent tumor cells.

These studies point out that in most experimental metastatic tumors, and also in human cancer metastases, the cell growth rate of both adenocarcinomas and squamous cell carcinomas is exceeded by the growth rate of their metastases. On the basis of analysis of 530 human tumors, a mechanical explanation suggests that cell exfoliation is much greater in the primary tumors than in their metastases (7). Also, an angiogenetic factor was isolated from tumors and was made responsible for tumor metastases (13). Studies show that cell population kinetics and the labeling index of transplanted and metastatic Lewis lung carcinoma, either as primary subcutaneous tumors or spontaneous lung metastases, decrease with increasing age or mass. Thus the metastatic tumors have a shorter doubling time (DT) than does the primary tumor. Also, the cell cycle and S (DNA synthesis phase) phase are shorter in metastatic tumors than in the primary tumors. The synthetic rate of the same amount of material (DNA, RNA, proteins) should be higher (1.5 to twofold) in the metastatic cells as compared to cells of the primary tumor. These autoradiographic studies clearly indicate that the metastatic cells are more rapidly dividing cells and have a shorter cell cycle, especially shorter S and G_1 phases, than do their parent somatic cells of the primary tumors (40,41).

Interestingly, S, G_2, and M-phase cells from the rapidly growing primary tumors produced more metastases (lung metastases) than G_1-phase cells. In vitro tissue culture studies showed that all cells from different cell cycle phases have the same clonogenicity, but the larger size of S, G_2, and M-phase cells or alterations on their cell surface, such as adhesiveness or deformability, could explain these differences in metastatic potential (44). This more rapid growth rate and cell kinetics of metastatic tumors can be related somewhat, according to the Gompertz function, to their smaller mass and age. The Gompertz equation, mathematically states that tumor growth is exponential at every instant but its growth constant is simultaneously decreasing exponentially. Thus reduction in tumor mass markedly shortens the doubling time (DT). All these data indicate that the metastatic cells having a shorter cell cycle and a more rapid cell growth rate are also more sensitive to the chemotherapeutic drugs. This sensitivity of metastatic cells can be related to the reduction in their mass (a quantitative factor), but a selective cell process with different biochemical and ultrastructural characteristic during the metastatic process cannot be ruled out. Therefore, the rapidly growing tumor cell population of metastases is more sensitive to antimetabolite drugs than the large and slower growing cell populations of the primary tumors.

According to the cell kinetics and cell cycle studies, the tumor cell populations at any certain time can be divided into three cell proliferative compartments: (I) dividing cancer cells, which are always in G_1 phase; (II) temporarily dividing cells, which can revert to (I) at any time from their G_0; or resting phase and (III) compartments of nondividing cancer cells, which have lost forever their proliferative capacity. Cells from the first compartment are always very sensitive to chemotherapeutic drugs, hormones or radiation; cells from the second compartment are only partially responsive to these drugs and the cells from the third compartment have completely lost their responsiveness. Recently it has been shown that cells from compartment IV are mainly composed of dying cells due to lyses or resorption by their neighbors, a phenomenon called apoptosis (from the Greek word apoptosis, "the dropping off of leaves from the trees") may play an important role in controlling tumor cell kinetics and homeostasis. Apoptosis can also be hormonally-induced (by glucocorticoids) and hormonally-controlled (52).

Thus, cancer drugs can be classified into two broad classes: (1) cell cycle specific (CCS) drugs, which act mostly during the cell cycle by interfering with the S phase (DNA synthesis) (however, there are CCS agents that are not cell cycle stage specific (CCSS) as well); and (2) drugs that are cell cycle nonspecific (CCNS) (antibiotics and alkylating agents). The first group kills cancer cells mostly when they are in the synthetic stage preparing for replication; the second group kills tumor cells whether or not they are in active metabolic stage, but dormant or resting cells as well. However, cytotoxic activity is greater than, but not rigidly correlated to, the cell cycle phases. For instance, CCS inhibits both DNA and RNA synthesis mostly in metabolically active cells, but is not restricted to cells in S, G_1, or G_2 phases; also, CCNS drugs are still more active during the metabolic activity than against resting cells. The difficult problem of metastasis treatment is first to detect the metastatic foci in their initial stage (micrometastasis) before they become clinically manifest (macrometastases). Also, the small fraction of nonkilled cells becomes more active and markedly increases the cloning efficiency. The presence of these inactivated (by drug or radiation) cells markedly increases or activates (by three- to fourfold) when suspended into a large, slow-growing population of cancer cells. This happens in many human tumors (cervical carcinoma, Hela cells) and in experimental transplanted tumors (Lewis lung carcinoma, B-16 melanoma, C_3H adenocarcinoma) in mice and hamsters after drug administration, radiation, or surgical manipulation (38). These findings also suggest that a regrowth can occur in radiologically, chemotherapeutically, or hormonally treated cancers, from this small portion of inactivated or still-viable cancer cells. This should be kept in mind when drugs, hormones, radiation, or immune factors are used for therapeutic purposes. Cells from compartment I are always dividing cells, and the proportion of dividing cells is higher when the tumor is small and when these are the only cells killed by CCS agents. Cells from compartment II are metabolically resting or inactive, but they retain the potential to resume cell division. Hence, when the dividing cell population from compartment I decreases to a subtotal radiation dose, incomplete surgical removal, or inadequate drug doses, cells move from compartment II into compartment I along with increasing cell proliferation and return of their sensitivity to CCS drugs. Cells from compartment III may be metabolically active but are incapable of cell division (they are progressing toward differentiated cells) and those of compartment IV (cell loss by lysis and resorption). Although cells from compartments III and IV are in the majority, representing most of the tumor mass, they are practically of no therapeutic value for radiation, drugs, or hormones, since they are nondividing cells and cannot resume their dividing activity (Fig. 7-4).

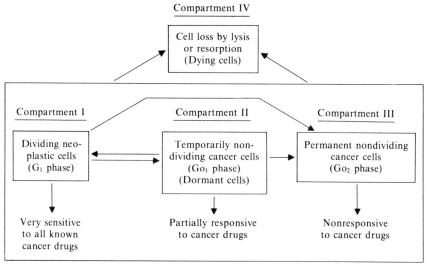

Figure 7-4 The proliferative compartments of cancer cells and their related sensitivity to cancer therapeutic drugs.

Clinical Metastases (Macrometastases): Strategies and Approaches for Treatment

Unfortunately, in spite of research and progress made in the last few decades, approximately 50 percent of all cancers are only detected in this advanced stage, when metastases are clinically manifest. Most micrometastases, especially those in lymph nodes, occur according to the examination of surgical specimens, even before therapy. In cases in which the disease is still localized, we have to (1) first eradicate the primary tumor, (2) thoroughly search for micrometastases, and (3) institute additional therapy in order to eradicate the micrometastases. When metastases are clinically manifest (i.e., macrometastases), we must treat the patient as we would for systemic disease. First, we have to reduce [at maximum] the surgical manipulations, in order to minimize the discharge of cancer cells from the primary tumor and their dissemination into circulation. Since some metastatic cells still retain their receptor site(s), these metastases are still responsive to the same drugs or hormones as are primary tumors. In this advanced stage, the clinician's attention should focus mainly on controlling metastases. The basis for the therapy of metastases is the higher growth fraction rate of cancer cells. Second, some metastatic cells are not as sensitive to the same drug as are the primary tumor cells. We must also make a distinction between the use of CCS drugs and CCNS drugs. Whereas CCS drugs can kill cancer cells at lower doses, hence are less toxic, the CCNS drugs always act according to a dose–response curve, which means that we have to use high, constant doses;

thus such patients are always exposed to high risks of toxicity. Combined or multiple use of therapeutic agents, such as chemotherapeutic drugs, radiation, or hormones, can reduce these risks. If the primary tumor is responsive to a drug, we have to try the same drug for its metastases, but if the primary tumor is not responsive to one drug, this does not deny its consideration for the treatment of its metastases. Always, when it is suspected after surgical removal for irradiation of the primary tumor, that metastases are present, chemotherapy, hormone therapy, or immunotherapy for the control of metastases should be started immediately.

Despite the progress and achievements made recently, the clinical oncologist is mostly confronted with an established stage of metastases—the most difficult situation in controlling the metastatic process. This stage is one of the most devastating causes of death, with 50 percent of human cancers having metastasized before clinical detection. The oncologist should corroborate with the endocrinologist, surgeon, radiologist, and immunologist in order to evaluate more accurately drug or hormone dependence and responsiveness and immune host–metastatic relationships. Of course, it is difficult to eradicate an entire population of cancer cells and thus eradicate the fatal disease, since it has been demonstrated that even a single cancer cell can proliferate and produce different neoplastic type cells. This monoclonal origin was established in most animal tumors tested with chemical carcinogens or in some myelomas of humans and animals originating from one cell and producing a single specific immunoglobulin. For instance, most advanced metastatic stages of human breast tumors, differentiated thyroid carcinoma, and prostatic cancers are partially responsive to the same drug or hormones as are the primary tumors. In this case, control of clinically manifest metastases should be started as soon as possible after eradication of the primary tumor, in an effort to prevent the dissemination of metastatic cells.

Despite the increased used of nonhormonal chemotherapeutic agents in recent years, the achievement of "cure" in advanced metastatic cancers is still a remote objective. In my opinion, practicing oncologists should be more realistic and more modest in their expectations and should rely mainly on the palliative methods that use drugs increasing the duration of survival and remission, providing a better tolerance and quality of life, with minimal untoward or toxic effects. For this reason, hormonal therapy alone or combined with nonhormonal agents still has a major role in the management of advanced breast metastatic cancer, prostate carcinoma, and thyroid carcinoma.

With improved radioimmunoassays for hormone receptors (estrogens, progesterone, androgens, and thyrotropin) on metastatic cancer cells and the development of new hormone agents, investigators are turning increasingly toward combined hormonal with nonhormonal therapeutic agents in treating this advanced metastatic stage of disease. The rationale for this therapy was to combine rapidly acting nonhormonal agents with slow-acting but less toxic hormonal agents. This additive therapy with nonhormonal agents, such as chemotherapeutic drugs, radiation, or immunotherapy, increases the duration of survival and remission, provides palliative effects, and minimizes untoward effects (alopecia, nausea, vomiting, hematotoxicity, neurotoxicity, oral ulcerations, and diarrhea). This combined therapy should always be attempted by oncologists, especially when a single therapeutic agent has failed. Clearly, the survival rate is considerably longer in patients with positive hormone receptor tests, reaching 50 to 60 percent in some advanced metastatic breast cancers. Furthermore, in nonresponders to endocrine therapy, such patients subjected to combined hormonal and nonhormonal therapy experience increased duration of survival and reduced recurrence, as compared with results with one therapeutic agent. Some advocates of this combined therapeutic procedure believe that the principal agents are the hormones and the nonhormonal agents used to support the hormonal therapy (5,22,38,42,49). The selection among chemotherapy, surgical removal, radiation therapy, hormone therapy, or immunotherapy of advanced metastatic disease resides mainly in the hands of the clinical oncologist, that is, in his or her competence in administering drug therapy, as well as skill in orchestrating these therapeutic procedures for each patient, thereby developing an individual treatment therapy. Also, in trials for new drugs, the clinical oncologist must be aware that some of these means may have a carcinogenic and metastatic potential.

COMMENTS AND CONCLUSIONS

Although most cancer patients (50 to 60 percent) die as a result of the metastatic process, and the malignancy of tumors is chiefly defined according to their tendency to invasion and metastasis, investigations have focused mainly on primary tumors. Since spontaneous metastases occur only seldom in experimental animal cancers, it is difficult to extrapolate data obtained from animals inoculated with cancer cells; hence we still lack a valid experimental model similar to that of human metastatic cancers. Nevertheless, significant progress has been made with the aid of modern methods, and it is now demonstrated that tumors are heterogeneous cell populations, or a mosaic of cells. Each tumor is composed of many cell subpopulations, or cell lines, which are different both qualitatively and (probably) quantitatively.

Metastatic cells are cells that exhibit different ultrastructural, cell-surface, and autoradiographic characteristics, thus exhibiting a high malignant potential and tendency to invasiveness. However, the metastatic process is more complex and cannot be explained by mechanical and biophysical characteristic of metastatic cells. Metastatic cells are neoplastic cells endowed with different biochemical, cell surface and molecular properties which make them more malignant, capable of invading, locating, and growing in a different local milieu or remote environment. They are super cells. The organ selection, organ specificity, or organotropism for different tumor metastases is another unresolved, poorly understood mechanism. The organ selection cannot be explained by seed and soil hypothesis alone. Metastatic cells, especially from micrometastases, are more rapidly dividing cells as compared with their parent somatic cells. However, they can remain for years in a latent or quiescent stage, in so-called dormancy. In some cases, an equilibrium is established between dividing and dormant cells that can at any time reenter the cell cycle and again proliferate. Hence, the metastatic process is more complex, and several factors can affect it. Recent data originating from studies on human cancers as well as on experimentally induced tumors strongly suggest that hormones can affect the invasiveness and metastasis formation of the cancer; also, organ specificity may be under some hormonal control. Thus the metastatic process is under endocrinologic regulation. Hormones act primarily as modulators on the metastatic process. They can increase the cell detachment by decreasing the intercellular connections, can act on dormant cells, can facilitate their reentry into the cell cycle (Fig. 7–1) of metastatic cells, ultimately inducing a local milieu favorable for location and growth of metastatic cells. Hormones and endocrinologic factors also have an important role in the treatment of advanced metastatic cancers. These patients should be treated as for systemic disease. Clinical oncologists should always be aware of the existence of micrometastases; a thorough search for their detection should be made, before any drugs, radiation, or other therapeutic agents are administered. Micrometastases are always more sensitive to cell cycle specific drugs than are their parent neoplastic cells. In patients in whom metastic cells still retain their hormone receptors, hormonotherapy should be tried first. In these cases, micrometastases and macrometastases are hormonoresponsive, and control of the metastatic process can be achieved in most instances. In cases in which metastatic cells have already lost their receptors, prognosis is poor, additive or combined therapy using a chemotherapeutic agent, radiation, and hormone therapy, should be instituted. This multiple, additive, or combined therapy reduces untoward or toxic effects and provides significant palliative effects. Since there is no statistical evidence that the use of highly toxic drugs, or so-called aggressive therapy, in advanced metastatic stages, can increase the duration of survival, significantly improving chances for "cure," I believe it is better to use a more conservative or palliative therapy. This approach provides similar effects, is less toxic, and offers patients a better quality of life. A realistic goal is not to attempt to "cure" the disease in the advanced stage, but to prolong the patient's survival and the quality of life. The clinical oncologist should not be so enthusiastic, but rather more modest and realistic in his judgments and decisions. Further research is still needed in order to clarify the biologic mechanisms of metastatic process and its controlling factors, namely endocrinologic modulation of metastases. In spite of intense research in this area, dissemination of cancer cells, cancer invasion, and the metastasizing process still remain the most intriguing events of cell biology of cancer cells. Data obtained from experimental tumor systems that correlate with or partially explain cancer invasion include the ameboid mobility of some cancer cells, decreased cell adhesiveness, cell-to-cell cohesion, release of lytic enzymes, lack of intercellular communications, and increased tumor tissue pressure owing to accelerated cell division of the central mass. However, few data relate directly to the mechanism(s) of metastatic process in humans. Of great therapeutic significance is the tumor cell dormancy and the presence of micrometastases. Tumor cells can persist in a dormant, nonproliferating or latent stage for many years, in symbiosis with the host organism. Thus distant metastases can appear many years after achieving an effective, permanent control of primary tumors in patients with breast carcinoma, prostate cancer, malignant melanoma, and hypernephroma. Several factors, such as mechanical (trauma), immunologic, and hormonal, can inhibit or accelerate the growth of these dormant cells. For instance, it has been demonstrated that trauma (surgical manipulation or partial hepatectomy) can enhance the growth of dormant cells from Walker 256 tumors in liver. Pulmonary dormant cells can grow to manifest clinical metastases when rats are immunosuppressed by the whole-body irradiation or thoracic duct drainage. Since this compartment of nonproliferating or dormant malignant cells represents a large pool of neoplastic cells, further research should be directed toward its controlling factors, particularly hormones and hormonelike substances.

Most advancements and improvements in knowledge that have been derived lately from the study of cellular kinetics and the cell cycle of neoplastic cells can direct our therapeutic strategies. Thus, as a tumor grows and its mass increases, the fraction of proliferating cells decreases, because many cells are leaving the proliferating phase of the cell cycle to enter a resting or dormant stage. Since most therapeutic agents (cytotoxic, radiation) exert their effects primarily on cells in the proliferating cycle, this can explain the resistance of tumors to chemotherapy or radiation therapy. However, we can manipulate tumor cell kinetics through the use of hormones, which stimulate the reentry into the proliferating cell cycle, thereby exposed these neoplastic cells again to therapeutic agents and increasing the effectiveness of chemotherapy or radiation therapy. This cell kinetic manipulation by hormones is an important factor in the treatment of cancer metastases. These CCS antimetabolites inhibit both DNA and RNA synthesis in actively dividing cells, but their activity is not strictly related to the cell cycle stage (S, G_1, G_2), hence they are far less demanding of a rigid treatment schedule in order to obtain an optimum therapeutic response, as compared with CCSS (cell cycle stage specific) drugs, for which these drugs should be used first.

Estrogens can stimulate the growth of dormant cells in several experimental tumors. It is possible that estrogens as other hormones exert their carcinogenic action not per se, but acting mainly on the dormant cells by enhancing their growth, and thus their reentry into the cell cycle from their G_0

phase. Hormones can also restrain the growth of dormant cells and hold the neoplastic cells at this stage for many years (Fig. 7–4). Thus hormones and hormonelike substances can markedly reverse the dormancy of neoplastic cells—this is a promising field for cancer research and for therapeutic implications as well. Since approximately 60 percent of all clinical cancers have metastases at the time of diagnosis, cancer should always be considered and treated as a systemic disease. Hence, research should be oriented toward the development of new adjuvant chemotherapy and hormonal agents for the sensitive metastatic cell strains. Hormone therapy should be used in all hormone-dependent cancers, as well as in many hormone-responsive tumors. In many patients with advanced metastatic cancers, hormones enhance the primary effects of chemotherapeutic agents, radiation therapy, or immune therapy and reduce their toxic effects, thereby reducing cancer invasiveness and prolonging the survival rate.

It is difficult, however, for the clinical oncologist to select a proper drug and dose and to predict the outcome of therapy in advanced cancer metastases. This difficulty arises from differences between cell kinetics and cell proliferation in the large masses of macrometastases, as compared with those of micrometastases. Hence, the drug response will be different in these large tumor masses. The effectiveness of a chemotherapeutic drug is dependent primarily on the size of a homogeneous kinetical cell population at the start of treatment; in order to ensure a "cell cure," population size should not exceed the total cell-kill capacity of the dose; if the population size exceeds this, no "cell cure" will occur. For this reason, it is better to start the treatment of micrometastases with CCS drugs that do not require high doses at the outset—CCNS drugs should be used in high doses, which will consequently increase the normal cell recovery from drug toxicity and will also have higher toxicity risks to vital normal cells, whereas CCS drug activity will be maximal at lower risk of toxicity to vital normal cells. Thus, in the case of drug resistance, we should recommend a combined therapy that can provide increased efficacy, as well as lower toxicity risks. At present, we do not know the intrinsic mechanism(s) of hormones on the metastatic neoplastic cells, for example, on DNA synthesis and replication, RNA and protein synthesis, cell surface and adhesiveness, cellular interconnection, or cell receptors. It appears that hormones act on more than one or two cell parameters. Even in patients with hormone-independent cancers, hormone therapy can provide significant palliative effects and a better quality of life. Various steroid hormones are used, such as corticosteroids and androgenic anabolic steroids to improve the feeling of well-being and increase the appetite and reduce the toxic reactions of cytotoxic agents. Recent experimental and clinical investigations, as well as the paraneoplastic effects of tumor, suggest that a hormonal milieu is important in the implantation and growth of metastatic cells in different organs; further studies are required to define this milieu and the role of hormones in modulating and controlling the cancer invasiveness and metastatic process. Hormones can modulate the growth rate of metastases as well as their organ specificity. For instance, cortisone can induce a shift in the metastase distribution from the lung in nontreated mice to the liver in cortisone-treated mice, enhancing the incidence of liver metastases. Also, in patients with advanced metastatic breast cancer, cortisone-treatment increases significantly the spleen metastases. Prostaglandins increase the bone metastase formation. These findings suggest that hormones are important factors in preparing the "soil and seeding" of the metastatic cells in a certain organ. It is interesting to mention that the same hormones (e.g., cortisone, estrogens) can exert opposite effects on the growth of primary tumor (by inhibiting or arresting it) and on metastases (by enhancing their growth rate, spreading and location). Further investigations are required in order to develop, by means of continuous cell selection and transplantability, new metastatic cell lines that will be more sensitive to hormones, radiation therapy, or antimetabolites. Such an accomplishment will be important for the treatment of advanced cancers with disseminated macrometastases. In many patients, hormones, whether alone or combined with radiation or antimetabolites, can act on and control the primary tumor and micrometastases, but are shown to exert poor action on macrometastases. We do not know why metastatic cells from macrometastase behave differently from their sister cells of micrometastases in terms of therapeutic response. These differences between micrometastatic and macrometastatic cells might be explained by a disequilibrium between the cell kinetics and proliferation in the three compartments, or macrometastatic cells might be more malignant and poorly differentiated cells as compared with micrometastatic cells.

We know that most micrometastatic cells are dividing cells that originate as the dormant neoplastic cells, still preserving, either totally or partially, their cellular characteristics, kinetics, and cell replication, as well as their receptor site(s), from their parent somatic neoplastic cells. However, the neoplastic cells from advanced disseminated and macrometastases are poorly differentiated cells that lost their receptor sites and that became more independent and autonomous in regard to growth and invasiveness. In spite of the many investigations in this field, we do not know why some tumors can grow without metastasizing for several years, and why others exhibit a highly metastatic potential and invasiveness from the outset. This is not related to tumor mass, but mostly to the cell lines, to their characteristic host–tumor immune defense mechanism, and to hormonal environment. For this reason, new animal models having greater sensitivity and accuracy should be developed if we are to extrapolate data from experimental oncology for use in clinical oncology.

The human model cannot be as easily manipulated as can the metastatic process of experimental animals. Do metastatic neoplastic cells represent a different mutant subpopulation derived by a clonal selection that can grow and multiply in a hostile environment—that is, are they some kind of super cell?

Since many cells detach and enter the circulation, but only few are able to locate and metastasize, it is natural to conclude that the metastatic cell is, in fact, a different mutant neoplastic cell. Electron microscopic, autoradiographic, and SEM studies also indicate that metastatic cells exhibit a peculiar and sometimes bizarre ultrastructural and cell surface pattern, having a rapid tendency and propensity to form colonies. Also, these cells are more rapidly dividing cells with a shorter cell cycle as compared with neoplastic cells from the original tumor. Clinical observations accumulated from surgical material (since the first surgical interventions were performed at the end of the last century in advanced metastatic cancers), also suggest a correlation between the rapidly growing tumors and their tendency to metastasize, as compared with slower growing tumors, most of which remain in a latent stage, without metastasizing.

An attempt to correlate the capacity to metastasize with the histologic type of primary tumor was also made. Studies of the cell kinetics of the resected specimens from the primary tumor, as well as from the latent micrometastasis, can be helpful for a good or poor prognosis for the patients with extensive metastatic thyroid cancers and for some with axillary metastasis of breast cancer. Thus, a rapidly dividing cell population would indicate a propensity of these cells for metastasis and poor prognosis; vice versa, slowly dividing cells are an indication for good prognosis. Hence, studies of cell kinetics and replication are good parameters for possibly distinguishing between latent micrometastases and those with an active growing potential and also between primary tumors which exhibit in most cases a high metastatic potential. Thus, cell kinetics studies can be better correlated with the metastatic potential than can tumor size or even histologic type.

The metastatic potential is directly related to special properties of tumor cells as well as to tumor–host interactions. A good latency period for the metastases of papillary thyroid carcinomas and some mammary carcinomas was established; only a few micrometastatic thyroid papillary carcinomas evolve toward clinically manifest metastases. Estimation of TSH receptors and the capacity of thyroid neoplastic cells to incorporate radioiodine and synthesize thyroglobulin are interesting parameters in establishing a good or poor prognosis and in making therapeutic decisions. Tumor transplantability experiments indicate that each tumor has a particular threshold. After the individual threshold dose is achieved, the transplantability and metastasizing capacity follows a dose–response curve. This tumor threshold depends mainly on various factors that can modulate tumor–host reactions, hence the environment in which neoplastic cells will disseminate.

Sometimes the primary tumor exerts inhibitory effects on the metastatic process. It is therefore important to minimize the use of such traumatic interventions as surgical removal of the primary tumor or other therapeutic or diagnostic procedures that can enhance the dissemination of tumor cells. A traumatic injury can be a good site for clinical metastases. Also, hormones and hormone-like substances can lower the tumor threshold and modulate the environment and thus can explain the occurrence of some unusual types of metastases.

However, many neoplastic strains that are sensitive to hormones or chemotherapeutic agents in vitro do not demonstrate sensitivity to the same agents in vivo. Unfortunately, most of these interesting findings are derived from experimental models that have certainly improved our knowledge regarding the biogenesis and mechanisms of metastatic process, but cannot be translated to human models.

In many cases the clinical oncologist is confronted with an established metastatic process. The classification of tumors in different stages on the basis of histologic structure remains arbitrary. Recent data demonstrate that the metastatic process is a complex one, of which histologic structure is only one parameter.

The extrapolation of data obtained from experimental models to the human metastatic process has failed in many cases, generally attributable to an unrealistic approach. It is easy to induce metastases in laboratory animals by injecting cell suspension, instead of studying spontaneous tumors and their metastases, which are closer to the human model. Modern methods such as electron microscopy and SEM should be used more often in investigating the morphologic events of the metastatic process. We do not know why human tumors have a low tendency to metastasize when transplanted in laboratory animals, as compared with their behavior in the clinical setting. Clearly, better experimental models for the study of metastases and therapeutic evaluation are needed. The role of hormones in cancer invasion and metastasis, as well as their therapeutic effects in many HDCs or in other HRTs should be thoroughly explored, since the immediate goal of oncologists is to prevent or arrest cancer invasion and the metastatic process.

The principal aim of this study is to indicate that the metastatic process is not a random process, but rather one that depends on many factors, including cellular factors, hormones, immunology, genetics, and vascular relationships. The pathophysiology of the metastatic process is still poorly understood. Most tumor cells exhibit greater mobility and migration as a result of defective synthesis of fibronectin (FN) and collagen-derived peptides (CDP). This defective FN and CDP synthesis can explain the initial phases of the metastatic process, as well as the predominant location of some metastases in organs rich in connective tissue.

In the last decade, it has been shown that collagen is a family of genetically distinct proteins. There are five types (I–V) of collagen. From these, type IV, primarily located in the basement membrane, is presumed to play an important role in tumor invasion and tumor-stromal reaction. Also, the enzymatic degradation of the basement membrane, which contains mostly collagen type IV, increases the incidence of metastases of murine tumor cell lines. Thus the metastatic potential can be well correlated with the destruction of basement membrane.

Hormones and hormonomimetic agents (prostaglandins, growth factors) may play an important role in the frequency as well as the location of metastases (organotropism) by influencing the environment or the soil in which the new cells, or "seeds," will be grown. Hormones, such as cortisone, significantly increase the incidence of lung metastases versus liver metastases in mouse mammary tumors, while hormonelike substances, such as prostaglandins, increase the frequency of bone metastases in both human and animal breast cancers. Thymus and pineal gland extracts exert an inhibitory effect on metastasis formation in transplanted sarcomas and carcinomas in rats. Conversely, thymectomy and pinealectomy increase metastasis formation, as well as their location. Pinealectomy increases the incidence of pancreas metastases, whereas thymectomy increases the incidence of liver metastases. Concomitant pinealectomy and thymectomy increases both pancreatic and liver metastases. (47) (See Chapter 3). Hence, hormones are important factors in metastatic formation and location; they should always be considered in the treatment and prophylaxis of advanced metastatic cancer.

REFERENCES

1. Agosin, M., Christer, R., Badinez, O., Gasic, G., Neghme, A., Pizarro, O. and Harpa, A.: Cortisone-induced metastases of adenocarcinoma in mice. *Proc. Soc. Exp. Biol. Med. 80*:128–131 (1952).
2. Agostino, D., and Clifton, E.: Trauma as a cause of localization of blood-borne metastases: Preventive effect of heparin and fibrinolysin. *Ann. Surg. 161*: 97–102 (1965).
3. Baserga, R. and Shubik, P.: Action of cortisone on disseminated tumor cells after removal of the primary growth. *Science 121*:100–101 (1955).
3a. Bauer, E., Uitto, J., Walters, R., and Eisen, A.: Enhanced collagenase production by fibroblasts derived from human basal cell carcinomas. *Cancer Res. 39*:4594–4599 (1979).
4. Bennett, A., Macdonald, A., Simpson, J., and Stanford, I.: Breast cancer, prostaglandins and bone metastases. *Lancet 1*:1218–1220 (1975).
5. Block, J., and Isacoff, W.: Adjuvant chemotherapy in cancer. *Sem. Oncol. 4*: 109–115 (1977).
6. Boeryd, B., and Suürkula, M.: Transplantability and metastasibility of an MCA-induced sarcoma in nude mice. *Acta Pathol. Microbiol. Scand. (A) 85*:745–750 (1977).
7. Charbit, A., Malaise, E., and Tubiana, M.: Relation between the pathological nature and the growth rate of human tumors. *Eur. J. Cancer 7*:307–315 (1971).
8. Cifone, M.: Correlation between bizarre colony morphology and metastatic potential of tumor cells. *Exp. Cell. Res. 131*:435–441 (1981).
9. Coman, D.: Decreased mutual adhesiveness, a property of cells from squamous cell carcinoma. *Cancer Res. 4*:625–629 (1944).
10. Eccles, S., and Alexander, P.: Immunologically-mediated restraint of latent tumor metastasis. *Nature 257*:52–53 (1975).
11. Fidler, I.: Cell heterogeneity and the biology of cancer invasion and metastasis. *Cancer Res. 38*:2651–2660 (1978).
12. Fisher, B., and Fisher, E.: Experimental evidence in support of the dormant tumor cell. *Science 130*:918–919 (1959).

13. Folkman, G., Merler, E., Abernathy, C., and Williams, G.: Isolation of a tumor factor responsible for angiogenesis. *J. Exp. Med. 133*:275–287 (1971).

14. Gasic, G., Gasic, T., and Murphy, S.: Antimetastatic effect of aspirin. *Lancet 2*: 932–933 (1972).

15. Gastpar, H.: Platelet-cancer cell interaction in metastasis formation: A possible therapeutic approach to metastasis prophylaxis. *J. Med. Clin. Exp. Theoret. 8*:103–107 (1977).

16. Glaves, D.: Metastasis: Reticuloendothelial system and organ retention of disseminated malignant cells. *Int. J. Cancer 26*:115–122 (1980).

17. Glaves, D., and Weiss, L.: Early arrest of circulating tumor cells in tumor-bearing mice. In Day, S., et al. (eds.): *Cancer Invasion and Metastases: Biologic Mechanism and Therapy* (New York, Raven Press, 1977), p. 175.

18. Glick, M.: Cell surface changes associated with malignancy. In Weiss, L. (ed.): *Fundamental Aspects of Metastasis*. (Amsterdam-Oxford, North-Holland, 1976), pp. 9–23.

19. Hanna, N.: Expression of metastatic potential of tumor cells in young nude mice is correlated with low levels of natural killer cell-mediated cytotoxicity. *Int. J. Cancer 26*:675–680 (1980).

20. Honn, K., Cicone, B., and Skoff, A.: Prostacyctin: A potent antimetastatic agent. *Science 212*:1270–1272 (1981).

21. Iversen, H., and Hjort, G.: The influence of corticoid steroids on the frequency of spleen metastases in patients with breast cancer. *Acta Pathol. Microb. Scand. (A) 44*:205–212 (1958).

22. Kaufman, R.: Advanced breast cancer: Additive hormonal therapy. *Cancer 47*: 2398–2403 (1981).

23. Kawaguchi, T., Endo, M., Yokoya, S., and Nakamura, K.: Influence of lodgement site on the proliferation-kinetics of tumor cells. *Experientia 37*:414–415 (1981).

24. Kinsey, D.: An experimental study of preferential metastasis. *Cancer 13*:674–676 (1960).

25. Lam, W., Delikatny, E., Orr, F., Wass, J., Varani, J., and Ward, P.: The chemotactic response of tumor cells: a model for cancer metastasis. *Am. J. Pathol. 104*:69–76 (1981).

26. Lupulescu, A.: Experimental squamous cell carcinoma: Ultrastructural and cell surface studies. In Bailey G. (ed.): *Proceedings of the Electron Microscopy Society of America*. (Baton Rouge, Claitor, 1979), pp. 216–217.

27. Lupulescu, A.: Ultrastructural and scanning electron microscopic studies of basal cell carcinomas. In Bailey, G. (ed.): *Proceedings of the Electron Microscopy Society of America*. (Baton Rouge, Claitor, 1980), pp. 728–729.

28. Moore, G., Kondo, T., and Oliver, R.: Effects of cortisone in tumor transplantation. *J. Natl. Cancer Inst. 25*:1097–1110 (1960).

29. Mortensen, J., Woolner, L., and Bennett, W.: Gross and microscopic findings in clinically normal thyroid glands. *J. Clin. Endocrinol. Metab. 15*:1270–1280 (1955).

30. Nichelson, G., and Brunson, K.: Organ specificity of malignant B_{16} melanomas: In vivo selection for organ preference of blood-borne metastasis. In Stansly, P., and Sato, H. (eds.): *Cancer Metastasis, Approaches to the Mechanism, Prevention and Treatment*. (Gann Mon. 20), (Tokyo, University of Tokyo Press, 1977), pp. 15–22.

31. Noble, R., and Hoover, L.: A classification of transplantable tumors in NB rats

controlled by estrogen from dormancy to autonomy. *Cancer Res. 35*:2935–2941 (1975).

32. Paget, S.: The distribution of secondary growths in cancer of breast. *Lancet 1*: 571–575 (1889).

33. Pomeroy, T.: Studies on the mechanism of cortisone-induced metastases of transplantable mouse tumors. *Cancer Res. 14*:201–204 (1954).

34. Poste, G.: The cell surface and metastasis. In Day, S., Stansley, P., Myers, W., Garattini, S., and and Lewis, M. (eds.): *Cancer Invasion and Metastasis: Biologic Mechanisms and Therapy*. (New York, Raven Press, 1977), pp. 19–47.

35. Powles, T., Easty, G., Easty, D., Dowsett, M., and Neville, A.: Factors influencing development of bone metastases. In Day, S., Stansley, P., Myers, W., Garattini, S., and Lewis, M. (eds.): *Cancer Invasion and Metastases: Biologic Mechanisms and Therapy*. (New York, Raven Press, 1977), pp. 425–429.

36. Powles, T., Easty, D., Easty, G., and Neville, A.: Inhibition by aspirin and indomethacin of osteolytic tumor deposits and hypercalcemia in rats with Walker tumor and its possible application to human breast cancer. *Br. J. Cancer 28*:316–321 (1973).

37. Roos, E., and Dingemans, K.P.: Mechanisms of metastasis. *Biochem. Biophys. Acta 560*:135–166 (1979).

38. Schabel, F.: Concepts for systemic treatment of micrometastasis. *Cancer 35*:15–24 (1975).

39. Shafle, S., and Liotta, L.A.: Formation of metastasis by human breast carcinoma cells (MCF-7) in nude mice. *Cancer Lett. 11*:81–87 (1980).

40. Simpson-Herren, L., Sanford, A., and Holmquist, J.: Cell population of kinetics of transplanted and metastatic Lewis lung carcinoma. *Cell Tissue Kinet. 7*:349–361 (1974).

41. Sugarbaker, E.: Cancer metastasis. In Hickey, R. (ed.): *Current Problems in Cancer*. (Chicago, YearBook, 1979), vol. 3, pp. 1–59.

42. Sugarbaker, E., and Ketcham, A.: Mechanisms and prevention of cancer dissemination: An overview. *Sem. Oncol. 4*:19–32 (1977).

43. Sugarbaker, E., Cohen, A., and Ketcham, A.: Facilitated metastatic distribution of the Walker 256 tumor and Sprague-Dawley rats with hydrocortisone and/or cyclophosphamide. *J. Surg. Oncol. 2*:227–231 (1970).

44. Suzuki, N., Frapart, M., and Gardine, D.: Cell cycle dependency of metastatic lung colony formation. *Cancer Res. 37*:3690–3693 (1977).

45. Taptiklis, N.: Dormancy by dissociated thyroid cells in the lungs of mice. *Eur. J. Cancer 4*:59–66 (1968).

46. Tarin, D.: Cellular interactions in neoplasia. In Weiss, L. (ed.): *Fundamental Aspects of Metastasis*. (Amsterdam, North-Holland, 1976), pp. 151–187.

47. Tyzzer, E.: Factors in the production and growth of tumor metastases. *J. Med. Res. 28*:309–333 (1913).

48. Watson, B.: Effects of cortisone and adrenalectomy on the growth rate of Ehrlich-ascites tumor in mice. *J. Natl. Cancer Inst. 20*:219–225 (1958).

49. Wheelock, E., Goldstein, L., Weinhold, K., Carney, W., and Marx, P.: The dormant state. In Day, S., Stansley, P., Myers, W., Garattini, S., and Lewis, M. (eds.): *Cancer Invasion and Metastasis: Biologic Mechanisms and Therapy*. (New York, Raven Press, 1977), pp. 19–47.

49a. Lupulescu, A.: Hormonal regulation of epidermal tumor development. *J. Invest. Dermatol. 77*:186–195 (1981).

50. Wood, J., Holyoke, E., Sommers, S., and Warren, S.: Influence of pituitary growth hormone on growth and metastasis formation of a transplantable mouse sarcoma. *Bull. Johns Hopkins Hosp. 96*:93–100 (1955).

51. Yogeeswaran, G. and Salk, P.: Metastatic potential is positively correlated with cell surface sialylation of cultured murine tumor cell lines. *Science 212*: 1517–1717 (1981).

52. Wyllie, A., Kerr, J., and Currie, A.: Cell death: The significance of apoptosis. *Int. Rev. Cytol. 68*:251–306 (1980).

Chapter 8

HORMONES AND TUMOR TRANSPLANTATION

GENERAL CONSIDERATIONS

In a broad sense, transplantation means the transfer of a tissue or cells from one person, or animal, to another, while preserving the functional integrity of the transplanted tissue in the recipient. Tumor transplantation is an important field for cancer research, providing interesting data in regard to tumor cellular kinetics and cytodifferentiation, biology, the host-tumor relationship, and the effects of hormones and drugs on tumor growth and progression.

The first successful transplantations of spontaneous tumors, reported at the beginning of this century, greatly expanded our knowledge of tumor behavior and transmissibility. For instance, Rous succeeded in 1910 in transplanting an avian neoplasm (sarcoma of the common fowl) that was histologically a spindle cell sarcoma of another hen. Transplantations were obtained serially for four generations in which young chickens were always more susceptible than adults (39). A few years later, other spontaneous tumors (lymphosarcoma and sarcoma) were transplanted into rabbits and

243

guinea pigs (42). At about the same time, a spontaneous adenocarcinoma of the mammary gland was successfully transplanted through eight successive series in guinea pigs. Transplantability was shown to increase with the number of passages, with metastases observed in some cases (20). A spontaneous sarcoma was also transplanted into guinea pigs. This tumor had a very slow rate of growth; no macroscopic metastases were observed, but a few micrometastases were seen in the lungs in the seventh tumor generation (28). All these first transplantations were performed in randomly selected (random bred) animals, with the cellular pattern remaining identical to that of the original tumor.

However, most transplanted tumors in the early experiments failed as a result of histocompatibility between tumor and recipient, that is, because of a failure of the immune defense mechanism(s) of the recipient. If these immune mechanisms are suppressed, by means of immunosuppressors, the tumor can grow and spread after it is transplanted. Once the immune mechanisms recover, however, the tumor will be destroyed. Thus, the survival of transplanted tumor depends on a deficiency or immunosuppression of the host–immune mechanism. A successful tumor transplantation is ensured in a host animal that is genetically immunodeficient or in which the immunodeficiency is experimentally induced by means of immunosuppressors. An ideal experimental model of immunodeficiency was found to be the nude mouse mutant or athymic nude mouse, that is, in which the thymus is absent. This congenitally immunodeficient animal is an ideal recipient for heterotransplantation (11,32).

A variety of human solid tumors (e.g., melanomas, breast cancers, osteosarcomas, basal cell carcinomas, lung cancers, and adenocarcinoma of colon) were successfully transplanted by two methods: using tumor fragments directly from biopsy material, or injecting subcutaneously tumor cell lines derived from human cancers into nude mouse (13,14,40,53). The effects of different chemotherapeutic drugs on human transplanted neoplasms, as well as their cell kinetics and cellular differentiation, were also studied.

Tumor transplantation in the clinical situation is obviously rare and has been limited chiefly to studies in consenting chronic debilitating patients with advanced and disseminated cancers. Transplantation of cancers in healthy patients is extremely rare—primarily the result of an accident during a cancer operation. Considerable evidence has accumulated during recent years from patients who received organ transplants, such as skin and kidney, from donors who had cancer. In most instances, experience in the clinical setting was found to duplicate observations made in experimental animals. The Denver Transplant tumor registry (through May 1980) has shown that among 79 patients who received organs from donors with cancer, cancer developed in 30 patients (38 percent). The transplanted tumors were identical to those in the original donors; in most cases, the tumor developed beyond the local homograph, and in 20 patients distant metastases were found. Also, a surprising increase in the incidence of cancer was observed in patients after clinical transplantation. The overall incidence of malignancy in a large series of transplant patients ranges from 2 to 13 percent. Most neoplasms occurring in organ transplant recipients are non-Hodgkin's lymphomas; skin cancers (squamous cell carcinomas, found at least 10 times higher in transplant patients than in the general population; and Kaposi's sarcoma, rising from 0.6 percent in the general population to 3.2 percent in transplant patients) (33).

The knowledge that many chemotherapeutic agents, hormones (corticosteroids, prostaglandins), and radiation therapy exert potential immunodepressor effects, has stimulated new research in this field. Also, a high incidence of malignancies has been observed in genetically immunodeficient patients with demonstrated congenital immunodeficient disease. All these experimental and clinical observations indicate that immunologic factors play an important role in the development and evolution of neoplasms (17,33). Recent data strongly suggest that hormones and hormone-like substances have a significant role in tumor transplantation. Thus, not all hormone-dependent cancers (HDCs) can be transplanted, nor can they survive and develop in hormone-deficient animals. The presence of hormones is indispensable for the growth and survival of transplanted tumors. If the hormonal supply is ensured, the tumor (e.g., thyroid, mammary, prostate, kidney) can be serially transplanted into animal recipients. If the recipients are hormone deficient, the tumor will regress and finally be destroyed.

Hormones are critical factors in the transplantation of HDCs. They also have an important role in the transplantation of other tumors. Hence, hormonal environment or hormonal milieu is required for the success of tumor transplantation (18,30,31).

TRANSPLANTATION OF EXPERIMENTAL CANCERS

Transplantation of chemically induced tumors in laboratory animals is an important area of cancer research. In the past, most of these experiments failed as a result of histocompatability differences between donor and recipient; most induced or spontaneous transplanted experimental animal tumors have been shown to immunize syngeneic recipient animals that developed antibodies only to the same tumor and not to normal tissues or to other types of tumors. These findings suggest the presence of specific antigens in tumor cells, but apparently not present in normal cells. These antigens are called tumor specific or, more accurately, tumor-associated transplantation antigens (TSTA). The occurrence of these tumor antigens during neoplastic transformation is well demonstrated in chemically carcinogen-induced tumors that develop specific antigens for each tumor, even with tumors induced by the same carcinogen (e.g., MCA or DMBA) and by virus-induced tumors, which sometimes show a cross-reactivity between tumors induced by the same virus. These TSTAs are well demonstrated in animal tumors and in some human cancers (malignant melanoma, osteosarcoma, Burkitt's lymphoma, and gastrointestinal tumors) (17,33). With the development of inbred strains of various species, this barrier was eliminated; the transplantability of cancer can be successfully accomplished in several species; thus, different transplantable tumor lines were obtained.

Experimental hepatomas, lung tumors, thyroid carcinomas, malignant melanomas, skin tumors (squamous cell carcinomas, basal cell carcinomas), pancreatic tumors, and mammary carcinomas can be successfully transplanted in different strains of mice, rats, and guinea pigs, providing useful information for cancer immunotherapy, hormonotherapy, and chemotherapy (2,19,21). Transplantation of experimental tumors can be performed by the use of sterile small tumor fragments or cell lines that grow locally and then metastasize, always preserving similar cell characteristics to the parent somatic cells of donors.

Recently, several transplantable tumor lines were developed, some of them hormone dependent; they make excellent experimental models for cancer research. In many instances, transplantability and metastability are two important parameters of neoplastic cell behavior; they are therefore studied together. Several lines of transplantable hepatomas induced by administration of diethylnitrosamine (DEN) were successfully obtained in syngeneic guinea pigs. They are used for the study of BCG immunotherapy of cancers. Both forms of hepatomas (original solid form and ascites variant) were transplanted into guinea pigs, presenting evidence that these chemically induced tumors are immunogenic. Immunization—either intramuscular or intradermal—produced significant protection against the growth of transplanted tumors (39). During successive transplantations of hepatomas, a subline arose that differed from original tumor in histologic pattern, transplantability, and chromosomal type, approaching adenocarcinoma (54).

Pancreatic acinar cell carcinoma induced by azaserine or by chronic treatment with clofibrate and nafenopin in rats was also studied. These studies demonstrated that only pancreatic acinar cell carcinomas induced by azoserine and nafenopin can be successfully transplanted and maintained in the transplantable form for several generations. Transplantable pancreatic acinar carcinoma provides an interesting model for the study of cell differentiation in neoplasms. Experiments using electron microscopy and radioisotopes (^{3}H-leucine) demonstrated that the neoplastic cells synthesize zymogen granules. Electron microscopic autoradiography indicates that protein synthesis begins at the ribosomes and membranes of rough endoplasmic reticulum, moves to the Golgi cisternae, and then forms mature zymogen granules. However, although these granules appear normal on electron microscopic examination, they exhibit a low discharge rate of incorporated radioactive material after administration of carbanylcholine. This study suggests a heterogeneous cytodifferentiation of neoplastic cells (52).

Mouse spontaneous reticulum cell sarcoma has also been successfully transplanted in syngeneic hosts by the intravenous, subcutaneous, and intracranial routes. The efficiency of transplantation depends on the route of administration, with the intravenous route being the most effective, and was also related to the number of cells received. The more concentrated cell suspensions were the most effective. Attempts to transplant the tumor by cell-free extracts failed (6).

Transplantation of HDCs (mammary carcinoma, thyroid carcinoma, and ovarian, kidney, uterine, and prostate tumors) was successfully carried out in several strains of rats, mice, guinea pigs, and hamsters; it was found to be completely dependent on hormonal secretion or supplementation. This experimental model is described below in the section on endocrine modulation of tumor transplantation. However, transplantation of chemically induced skin tumors (squamous cell carcinoma, basal cell carcinoma, fibrosarcomas, and melanomas) has proved one of the most widely used and effective instances, providing an excellent experimental model for the study of neoplastic transformation, cell biology, and cytodifferentiation of cancerous cells.

Squamous cell carcinomas, differentiated as well as highly dedifferentiated, were transplanted into mice. Most of these tumors are chemically induced by long-term administration of 3-methylcholanthrene. Transplantability of these tumors can be maintained for several generations (2). With the subcutaneous route and small tumor fragments kept under sterile conditions, several laboratories, including ours, were able to transplant this tumor and use this model in studying cytodifferentiation, cell division, and the hormone responsiveness of neoplastic transplanted cells. The transplantability of squamous cell carcinomas was facilitated and the yield of transplanted tumors greatly increased in immunosuppressed animals—either drug induced (azothiopurine, methotrexate) or congenitally (athymic nude mice)—in hormone treated mice, and in neonatally thymectomized mice (29). Fibrosarcomas induced by 3-methylcholanthrene can also be transplanted in guinea pigs. Most of these experiments have proved successful in syngeneic animals; thus several syngeneic lines have been obtained (i.e., J_4, H_{10}, H_{12}, and H_9A); in addition, allogenic sublines have been established for mice, rats, and guinea pigs. (21).

Basal cell carcinomas chemically induced by 3-methylcholanthrene in rats were more difficult in transplantation. We succeeded only in very few instances, namely, in syngeneic rats. However, basal cell carcinomas were successfully transplanted in such remote areas as the uterus of estradiol-treated virgin inbred adult rats (5). Both squamous cell carcinomas and basal cell carcinomas induced by methylcholanthrene are similar to those in human cancers. Spontaneous squamous cell and basal cell carcinomas are unknown in common laboratory animals.

It is interesting to note that cytodifferentiation of squamous cell and basal cell carcinomas is markedly altered under various hormonal treatments. Prostaglandin administration (i.e., PGE_2, $PGF_{2\alpha}$) but mostly $PGF_{2\alpha}$, significantly increases the transplantability of methylcholanthrene-induced squamous cell carcinomas and enhances their cellular atypicality. Our experiments showed an increase in transplantability from 40 percent in nontreated to 87 percent in prostaglandin-treated mice. The cellular atypicality is also greatly increased, from type I to type IV (anaplastic squamous cell carcinoma), according to Broder's system (3,25).

Also, in transplanted basal cell carcinomas, histologic examinations indicate that basal cells change into larger prickle cells of benign appearance, which form keratinizing foci and cysts that spread over the surface of the uterine lumen, replacing the columnar epithelium (5). Investigators have suggested that this model can be used for the study of reconversion of neoplastic cells from a malignant stage to a relatively benign behavior. A successful model of serially transplanted melanoma and plasmocytoma was developed by Fortner et al. in Syrian hamsters (12). Several lines of hamster plasmocytomas were used to study the sensitivity of these tumors to various chemotherapeutic drugs. The tumor response of plasmocytoma was found to exhibit altered sensitivity to cytosine arabinoside and to decline with increasing size in tumor cell population; however, this sensitivity will be restored with the reduction of a viable cell population. Thymidine indices also indicate a heterogeneous cell population, especially of the proliferative compartment, explaining this altered sensitivity (16). Thus, these transplanted animal tumor models can be used in studying cell kinetics and the therapeutic evaluation of anticancer drugs.

TRANSPLANTATION OF HUMAN CANCERS

Studies regarding the autotransplantation and homotransplantation of human cancers were performed in patients debilitated with advanced and disseminated tumors. Thus, subcutaneous autotransplantation of human cancer cell suspension (from adenocarcinomas, epidermal tumors, and sarcomas) was performed in 35 patients with advanced cancer, but only six had evidence of the growth of transplanted tumors after 3 weeks. Quantitative evaluation of these experiments is difficult, because a large number of viable cancer cells are necessary—more than one million—and also because the proliferation of implanted cancer cells is restrained by the host-defense mechanism. Similar observations made in homotransplanted patients with tissue-cultured cancer cells suggest a parallelism between autotransplantation and homotransplantation; possibly, the same mechanisms operate against both homologous and autologous cells (45).

ATHYMIC NUDE MOUSE:
A MODEL FOR TUMOR TRANSPLANTATION

Flanagan described the nude hairless mouse mutant (BALB/c nu/nu) (11), later found by Pantelouris to be congenitally thymus deficient (32). The fact that the thymus is never present in this immune-deficient animal, makes the nude mouse an ideal recipient for heterotransplantation—an important step in experimental oncology and immunology. Until now, most heterotransplantation of neoplastic tissue from one animal species to another was followed by rejection of the graft, except when the host was rendered immunodeficient by administration of immunosuppressors. The availability of nude mouse provides an important experimental model in which human malignant tumors, as well as experimental tumors, can grow indefinitely and invasively; several tumors can thus be harvested in this animal, permitting the role of hormones and antineoplastic drugs to be studied.

The only apparent problem in using the nude mouse on a wide scale in tumor transplantation was its short life-span under conventional conditions. It was recently found, however, that kept under appropriate pathogen-free conditions, the nude mouse can enjoy dramatically increased health and life-span. These long-lived nude mice have eliminated many of the previous obstacles, permitting several types of human cancers to be successfully heterotransplanted.

The first successful experiments regarding the transplantation of human cancer directly from the patient into a nude mouse were recorded about 10 years ago (40). Since then, several human malignant tumors were successfully transplanted into nude mice. Thus, human amelanotic melanomas were transplanted into nude mouse, one of which metastasized to the lungs. Human melanomas grown in tissue culture were also transplanted by intradermal or subcutaneous inoculation into thymus-deficient nude mice, and invasive tumors were produced by melanomas at the site of injection. Most of these tumors metastasized to the lymph nodes, and a few to the lungs. Karyotypic analysis of these metastatic tumors identified them as human cancers. These findings suggest that human tumors transplanted into the nude mouse reproduce the original histologic pattern, which they follow in their natural host (14).

A variety of human tumors, such as lung carcinomas (squamous adenocarcinoma, alveolar cell carcinoma, undifferentiated carcinoma and carcinoid), pleural mesothelioma, adenocarcinoma of colon, carcinoma of the breast, osteosarcoma, melanoma, and basal cell carcinoma have all been grown rapidly in the nude mouse. It has also been found that human benign neoplasms (epithelial polypi of the colon) can survive and grow in the nude mice, but the rate of growth is much slower as compared with that of malignant neoplasms.

Despite the growth and proliferation of many malignant tumors, no metastatic growth has been observed (53). It is interesting that the growth and survival of human cancers transplanted into nude mice is prevented by previous thymus implantaton. Also, implantation of thymus into mice with established tumors results in increased animal survival and, in some cases, complete tumor regression (41). The restoration of tumor regression or inhibition is attributable to the presence of T cells or thymus lymphocytes, which play an important role in immune host-defense mechanisms.

Large numbers of human cancers—more than 200—have been successfully transplanted into nude athymic mice. These tumors grow and remain human tumors, as proved by isoenzyme and karyotype analysis. Also, a histopathologic comparison demonstrated a striking similarity between the original human cancers and their transplanted fragments in mice. Most of these tumors can be serially transplanted from mouse to mouse. However, breast carcinoma is still the only major human type of tumor that is serially transplanted only with difficulty. The incidence of metastases from these transplanted tumors remains low and does not represent a valid explanation for this phenomenon (13).

Recently, the nude mouse was used extensively in testing the effect of new anticancer drugs—alone or in combination with hormones—on the evolution of neoplasms, with very encouraging results.

ENDOCRINOLOGIC MODULATION OF TUMOR TRANSPLANTATION

Experimental investigations demonstrate that some transplanted tumors require a hormonal environment for their development and metastasis. Transplantation of HDCs succeeds only when this hormonal environment of hormonal milieu is present; in the absence of this hormonal environment, tumor implantation has failed. Hormones can facilitate the transplantation of other non-HDCs (Fig. 8–1) or HITs. Hormones are therefore, modulating factors of tumor transplantation. Several transplantable HDT lines have been established (31,43,50). The transplantable HDT lines can be distinguished from the HIT and anaplastic tumors (AT) through the use of sensitive biochemical methods, such as estimation of hormone receptors. In HDT lines, the hormone receptors are always present, whereas they are lacking or poorly developed in HID or AT lines. Thus, it is possible to distinguish between HDT and HID or AT of most transplantable mammary carcinomas, thyroid tumors, and prostate tumors (4,18).

Cortisone, estrogens, androgens, pituitary hormone, insulin, progesterone, and thyroid hormone can markedly affect the development and evolution of transplanted tumors, including human cancers. Irrespective of the mechanism of carcinogenesis (chemical, viral, or hormonal), the hormonal requirement is always retained in HDCs. Although the work of

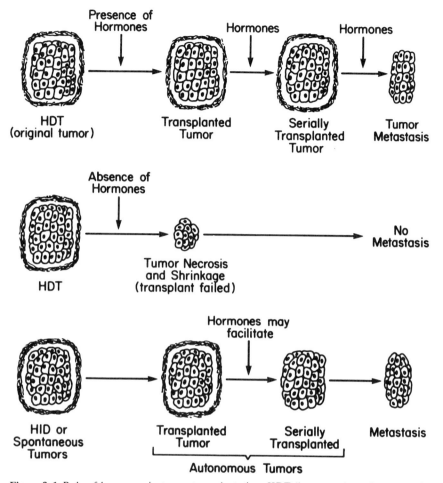

Figure 8-1 Role of hormones in tumor transplantation. HDT (hormone-dependent tumors), HID (hormone-independent tumors).

Huggins, Furth, and Dunning has led to a number of transplantable tumor lines in widespread use, the role of hormones on tumor transplantation is not yet fully understood. It seems that a variety of tumors that are not hormone dependent still require a particular hormonal milieu for their implantation, development, and propagation (metastasis).

Cortisone

Chronologically, cortisone was the first hormone described as an active agent affecting tumor transplantation (19). Transplantation of tumors was shown to succeed only if the capillary invasion that nourishes the graft and the stromal reaction occur. When capillaries do not invade and there is an accumulation of lymphocytes, the transplanted tumor fails to grow as a result of partial necrosis. This early work suggests that pretreatment with cortisone enhances the tendency for homologous transplantation when the host is not too resistant. Thus, parenteral administration of cortisone improves the possibility of homologous transplantation of several types of tumors (fibrosarcomas, mesenchymomas, and rhabdomyosarcomas) in Swiss mice. Also, cortisone increases the number of successful transplantations of methylcholanthrene-induced tumors (squamous cell carcinoma, sarcoma). Possible explanations for this enhancement of tumor transplantation after cortisone pretreatment include the appearance of many blood vessels, particularly veins over the tumor surface, as well as by suppression of the allergic immune reactions, which are partially responsible for the absorption of the transplanted tissue.

Several human neoplasms (sarcoma, epidermoid carcinoma, and embryonal rhabdomyosarcoma) have been successfully transplanted and maintained for several generations in cortisone-treated laboratory animals. Thus, several transplantable lines, H.S. #1, (human soft sarcoma), H.Ep. #1, H. Ep., #2, and H. Ep. #3—all human epidermoid carcinoma and H. Emb. Rh. #1 9 human embryonal rhabdomyosarcoma—were established (50).

Some human transplanted tumors appear to grow better in animals than they do in their donor—possibly because of the immune-defense mechanism of the host or because of stromal reactions, which can be different in human subjects than in rats. Some human neoplasms can be maintained for more than 16 months in cortisone-treated rats. Hamsters are even more responsive to human tumor transplantation. Thus, a single cortisone injection is sufficient to ensure the growth of human sarcoma and squamous cell carcinoma in hamsters. None of the human tumors has grown in untreated or normal hosts. Effects of cortisone on tumor transplantation have been shown by other investigators (27), who confirmed earlier observations that pretreatment with cortisone effectively aids the growth of transplanted sarcoma 180, Krebs-2, and Ehrlich ascites tumor cells. Pretreatment with cortisone also significantly reduces the number of cells required in establishing tumor implants. It is important to note that the effects of cortisone on transplanted tumors are both dose related and time dependent. For instance, only cortisone given before tumor inoculation functions as a tumor growth promoter. However, if the cortisone or corticotropin (ACTH) is given in large doses after transplantation of mammary carcinoma, the growth of the transplanted tumor is inhibited and the survival of animals prolonged. Neither product inhibits the growth of an ascite-producing sarcoma (15).

Estrogens

The role of other hormones, particularly of estrogens, has also been thoroughly investigated in tumor transplantation. For example, tumors occurring in rats of the Nb strain, either spontaneously or after long-term treatment with estrogens, were transplanted in the same Nb rats. Whereas all spontaneous tumors were shown to be autonomous or hormone-independent when transplanted, tumors arising in estrogenized rats require the presence of hormones to maintain growth after transplantation. A large number of estrogen-induced tumors, some occurring in hormone-dependent tissues, such as mammary carcinoma, adrenal cortex tumors, pituitary tumors, ovarian (thecomas), uterine (leiomyomas), vagina (fibrosarcoma), and Leydig cell tumors of the testis, or in non-hormone-dependent tissues, such as thymus, pancreas, salivary glands, orbital glands, liposarcoma, and lymphoma, continue to require hormones after transplantation. All estrogens, including estriol, are active in this respect. The incidence of more common tumors of the breast, adrenal gland, or pituitary is greatly increased in estrogen-treated animals as compared with controls. These findings are explained by the fact that estrogens are not carcinogenic per se, but that they stimulate the already altered cells and that the hormonal requirement is retained after tumor transplantation (30). Also, testosterone can induce tumors when administered to rats pretreated with estrogens. Transplants from spontaneous tumors always grew faster than that of hormone-dependent tumors. Most transplanted adrenal cortex carcinomas and mammary carcinomas are hormone dependent during serial transplantation. Other tumors, such as pituitary adenomas and thyroid adenomas, or thyroid well-differentiated carcinomas, are also hormone dependent and require the presence of hormones for transplantation. Most of these tumors are hormone secreting tumors and can produce important biologic changes in the host. However, after successive transplants, some of these tumors can lose their hormone dependency and become autonomous tumors, displaying a more undifferentiated or anaplastic pattern. Interestingly, some tumors that occur in such organs as the pancreas, salivary glands, lymphoid, and adipose tissue can become hormone dependent. Since most of these tumors exhibit a striking similarity in morphology to that of human tumors, it seems likely to assume the role of estrogens in their etiology and pathogenetic mechanism, and some of these data can be extrapolated to human cancers. Overall, these findings demonstrate that hormones are important not only as causative factors in carcinogenesis, but also as active factors in tumor behavior after transplantation, hence in host-defense mechanism and in cancer control. Many transplantable tumor lines in estrogen-induced tumors can be established in Nb rats, including tumors of breast, adrenals, salivary glands, and pancreas, as well as lymphoma and liposarcoma. Tumor growth after transplantation was dose related. Intermittent estrogen administration is less effective, and tumor growth takes place more slowly. The growth rate of hormone-dependent adrenal carcinomas is also dose related. Mammary carcinomas require the largest amount of estrogens for growth. The growth rate in conditioned hosts of most transplanted tumors can be maintained as hormone dependent over 10 years, and is increased during successive generations.

Progression of these hormone-dependent tumors towards an autonomous or more anaplastic pattern after successive transplantations is slower in contrast to transplanted DMBA-induced mammary carcinomas, which rapidly progressed towards autonomous or anaplastic pattern (31). The growth behavior of transplanted tumors (transplants were made from tumor cell homogenates) has led to a classification of five types or lines of estrogen-dependent tumors.

All these tumor lines, when transplanted, grew successfully in almost 95 percent of rats. It is interesting that some of transplants can remain dormant for many years until the cells are triggered by surgical operation or estrogens. Thus, when tumor cells are transplanted to untreated animals, they can remain for many years viable but dormant, and they do not grow until they are stimulated again by estrogens. The animals bearing the dormant tumor transplants have a normal life-span, and they are not distinguishable from control animals. However, when hormones, especially estrogens, are added, the tumor growth restarts. Thus, some of these transplanted tumors can be reverted to hormone-dependent tumors. In the absence of hormones, many of these tumors are undergoing a spontaneous progression, still gradually, toward autonomous tumors. Hence, tumor transplantability can be manipulated by hormonal changes in the hosts.

Hormone dependency of serially heterotransplanted human breast cancer (BR-10) was also demonstrated in nude mice. Thus, the human breast cancer (Br-10) serially transplanted to nude mice (BALB/c-nu/nu) grows well in female but very slowly or not at all in untreated male mice or female mice treated with testosterone. The tumor growth was arrested by ovariectomy in female mice and was accelerated by estradiol administration to male mice. Histologically, tumors of female and estrogenized male mice retained the original pattern of duct carcinoma, whereas tumors in ovariectomized female or androgenized females markedly changed their histologic pattern toward more dilated lumina and arrangements, predominantly as lobular patterns. Thus, hormones affect the growth of transplanted tumors as well as their cytodifferentiation. Estimation of hormone receptors indicates the presence of high-affinity 8S and 4S estrogen receptors in tumors transplanted into female nude mice, but no progesterone receptors were detected.

These findings suggest the hormone dependency of human breast cancer and particularly the role of estrogens and androgens in the regulation of growth and cytodifferentiation of transplanted tumors (18). It is also possible that in serially transplanted tumors more highly hormone-dependent clones can occur by a selection process that can explain the variation in their growth from one passage to another. Estrogens and androgens can act on transplanted tumors through their specific cytoplasmic receptors. In addition to cortisone, ACTH, estrogens, and androgens, pituitary hormones can strongly affect the rate of tumor growth in transplanted animals. Administration of pituitary growth hormone (GH) to C_3H mice bearing a transplantable mammary adenocarcinoma induced a significant increase of body weight and an acceleration of growth of transplanted tumors. In both sexes the tumor weight at the end of experiments (27 days of GH administration) was significantly greater than that in the control mice (44).

Transplanted human mammary cancer can also become an ideal experimental model for the study of hormones on cancer biology and tumor transplantability. The hormonal environments are required for the human breast cells (MCF-7) to produce solid tumors in nude mice. Thus, a 100 percent transplantation was obtained within 7 days after inoculation of actively growing (log-phase) MCF-7 cells into the mammary fat pads of intact, athymic BALB/c nude mice. Some tumors failed to develop in ovariectomized mice or in mice made diabetic by streptozotocin and observed 90 days after cell inoculation. A 100 percent tumor development was obtained again in hypophysectomized mice or diabetic mice which received insulin. The same 100% tumor incidence was obtained in ovariectomized mice that received 17β-estradiol as subcutaneously pellets concomitantly with cell inoculation. Palpable tumors also developed in ovariectomized mice treated with prolactin, estrone or estriol but no tumor development was observed in ovariectomized mice treated with progesterone, 5β-dihydrotestosterone or cortisol. A stimulation of tumor growth (MCF-7) five- to sixfold in both intact and hypophysectomized mice was obtained that each received 17β-estradiol pellets. When 17β-estradiol was removed, tumors failed to develop in ovariectomized mice. However, tumors which continued to grow in ovariectomized mice regressed by 50 percent or more when tamoxifen (antiestrogen) was injected. When tamoxifen was replaced by cyclic AMP (cAMP) and theophylline, a tumor arrester, was observed within 2 to 3 weeks' treatment period. Streptozotocin-induced diabetes in tumor-bearing mice always resulted in complete tumor regression (43). Therefore, a hormonal environment or hormonal milieu is necessary for tumor development and cellular evolution of transplanted tumors. The role of hormones in tumor transplantability is summarized in Figures 8-1a, b and 8-2. These transplantable tumor lines can be used as excellent experimental models for the study of antineoplastic drugs, hormones or immune factors in human cancers.

ROLE OF PROSTAGLANDINS IN TUMOR TRANSPLANTATION

Special emphasis was recently made regarding the role of prostaglandins in carcinogenesis (7). Recent studies demonstrate that prostaglandins (PG) particularly F_2 ($PGF_{2\alpha}$) and E_2 (PGE_2) can significantly influence tumorigenesis, thus they enhance the development of squamous cell carcinoma in mice (24). Some investigators also suggest that prostaglandins can play a key role in the tumor–host immune competence and the cellular immune

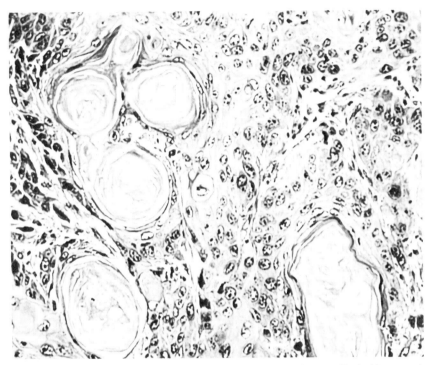

Figure 8-2 Transplanted squamous cell carcinoma in a nontreated mouse. Typical horn pearls can be seen. Paraffin section, H & E stained, ×400.

mechanisms by suppressing the body's defense mechanism(s) to cancer via cyclic nucleotides (cAMP, cGMP) (26,34,36). Our studies demonstrated that administration of $PGF_{2\alpha}$ and PGE_2 to syngeneic mice transplanted with squamous cell carcinoma 3-methylcholanthrene-induced from the same species (allograft) markedly enhanced the transplantability and cellular atypicality of tumors. Thus, large, invasive tumors with an atypical cellular pattern, anaplastic squamous cell carcinoma (grade IV, according to Broder's or fibrosarcoma) (3) occurred in approximately 87 percent of mice transplanted with squamous cell carcinoma, grade I and treated with $PGF_{2\alpha}$.

Similar transplanted tumors in syngeneic nontreated mice grew to a much lesser extent and always remained squamous cell carcinoma, grade I, as original tumor. The original tumor was obtained in male albino Swiss COBS (cesarean-originated, barrier sustained) mice by topical application of 0.4 percent acetone solution of 3-methylcholanthrene on their dorsal skin, three times weekly for 4 to 6 months. After the histologic diagnosis of squamous cell carcinoma (grade I) was made, small tumor fragments were removed, soaked in 0.9 percent sodium chloride and penicillin, and then transplanted into the interscapular area. Some transplanted animals were treated with $PGE_{2\alpha}$ at a dose of 10 μg, intramuscularly three times weekly and observed for 6 weeks;

others were treated similarly with $PGF_{2\alpha}$, also for 6 weeks, and the third group was only transplanted but not treated. The results, summarized in Table 8–1, show the tumor incidence and its average weight as compared with nontreated mice. Thus, prostaglandin-treated and -transplanted mice, particularly $PGF_{2\alpha}$ treated, developed large, invasive tumors, weighing 3850 g, as compared with only 721 g in transplanted but not treated mice. The incidence of transplanted tumors or "takes" was also high, approximately 87 percent as compared with only 40 percent, which occurred in transplanted but not treated mice. Autopsy indicated that tumors from PG-treated mice had a solid, meaty consistency, as compared with the much smaller tumors of soft consistency. The findings are similar to those of transplanted and estrogen-treated mice (Table 8–1). This last group of transplanted and estradiol-treated mice was studied for comparison to that of PG-treated, transplanted mice. Estradiol propionate was given intramuscularly twice weekly, a dose of $50\mu g$ per animal, also for 6 weeks.

Light microscopic observations demonstrated a characteristic histologic pattern of well-differentiated squamous cell carcinoma (grade I) with horn pearls in transplanted but not treated animals (Fig. 8–2). A bizarre histologic pattern was seen in mice transplanted and prostaglandin-treated mice. This pattern is mostly anaplastic, with spindle-shaped, disorderly arranged cells devoid of intercellular bridges. No epidermal or horn pearls were visible, and the keratinization process was absent. Mitoses were frequently seen. This tumor resembled invasive fibrosarcoma or anaplastic squamous cell carcinoma, grade IV (Fig. 8–3). The estradiol-treated and transplanted tumors still preserved their original histologic pattern, despite the fact, that the tumor incidence and growth are similar to those of PG-treated animals.

Light microscopic autoradiograms (using ^{3}H-thymidine) showed a significant increase (six- to sevenfold) of autoradiographic reaction in transplanted and PG-treated tumors. A similar increase is seen in estradiol-treated and -transplanted tumors (Table 8–2). The autoradiographic reaction is predominantly located in the basal layers or so-called proliferative compartments of squamous cell carcinoma.

Ultrastructural studies demonstrate the predominance of typical squamous cells separated by widened intercellular spaces and desmosomes. Cytoplasm contains tonofilaments, polysomes, and dense granules, possibly dyskeratotic material and enlarged nuclei with two to three nucleoli. A different ultrastructural pattern is seen in transplanted tumors and treated with $PGF_{2\alpha}$. Most of these cells are anaplastic cells resembling atypical fibroblasts that exhibit an abundant rough endoplasmic reticulum (RER), polysomes, few dense granules, and nuclei rich in chromatin. No tonofilaments and desmosomes can be seen. Neoplastic cells are separated by enlarged intercellular spaces and can synthesize collagen fibers. Some original squamous cells can be seen, indicating that atypical fibroblasts originate in squamous cells (Fig. 8–4). Thus the cellular evolution is shifted in trans-

Table 8-1 THE INCIDENCE AND AVERAGE WEIGHT (MEAN ± SEM) OF TRANSPLANTED TUMORS IN MICE AFTER PGE_2, $PGF_{2\alpha}$, AND ESTRADIOL ADMINISTRATION[a,b]

GROUP	TREATMENT (TRANSPLANTED 6 WEEKS)	NUMBER OF MICE	TYPE OF TUMOR	AVERAGE WEIGHT OF TUMORS (MG)	% OF TUMORS
1	Squamous cell carcinoma + solvent	15 (6)	Squamous cell Ca (grade I)	721 ± 70	40
2	Squamous cell Ca + PGE_2	15 (11)	Invasive fibrosarcoma (squamous cell Ca, grade IV)	3015 ± 178	73
3	Squamous cell Ca + $PGF_{2\alpha}$	15 (13)	Invasive fibrosarcoma (squamous cell Ca, grade IV)	3850 ± 201	87
4	Squamous cell Ca + estradiol	15 (12)	Squamous cell Ca, grade I	3675 ± 300	85

[a]Data presented are based on count of tumors visible to the naked eye, as well as on diagnosis made by light microscopy.
[b]Numbers in parentheses represent mice with tumors.

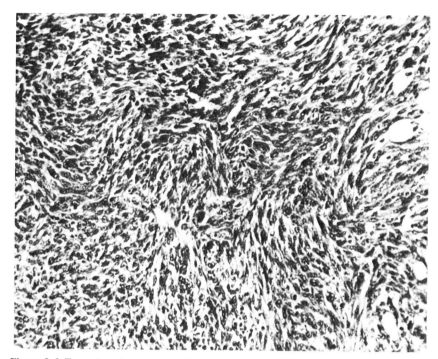

Figure 8-3 Transplanted squamous cell carcinoma in a $PGF_{2\alpha}$-treated mouse. A bizarre pattern resembling fibrosarcoma with several spindle cells can be seen. Paraffin section, H & E stain, ×400.

Table 8-2 QUANTITATIVE ESTIMATION OF AUTORADIOGRAMS WITH ^{3}H-THYMIDINE IN CONTROLS, PROSTAGLANDINS, AND ESTRADIOL-TREATED TRANSPLANTED TUMORS IN MICE

GROUP	TREATMENT	NUMBER OF LABELED CELLS/ TOTAL NUMBER OF CELLS	%
1	Controls + solvent	170/2100	8.09
2	Transplanted squamous cell Ca + solvent	850/2890	29.41
3	Transplanted Squamous cell Ca + PGE_2	1100/2630	41.82
4	Transplanted squamous cell Ca + $PGF_{2\alpha}$	1205/2430	49.58
5	Transplanted squamous cell Ca + estradiol	1250/2720	46.0

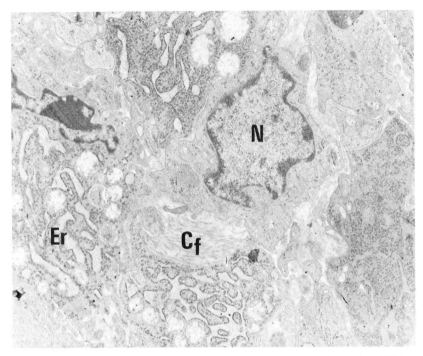

Figure 8-4 Electron micrograph of a transplanted squamous cell carcinoma in a $PGF_{2\alpha}$-treated mouse. Predominance of fibroblastlike (atypical fibroblast) cells with abundant endoplasmic reticulum (Er), nuclei (N), and collagen fibers (Cf). Epon, uranyl acetate, and lead citrate, $\times 10,000$.

planted and Pg-treated mice, toward atypicality with large fibroblasts (fibrosarcomas, or grade IV). However, the cellular evolution is similar to that of original tumors in transplanted and estrogen-treated tumors. Thus, prostaglandins, particularly $PGF_{2\alpha}$, markedly increased the transplantation of chemically induced tumors and enhanced their cellular evolution toward cellular atypicality (25).

It is possible that prostaglandins decreased the immunologic competence of host animals and their surveillance mechanism, by suppressing the lymphocytes and macrophages, and thus increased the tumor transplantability. It was recently found that certain tumor cell lines can synthesize excessive amounts of PGE_2 and $PGF_{2\alpha}$ (7). It was also found that the addition of PGE_2 to in vitro cultures of cancerous and spleen cells induced immunosuppressive effects; this immunosuppressive effect might explain the enhancement of tumor transplantability and atypical cellular evolution of transplanted tumors. It seems likely that prostaglandins can also act by affecting DNA synthesis; our autoradiographic investigations support this view.

Thus, prostaglandins, which are local or tissue hormones, significantly increase tumor transplantability and alter the morphology of transplanted tumors from squamous cell carcinomas into fibrosarcoma. Accordingly, prostaglandins can play an important role in tumor transplantation and cellular immune–host defense mechanisms.

However, when tumor cells obtained from a chemically induced tumor and maintained by serial passages were suspended in prostaglandin solutions (PGA_2, E_2, and F_2) and inoculated subcutaneously in weaning rats, a moderate inhibition of tumor growth was observed, especially in rats treated with PGA_2. Tumor cells were assumed to secrete a prostaglandin antagonist that can induce a PG deficiency, and consequently an immunologic paralysis in the tumor vicinity; this allergic reaction inhibits tumor implantation. Prostaglandins do not exert a direct cytopathic effect on tumor cells, since the same suspension of neoplastic cells in PGA_2, F_2, and E_2 grows well when inoculated intramuscularly. However, when tumors reach a certain size, prostaglandins do not exert any effect. PGA has been postulated as being more stable than other prostaglandins, possibly explaining its more favorable results (46).

OTHER FACTORS THAT CAN AFFECT TUMOR TRANSPLANTATION

In addition to hormones and hormonelike substances, pretreatment with irradiation also favors the growth of transplanted cells. Epidermal chalones and epidermal growth factor also exert significant effects on transplantability and cellular evolution of tumors. Thus when effects of epidermal chalones (G_1, G_2) and epidermal growth factor (EGF) were studied on transplantable nonkeratinizing epidermal carcinoma (Hewitt) in mice, it was found that epidermal G_1 chalones do not inhibit either DNA synthesis or tumor growth of transplants, whereas crude skin extracts suppress DNA labeling (probably because of cytotoxic effects). Consequently, repeated injections of extracts containing epidermal G_1 chalone do not prolong the survival rate of tumor-bearing animals.

Extracts made from normal mouse epidermis exhibit a strong inhibitory effect on epidermal DNA labeling, whereas extracts made from tumor tissue do not show any G_1 chalone activity. Despite the fact that transplanted tumors are resistant to epidermal G_1 chalone, the carcinomas are susceptible to skin extracts containing the epidermal G_2 chalone. G_2 chalones, because of their antimitotic effect, inhibit the growth and development of transplanted epidermal carcinoma. Epidermal growth factor exhibits a significant stimulatory effect by doubling the DNA labeling in the transplanted tumors and their growth.

It is assumed that epidermal chalone G_1 controls only the proliferation of stem cells in a more advanced stage of differentiation, whereas epidermal G_2

and epidermal growth factor affect cell proliferation in a more primitive stage (1,8).

The role of immune factors and the immune surveillance mechanism are also important in transplantation tumors. Despite the fact that some spontaneous tumors can be transplanted in so-called nonconditioned or normal animals, most tumors can grow, survive and spread only in immunosuppressed animals. If the immunosuppressive therapy is discontinued, the immune system will recover and can destroy the transplanted tumor. There is experimental and human evidence that immunosuppression enhanced the transplantability of tumors. Thus a variety of chemically induced tumors (e.g., 3-methylcholanthrene, DMBA), such as squamous cell carcinoma, sarcoma, Ehrlich carcinoma, fibrosarcoma, and liposarcoma) can be successfully transplanted in immunosuppressed animals by azothiopurine (29). Also, other immunosuppressors, such as corticosteroids, cyclophosphamide, and antilymphocyte globulin, facilitate the transplantability and oncogenicity of tumors induced by chemical, viral, or physical carcinogens.

The discovery of a nude or hairless mouse that is congenitally athymic and immunodeficient strongly supports this hypothesis. This also proves that immune surveillance mechanism acts through the small thymic lymphocytes or T lympocytes (T cells). Also, clinical transplantation shows an increased incidence in malignant tumors (lymphomas, common skin cancers, Kaposi's sarcoma, and carcinoma in situ of the cervix of the uterus) in transplant patients treated with immunosuppressive agents (e.g., azothiopurine). Also, a high incidence of malignant tumors is seen in patients with congenital immunodeficiencies.

Since many immunosuppressive drugs are used as chemotherapeutic drugs for cancer treatment, it is interesting to speculate whether these chemotherapeutic agents can increase the transplantability of cancer cells from original tumor by inducing a weak immune defense mechanism of the host, thus increasing the incidence of metastases. There is an increased evidence of occurrence of second malignancy (acute leukemia) in patients with carcinoma of the breast, carcinoma of the ovary, and multiple myelomas, treated with chemotherapeutic drugs. This incidence is even higher in cancer patients treated with a combination of chemotherapy and intensive radiotherapy. It is also possible that ionizing radiation acts indirectly, by inducing immunosuppression.

Topography of tumor vascularization can also influence the growth and cellular orientation of transplanted tumors (49).

CELLULAR EVOLUTION (CYTODIFFERENTIATION) OF TRANSPLANTED TUMORS

While most transplanted tumors preserve their original cellular pattern, being similar or identical to that of original tumor, tumors undergo a heterogeneous cytodifferentiation during serially transplantation. The cell structure of most transplantable tumors has seldom been investigated, mainly by light micro-scopy; the more accurate details regarding the cytodifferentiation of trans-planted tumors are lacking.

Modern methods, such as electron microscopy, autoradiography, scan-ning electron microscopy, and receptor estimation, should often be employed for the study of fine structural changes, autoradiographic distribution of ^{3}H-thymidine-labeled neoplastic cells, and surface changes during their prolifer-ative, dormancy, or autonomous stage. It is clearly demonstrated that hor-mones or hormonelike substances have an important role in preserving the cellular evolution during transplantation of hormone-dependent cancers. Thus, mammary carcinoma, thyroid neoplasms, and prostate tumors require a certain hormonal environment; in the absence of these respective hormones (estrogens, TSH, androgens), these tumors lose their well-differentiated pattern, and their cellular evolution is shifted toward a poorly differentiated anaplastic cellular pattern. Thus, losing their hormone dependency and moving towards autonomy, they also lose their cellular differentiated pattern, becoming more anaplastic and poorly differentiated.

Autoradiographic studies from our laboratory show different cell compartments of transplanted tumors: an active, proliferative, or growth fraction, a dormant state (transplanted tumor fragments can be silent or dormant cells, but still responsive as soon as the original stimulus is added), and a large cell population undergoing cytolysis or necrosis. We should keep in mind that most hormones, antineoplastic drugs, or immune factors act primarily on the proliferative or growth fraction or on dormant cells, but they do not affect the large cell population of dying or necrotic cells.

It is interesting to note that hormones or hormonelike substances can significantly influence the cellular evolution and cytodifferentiation of transplantable tumors. Thus, methylcholanthrene-induced basal cell carci-nomas in rats resembling those of human skin (a tumor that cannot be transplanted under normal conditions) can be transplanted successfully in the estradiol-treated uterus of the same strain. When tumor fragments are transplanted into the uterus of the estradiol-treated virgin females, the cellular evolution and cytodifferentiation of these tumors is shifted or reconverted from a malignant to a benign state. Thus, the small basaloid neoplastic cells are progressively changed into larger prickle cells of benign behavior, forming keratinizing foci and cysts and between 4 and 6 weeks after implantation; no nodular tumor growth and malignant cells were found, and the uterine lumens were covered primarily by a stratified epithelium resembling the normal skin implants. Estradiol can influence the cytodifferentation of basal cell carci-nomas (5).

Our investigations have also demonstrated that prostaglandins (PGE$_2$, PGF$_{2\alpha}$) can significantly change the cellular evolution of methylcholanthrene-induced squamous cell carcinomas in mice from a more benign and well-differentiated stage toward a more malignant, anaplastic stage, when this tumor was transplanted subcutaneously in the syngeneic and PG-treated mice. Electron microscopic studies have shown that the cellular evolution is shifted toward a more atypical anaplastic cell pattern, predominantly atypical of fibroblasts that can synthesize and release the collagen extracellularly. Intermediate stages between squamous neoplastic cells and fibroblasts can be detected, indicating that these atypical fibroblasts originate from the squamous cells. Autoradiography using ^{3}H-thymidine demonstrated that these atypical fibroblasts exhibit several mitoses and a higher thymidine-labeling index as compared with neoplastic squamous cells of transplanted but not PG-treated tumors. Thus, prostaglandins enhanced the cellular atypicality of transplanted tumors from a well-differentiated type tumor (grade I) to a more anaplastic or fibrosarcoma (grade IV) (25).

Microscopic examination showed also an increased cellular atypicality with predominant malignant cells in transplanted skin tumors induced by methylcholanthrene and Ehrlich carcinoma in mice made immunosuppressive by azothiopurine or in athymic nude mice (2,21,29). Estradiol reverses the cellular evolution of neoplastic cells of methylcholanthrene-induced basal cell carcinomas in rats and transplanted in uterus from malignant to more benign cells, probably by acting on tumor stromal reaction, which can prevent their neoplastic proliferation. By contrast, prostaglandins enhanced the cellular atypicality from a more benign and well differentiated toward a more malignant type of tumor, by acting mainly on DNA synthesis in transplanted tumor cells. Estrogens can also stimulate or reactivate the dormant cells of transplanted tumors and their reentry to the cell cycle, and thus to a proliferative phase. It is postulated by some investigators that estrogens and possibly other hormones influence the neoplastic transformation by acting on dormant cells and shifting them to cell proliferation, and not being carcinogenic per se (10,31).

Cell proliferation in transplanted tumors is also dependent on blood supply and oxygen in the vascular system. Thus, transplanted tumor fragments originating from a moderately differentiated spontaneous mammary adenocarcinoma were found to decrease their cellular proliferation and both mitotic and labeling indices with increasing distance from the axial blood vessels in transplanted mice. Oxygen was found to play a major role in controlling the rate of cellular proliferation acting on growth fraction of transplanted tumors. Two cell types were described: type A with a high cytoplasmic nucleotide content, close to the blood vessels and type B with a low cytoplasmic nucleotide content and close to the regions of necrosis. Type A cells are characterized by a higher rate of protein synthesis and proliferation than are type B cells (49).

Using electron microscopic autoradiography, a heterogeneous cytodifferentiation was found in transplanted pancreatic acinar carcinoma in rats. Thus, electron microscopic autoradiography with ^{3}H-leucine and administration of carbamylcholine (a secretagogue) indicated that the acinar cells of transplanted pancreatic carcinoma exhibit a low rate of radioactive protein discharge following carbamylcholine administration as compared with normal acinar cells (52). Scanning electron microscopy also provides interesting findings regarding the cell surface changes and morphology of transplanted human colon carcinoma in the peritoneal cavity of BALB/c mice. Thus a quantitative estimation of multicellular tumor spheroids of HT-29 human colon carcinoma cells showed little damage to spheroids during the initial 4 days after implantation, but a complete destruction occurred between 4 and 7 days owing to a concomitant host-cell infiltration (23).

Electron microscopy and scanning electron microscopy reveal also interesting changes in cytodifferentiation of original and transplanted tumors after hormone administration, such as increased keratinization, cord tumor cells, and sclerosis.

COMMENTS AND CONCLUSIONS

Why some experimental and human tumors are easier to transplant or take better than others in the animal hosts is as yet unknown. Experimental and clinical observations strongly suggest a hormonal modulation or manipulation of tumor transplantability.

The mechanism by which hormones can act on transplanted tumors are complex: they can act directly through their receptors by interferring in the DNA synthesis, acting on dormant cell populations or on cell-mediated immune mechanisms. Since the transplantability and metastability process are quite similar, metastasis being a transplanted cell tumor in the same patient (autotransplantation); the effects of controlling factors, including hormones, are also similar. Transplanted tumors can be an ideal model for the study of human cancer biology and therapeutic trials. Experimental investigations indicate individual differences between species and even between animals from the same strain, as regards the evolution of transplanted tumors. Also some tumors can be serially transplanted over hundreds of passages without great difficulty, whereas others are immediately rejected. There are factors that can be controlled or modified and thus the tumor transplantability is markedly influenced. For instance, we have no control over such factors as heredity, sex, and strains; however, we can significantly enhance or arrest the tumor transplantation by changing the host immune defense mechanisms or its hormonal environment hormonal milieu. Several transplantable tumor lines are now established by manipulating these factors, and a new model, the hairless (or nude) athymic mouse, was discovered. This is a mutant BALB/c (nu/nu) which is congenitally thymus-deficient and becomes an ideal experimental model for tumor transplantation being extensively used for the transplantation of a variety of human cancers or experimentally induced tumors. Despite the fact that the mutation nude apparently has no effect on the induction of tumors induced by methylcholanthrene (nu/nu mice had the same susceptibility to tumor induction by methylcholanthrene as controls and the latent period is similar in both groups), viral oncogenesis is profoundly affected; also, transplantation of chemically or viral induced tumors is greatly increased (47).

The use of nude mice is superior to that of immunosuppressed animals (e.g., azothiopurine). Thus, the effects of several hormones or chemotherapeutic drugs are more accurately studied on transplanted tumors in nude mice. Also, a great deal of knowledge regarding the basic mechanisms of tumor transplantability is derived now from human experience. Autotransplantation of human neoplasms is very rare, occurring only by accident and still inconclusive. However, ample evidence recently emerged from heterotransplantation of human cancers in nude mice. The several transplantable cell lines of human cancers that have been established are frequently used for the study of effects of hormones and chemotherapeutic drugs on tumor behavior and their susceptibility to these agents. These became ideal experimental models for the study of chemotherapeutic drugs and hormone dependency without exposing the patients at risk, and the preliminary results are very encouragng. Cytologic studies revealed that nude mice have normal thymocyte precursors but the differentiation of thymocytes into mature cells is defective (9,17).

The human experience duplicated in most instances the observations made on experimental animals. Transplantation or inoculation of human cancer cells is very rare and successful only in chronic debilitating patients, in whom the immune defense mechanisms are impaired. Thus an increased malignancy was observed in both immunosuppressed human subjects and animals. A higher incidence of malignant tumors was also observed in patients who received the transplant organs (skin, kidney) from donors with cancers. Hence, experimental and clinical transplantation provides interesting findings regarding the basic mechanisms governing the transplantation process, particularly cell mediated immunity, tumor antigenicity and immune surveillance. Also, an increased incidence of human cancers was observed in patients with congenital immunodeficiency.

Thus, surveillance against neoplastic cells is one of the most important functions of the immune system. These findings suggest that immune factors play an important role in tumor transplantability; however, it is not certain if the immune factors play a similar role in the occurrence and development of spontaneous neoplasms (17,33). We should keep in mind that some immunosuppressor agents are also used in cancer chemotherapy as antineoplastic drugs; their chemical configuration is quite similar. Thus they can increase the incidence of secondary malignancy.

Clinical and experimental observations strongly suggest that hormones and hormone like substances play an important role in transplantation process. In order for a transplanted and hormone-dependent tumor to grow and survive, a hormonal environment or hormonal milieu is essential. If this hormonal milieu is lacking, the transplant failed and the tumor is resorbed. Empirical observations indicate that some animal strains are more susceptible to transplants; the tumor can grow and reach huge size as compared with original tumor, whereas others are more resistant. There is also a great variability among the animals from the same strain. Also some spontaneous tumors, chemically or virally induced tumors can be easily transplanted, whereas others have failed.

Inasmuch as we have no controls over such factors as heredity, sex, and strain, we can control other factors, such as immune factors, hormones, and diet. Transplanted tumoral cells have to grow and survive in a hostile environment; therefore, through a cellular selection process, only the most gifted cells can compete and grow in this new and hostile environment. Hormones can modulate this hostile environment and thus facilitate the tumor transplantability. Hence, hormones are important modulator factors of transplantation. In hormone-dependent cancers, they are critical factors; tumor transplants cannot grow and survive in the absence of hormones. In animals deprived of their natural hormones, tumors cannot be transplanted unless the respective hormone is supplemented. In this case, tumors can be transplanted over several generations. This phenomenon is more evident in the transplantation of mammary carcinomas, prostate tumors, thyroid carcinoma, some kidney tumors, ovarian tumors, and pituitary tumors. Recently, several hormones, such as estrogens, androgens, cortisone, ACTH, TSH, GH, and insulin, were investigated concerning their effects on transplanted tumors; also the effects of hormonelike substances, such as prostaglandins, chalones, and epidermal growth factor, were thoroughly examined. The role of hormones on tumor transplantation is more complex.

It is possible that hormones can act directly on transplanted neoplastic cells by enhancing their DNA synthesis and consequently modifying cellular multiplication and differentiation; by increasing vascular permeability, on cell-mediated immunity, and consequently on immune host defense mechanism, by enhancing or inhibiting antibody formation against neoplastic cells; and by modifying the stromal barrier reactions (or stromal environment). Hormones can affect the receptor site(s) on the cell surface or nucleus. These are cytoplasmic hormonal and nuclear receptors.

Through the use of such modern methods as electron microscopic autoradiography, scanning electron microscopy, and enzyme–receptor estimation, we can detect the hormone-intrinsic mechanism of action. The effect of hormones on tumor transplantation can be better investigated in the athymic nude mouse, in which the immune defense mechanism is deficient, owing to a lack of T cells. Several investigations were carried out as regards the role of hormones on mammary cancer, prostate tumors, and thyroid carcinomas. Autoradiographic studies demonstrate that the neoplastic cell population of transplanted tumors can be divided first into two compartments: (1) one of dividing cells, which represents the growth fraction; and (2) one of dormant cells, represented by the temporarily nondividing cells, or silent cells; and later (see below) into (3) one of differentiated cells. This rather large cell population is in a quiescent or "dormant stage," but can be reactivated at any time by various factors, primarily hormones, into dividing cells. The growth and survival of transplanted neoplasms are largely dependent on an equilibrium between these two compartments. Hormones act primarily on the dormant cell population by reactivating these silent neoplastic cells from their stage of dormancy toward rapidly dividing cells. Thus hormones enhanced the reentry of dormant cells into the cell cycle. Some investigators have postulated that hormones are not carcinogenic per se, but that they can modulate or modify (via modulators or modifying factors) the tumor transplantability, by acting chiefly on dormant cells (31).

Electron microscopic studies from different laboratories, including our own, have shown original tumors to exhibit a heterogeneous cell population or mosaic of cells (25,35). During transplantation, these cells can evolve in different cell lines. These transplantable tumor cell lines or sublines during several passages by a selection process can become more hormone responsive or move into the third compartment: differentiated cells. Thus, neoplastic cells as a population not only divide and proliferate, but differentiate as well; a fascinating phenomenon, the so-called "self-cure of cancer by cell differentiation," can occur during neoplastic transformation and transplantability. Hormones can also influence the differentiation of neoplastic cells from a malignant to a more benign stage (35). Hence, the behavior of neoplastic cells is largely dependent on their new environment, which can be modified as well. Therefore, hormones have an important role in modulating the behavior of transplanted neoplastic cells and their cytodifferentiation. Hormonelike substances, such as prostaglandins, can also significantly affect the cellular evolution of transplanted tumors. Early experimental observations indicate that most neoplasms retain their original cellular pattern during transplantation.

Administration of prostaglandins, especially $PGF_{2\alpha}$, to transplanted tumor animals, markedly enhanced their cellular atypicality, shifting their cellular evolution from a benign or well-differentiated stage (squamous cell carcinoma, stage I) to a more undifferentiated or atypical and malignant tumor (atypical fibrosarcoma, stage IV).

Ultrastructural studies can better visualize all intermediate steps between original squamous neoplastic cells and atypical fibroblasts. These changes of transplanted neoplastic cells are accompanied by marked changes in their DNA synthesis (25). Another exciting and fruitful field of research is the role of thymus and hormones in cell-mediated immunity and surveillance mechanism(s) of transplanted neoplastic cells, which can lead to the graft rejection.

All relevant studies to date indicate a regulatory mechanism in the hypothalamus–pineal–pituitary neuroendocrine axis in relationship to the thymus. These thymic–neuroendocrine interactions may play an important role in tumor transplantation. Thus growth hormone and insulin have been shown to act preferentially on T-cell-dependent immune functions, whereas thyroxine and sex hormones act on both T and B cells (9).

Hormones can also influence the balance or equilibrium between different T cell subpopulations. There are at least two T cells: (1) T_1 cells, which are predominantly thymic small lymphocytes that control the antibody formation and antibody responses; and (2) T_2 cells (amplifier cells), helper T-cells, occurring predominantly in lymph nodes. Hormones can control T cell differentiation and T-cell biology. On the other hand, evidence is accumulating to indicate that thymus, by its hormone thymosine, can modulate hormonal levels.

The central nervous system can also play an important role in transplantation and graft rejection. Thus stress and other psychologic factors can influence skin graft rejection and antibody responses. Lesions in the anterior basal hypothalamus, but not in posterior or median hypothalamus, can reduce the severity of anaphylactic reactions and depress delayed hypersensitivity. Owing to the process of thymus atrophy and involution, the immune systems and most defense mechanism are decreasing in old animals. Early observations indicate that younger animals are more susceptible to tumor transplantation than are adults (20,39,42). This hypothesis is confirmed by the mutant athymic nude mouse, which is congenitally immunodeficient and becomes an ideal experimental model for the tumor transplantation of several human cancers or experimentally induced tumors. In this animal the precursors of T cells persist, but they are unable to differentiate into mature T cells. Recently purified plasma membranes were obtained from transplantable human tumors (astrocytoma, oat cell carcinoma, and melanomas) and were studied for their enzyme content.

A diversity of plasma membranes from different tumors and between tumors from the same type was found. Thus, low nucleotidase activity was found in the membrane of oat cell carcinomas, in contrast to large amounts of NAD pyrophosphatase in the plasma membranes of melanomas and large amounts of acid phosphatase in the plasma membranes of astrocytoma (22).

Significant fluctuations in lysosomal enzyme activity in the interstitial fluids of transplanted mouse solid tumor were also found (48). Studies of cell surface, particularly their enzyme distribution, provide more accurate details as regards the transplantation process, as well as the neoplastic transformation of normal cells into malignant cells in general. Some transplantable tumors have maintained their hormone-dependency over several generations (mammary carcinoma, adrenal carcinomas, thyroid carcinomas) and exhibit only a very slow progression to autonomy when the respective hormone is supplemented, whereas others, such as transplantable prostatic adenocarcinoma of rats split into hormone-dependent tumors (HDT), hormone-independent tumors (HID), and anaplastic tumor (AT) sublines. This different tumor behavior during transplantation could be attributable to a specific distribution of cytoplasmic androgen receptors and some enzymes (protein kinases) and cyclic AMP during propagation (4).

Overall, the ultrastructural, autoradiographic, and biochemical data have permitted us to distinguish different types or lines of transplantable tumors:

1. *Hormone-dependent tumors (HDT):* Always require the presence of respective hormone; in its absence, these tumors fail to grow and survive.
2. *Hormone-responsive tumors (HRT):* Growth rate and transplantability are facilitated or increased in the presence of hormones.
3. *Hormone-independent tumors (HID):* Can be transplanted and grown in the absence of hormone, most of which are spontaneous tumors.
4. *Anaplastic tumors (AT):* Can grow indefinitely and metastasize in different organs without hormone supply.

Another important factor that can modulate the transplantability of human cancers and experimentally induced tumors is the stromal environment (37,51). This stromal environment can explain why some tumors cannot be transplanted as homologous or autologous transplants, but can be heterologously transplanted in animals. Thus, several human epidermal cancers grow and retain their original histologic pattern when transplanted with their intact stroma. However, when the same tumors are transplanted without stroma (pure epithelium), they either do not survive at all or change their morphology and resemble those of normal epithelium. Thus, transplantation of tumors succeeds only when the stromal reaction occurs and the transplanted tissue acquires a new blood supply. This stromal reaction is mainly a mesenchymal proliferation and new capillary formation. In these cases, stromal environment facilitates the tumor transplantation, whereas in other cases (basal cell carcinoma), tumor stroma can release inhibitory stimuli, preventing transplantation and cellular maturation; however, when this stromal environment is changed (tumor being transplanted into a normal stromal environment), they express their differentiation potential.

Hormones can influence the tumor transplantations by acting on stromal environment and significantly changing these stromal barriers. Thus, cortisone inhibits the initiation of stromal reaction, namely, the mesenchymal proliferation, thereby aiding in tumor propagation. Also, cortisone has developed the neoformation of blood vessels. Estrogens can affect the stromal environment by increasing the content of mucopolysaccharides in the connective tissue, as well as the neoformation of blood capillaries. Thus, successful intrauterine transplantation of chemically induced basal cell carcinoma has been achieved only in female rats treated with estradiol (5). Hence, tumor transplantation and propagation are largely dependent on stromal environment. It is possible that tumoral stroma exert inhibitory effects and prevent the transplanted tumor from expressing its growth and differentiation potential, whereas the same tumor transplanted into a normal stromal environment can grow and survive. Hormones acting on the stromal environment can modulate the tumor transplantation. All these investigations provide interesting material whereby our understanding of tumor biology and of the controlling mechanisms of transplantation can be improved. An interesting model for the study of growth and progression of transplanted tumors is provided by hormonally induced tumors in Nb rats. When hormonal stimulus (estrogens) was removed, tumor regression usually occurred. Such a regressed tumor can always regrow if estrogen treatment is added, indicating that tumor maintains its hormone dependency. However, when a spontaneous regrowth occurs in the absence of estrogen stimulus, these tumors always progress toward autonomy. Although regression per se was not obligatory for autonomous changes, the paradox was evident that progression toward autonomous growth was accelerated by procedures used to check tumor growth; conversely, it was minimal with procedures to accelerate it. Thus, liver metastases of hormone-dependent adrenal carcinoma continued to grow and were not influenced by estrogen removal, although the primary transplant regressed when such metastases were transplanted, yet they retained hormone dependency without progressing toward autonomy. Progression is independent of tumor growth and is more influenced by homeostatic mechanism, especially by fluctuations in hormonal milieu, whereas regression is more sensitive to abrupt changes. Heterogeneous tumor cell populations can be differently affected by hormones. Thus, repeated stimulation and regression enhance the selection cellular process and result in a rapid progression to autonomy. Also, old age is associated with changes in hormonal levels, and such changes can elicit outgrowth of hormone-unresponsive tumor cell clones. A tendency to autonomous growth of spontaneous and hormonally induced tumors increases in older animals (9,31). Work from our laboratory suggests that hormones act on this heterogeneous cell population of transplanted tumors, which contains a wide gamut of cellular clones, some of well-differentiated, hormone responsive clones, others of poorly differentiated, hormone-unresponsive clones. Hormones and hormonelike substances (prostaglandins, epidermal growth factor, and chalones) can elicit the growth of hormone-responsive clones, and the tumor transplant will retain its hormone dependency or, in some cases, can enhance the outgrowth of poorly differentiated cells and hormone-unresponsive clones; consequently, the transplanted tumor will become an autonomous growth. Thus, tumor transplantation provides us with an ideal experimental model for the study of hormone dependency and autonomous growth and their cellular evolution. Hormones act similarly on the growth and cellular evolution of transplanted tumors, regardless of their origin (chemical, viral, ionizing radiation, or spontaneous). The mechanism of action of hormones on transplanted tumors is more complex; they can act by interfering with DNA, RNA, and protein synthesis; or on tumor cell population, especially dormant cells, or on stromal environment. Whether hormones influence in one or other of these ways is somewhat dependent on genetic factors, sex, the host-immune defense mechanism, and age of tumor recipients.

Furthermore, tumor transplantation also becomes an interesting model for the study of human cancers and their behavior, as well as for the study of various chemotherapeutic drugs on the neoplasm. Since cytologic, chromosomal, and enzyme studies have demonstrated that human cancers always retain their original cellular pattern when transplanted in athymic nude mouse, several human cancers were heterotransplanted; thus this model can be easily manipulated (by injecting either human cell lines or tumor fragments); in particular, many data obtained in long-lived nude mice can be extrapolated to humans. Therefore, a variety of chemotherapeutic or antineoplastic drugs (Cytoxan (cyclophosphamide, U.S.P.), 5-FU, Alkeran (Melphalan, U.S.P), methotrexate, vincristine, and adriamaycin) were tried alone or combined with hormone therapy or radiotherapy and the cell sensitivity and therapeutic value of each agent was more accurately evaluated.

All these data strongly suggest that hormonal environment or hormonal milieu exerts an important role in transplantation biology. However, this hormonal environment is more complex in vivo than in vitro. Therefore, not all data obtained in transplanted cell lines can be extrapolated to human cancers in vivo.

Transplantation and tumor growth are also dependent on the age of the animals. Transplanted mammary tumors grow more slowly, with a longer latent period in younger mice as compared with that of older animals. The fraction of necrobiotic cells, after tumor radiation is always higher in aging animals. This difference can be attributable to their immune systems.

Thus most present data strongly suggest that hormones have an important role in tumor transplantation. Some transplantable tumors are definitely dependent on the hormonal status and their transplantation always requires hormonal pretreatment of the host or ablative endocrine surgery (castration). The transplanted tumors can also synthesize and secrete their own hormones, which alter the anatomic structure as well as the hormonal milieu of the host.

However, our understanding of this hormonal milieu is still incomplete.

REFERENCES

1. Bertsch, S., and Markes, F.: Effects of epidermal chalone and epidermal growth factor on a transplantable epidermal carcinoma (Hewitt) of the mouse in vivo. *Cancer Res.* *39*:239–243 (1979).

2. Boeryd, B., and Suurkula, M.: Transplantability and metastability of an MCA-induced sarcoma in nude mice. *Acta Pathol. Microbiol. Scand. (A)* 85:745–750 (1977).

3. Broders, A.: Practical points on the microscopic grading of carcinoma. *N. Y. State J. Med.* 32:667–671 (1932).

4. Chung, L., Thompson, T., and Breitweiser, K.: Sensitive biochemical methods to distinguish hormone dependent and independent Dunning Tumors of prostatic origin. *Proc. West. Pharmacol. Soc.* 24:305–310 (1981).

5. Cooper, M., and Pinkus, H.: Intrauterine transplantation of rat basal cell carcinoma as a model for reconversion of malignant to benign growth. *Cancer Res.* 37:2544–2552 (1977).

6. Covelli, V., DiMajo, V., Bassani, B., and Siline, G.: Cell and cell-free transplantation experiments with a mouse reticulum cell sarcoma. *Tumori* 67:1–7 (1981).

7. Curtis-Prior, P.: Cancer and prostaglandins. In Curtis-Prior, P. (ed.): *Prostaglandins: An Introduction to Their Biochemistry, Physiology and Pharmacology.* (Amsterdam, North-Holland, 1976), pp. 145–149.

8. Elgio, K., and Hennings, H.: Epidermal chalone and cell proliferation in a transplantable squamous cell carcinoma in hamsters. I. In vivo results. *Virchows Arch. (Cell Pathol.)* 7:1–7 (1971).

9. Fabris, N., and Piantanelli, L.: Hypopituitary dwarf and athymic nude mice and the study of the relationship among thymus, hormones and ageing. In Bergsma, D., and Harrison, D. (eds.): *Genetic Effects on Ageing.* (New York, Alan R. Liss, 1978) pp. 315–333.

10. Farber, E.: Carcinogenesis—Cellular evolution as a unifying thread. *Cancer Res.* 33:2537–3550 (1953).

11. Flanagan, S.: "Nude," a new gene with pleiotropic effects in the mouse. *Genet. Res.* 8:295–309 (1966).

12. Fortner, J., Mahy, A., and Cotran, R.: Transplantable tumors of the Syrian (golden) hamster. II. Tumors of the hematopoietic tissues, genitourinary organs, mammary glands and sarcomas. II. *Cancer Res.* 21 (6) (suppl): 199–234 (1961).

13. Giovanella, B., Stehlin, T., Williams, L., Lee, S., and Shepard, R.: Heterotransplantation of human cancers into nude mice. *Cancer* 42:2269–2281 (1978).

14. Giovanella, B., Yim, S., Stehlin, J., and Williams, L.: Metastases of human melanomas transplanted in "nude" mice. *J. Natl. Cancer Inst.* 50:1051–1053 (1973).

15. Gottschalk, R., and Grollman, A.: The action of cortisone and ACTH on transplanted mouse tumors. *Cancer Res.* 12:651–653 (1952).

16. Griswold, D., Simpson-Herren, L., and Schabel, F.: Altered sensitivity of a hamster plasmocytoma to cytosine arabinoside (NSC-63878). *Cancer Chemother. Rep.* 54:337–346 (1970).

17. Haughton, G., and Whitmore, A.: Genetic control of tumor immunity. In Waters, H. (ed.): *The Handbook of Cancer Immunology*, vol. 1. (New York, Garland STPM Press, 1978) pp. 96–132.

18. Hirohashi, S., Shimosato, Y., Kameya, T., Nagai, K., and Tsunematsu, R.: Hormone dependency of a serially transplanted human breast cancer (Br-10) in nude mice. *Cancer Res.* 37:3184–3189 (1977).

19. Howes, E.: Cortisone and homologous transplantation of tumors. *Yale J. Biol Med.* 23:454–461 (1951).

20. Jones, F.: A transplantable carcinoma of the guinea pig. *J. Exp. Med.* 23:211–218 (1916).

21. Kataoka, T., and Tokunaga, T.: Transplantable sarcomas induced by 3-methylcholanthrene in inbred guinea pigs of JY-1 and Hartley/F strains. *Gann* 67:25–31 (1976).
22. Knowles, A., Leis, J., and Kaplan, N.: Isolation and characterization of plasma membranes from transplantable human astrocytoma, oat cell carcinomas and melanomas. *Cancer Res.* 43:4031–4038 (1981).
23. Lees, R., Sordat, B., and MacDonald, H.: Multicellular tumor spheroids of human colon carcinoma origin. *Exp. Cell Biol.* 49:207–219 (1981).
24. Lupulescu, A.: Enhancement of carcinogenesis by prostaglandins. *Nature* 272:634–636 (1978).
25. Lupulescu, A.: Effects of prostaglandins on tumor transplantation. *Oncology* 37:418–423 (1980).
26. Mertin, J.: Polyunsaturated fatty acids and cancer. *Br. Med. J.* 4:357 (1973).
27. Moore, G., Kondo, T., and Oliver, R.: Effect of cortisone in tumor transplantation. *J. Natl. Cancer Inst.* 25:1097–1110 (1960).
28. Murray, J.: Transplantable sarcoma of the guinea pig. *J. Pathol. Bacteriol.* 20:260–268 (1916).
29. Nemato, N., Kato, N., Mizuno, D., and Takayama, S.: Progressive development of chemical carcinogen-induced skin tumor and of a transplantable carcinoma with an immunosuppressor. *Gann* 62:293–300 (1971).
30. Noble, R., Hochachka, B., and King, D.: Spontaneous and estrogen produced tumors in Nb rats and their behavior after transplantation. *Cancer Res.* 35:766–780 (1975).
31. Noble, R., and Hoover, L.: A classification of transplantable tumors in Nb rats controlled by estrogen from dormancy to autonomy. *Cancer Res.* 35:2935–2941 (1975).
32. Pantelouris, E.: Absence of thymus in a mouse mutant. *Nature* 217:370–371 (1968).
33. Penn, I.: Some contributions of transplantation to our knowledge of cancer. *Transplant. Proc.* 12:676–680 (1980).
34. Perrin, L.: Les prostaglandins et la réponse immunitaire. *Rev. Fr. Allerg.* 14:213–217 (1974).
35. Pierce, G., and Wallace. C.: Differentiation of malignant to benign cells. *Cancer Res.* 31:127–134 (1971).
36. Plescia, O., Smith, A., and Grinwich, K.: Subversion of immune system by tumor cells and role of prostaglandins. *Proc. Natl. Acad. Sci. USA* 72:1848–1851 (1975).
37. Pinkus, H.: Premalignant fibroepithelial tumors of the skin. *Arch. Dermatol.* 67:598–615 (1953).
38. Rapp, H., Churchill, W., Kronman, B., Rolley, R., Hammond, E., and Borsos, T.: Antigenicity of a new diethylnitrosamine-induced transplantable guinea pig hepatoma: Pathology and formation of ascites variant. *J. Natl. Cancer Inst.* 41:1–11 (1968).
39. Rous, P.: A transmissible avian neoplasm (sarcoma of the common fowl). *J. Exp. Med.* 12:696–705 (1910).
40. Rygaard, J., and Povlsen, C.: Heterotransplantation of human malignant tumor to "nude" mice. *Acta Pathol. Microbiol. Scand. A* 80:713–717 (1972).
41. Schmidt, M., and Good, R.: Transplantation of human cancers to nude mice and effects of thymus grafts. *J. Natl. Cancer Inst.* 55:81–87 (1975).
42. Schultze, W.: Beobachtungen an einem transplantablen kanninchensarkom. *Verhandl. d. Deutsche. Pathol. Geselsch.* 16:358–363 (1913).

43. Shafie, S., and Grantham, F.: Role of hormones in the growth and regression of human breast cancer cells (MCF-7) transplanted into athymic nude mice. *J. Natl. Cancer Inst. 67*:51–56 (1981).
44. Smith, M., Slattery, P., Shimkin, M., Li, C.H., Lee, R., Clarke, J., and Lyons, W.: The effect of pituitary growth hormone (somatotropin) on the body weight and tumor growth in C_3H mice bearing a transplantable mammary adenocarcinoma. *Cancer Res. 12*:59–61 (1952).
45. Southam, C., and Brunschwig, A.: Quantitative studies of autotransplantation of human cancer. *Cancer 14*:971–978 (1961).
46. Stein-Werblowsky, R.: The effect of prostaglandins on tumor implantation. *Experientia 30*:957–959 (1974).
47. Stutman, O.: Tumor development after 3-methylcholanthrene in immunologically deficient athymic nude mice. *Science 183*:534–536 (1974).
48. Sylven, B.: Lysosomal enzyme activity in the interstitial fluid of solid mouse tumor transplants. *Eur. J. Cancer 4*:463–468 (1968).
49. Tannock, I.: The relation between cell proliferation and the vascular system in a transplanted mouse mammary tumor. *Br. J. Cancer 22*:258–278 (1968).
50. Toolan, H.: Transplantable human neoplasms maintained in cortisone-treated laboratory animals: H.S.#1; H.Ep.#1; H.Ep.#2; H.Ep.#3 and H. Emb. Rh.#1. *Cancer Res. 14*:660–666 (1954).
51. Van Scott, E. and Reinerston, R.: The modulating influence of the stromal environment on epthelial cells studied in human autotransplants. *J. Invest. Dermatol. 36*:107–117 (1961).
52. Warren, J., and Reddy, J.: Transplantable pancreatic acinar carcinoma. *Cancer 47*:1535–1542 (1981).
53. Wynn-Williams, A., and McCulloch, P.: Human cancer and other transplants in the "nude" mouse. *J. Pathol. 122*:225–228 (1977).
54. Zbar, B., Wepsic, H., Rapp, H., Whang-Peng, J., and Borsos, T.: Transplantable hepatomas induced in strain-2 guinea pigs by diethylnitrosamine: Characterization by histology, growth and chromosomes. *J. Natl. Cancer Inst. 43*:821–831 (1969).

Chapter 9

CANCER AND ECTOPIC HORMONES: CLINICAL AND BIOLOGICAL ASPECTS

GENERAL BIOLOGICAL CONSIDERATIONS

During the last two decades, there has been an explosion of knowledge concerning the synthesis and secretion of several hormones by nonendocrine cells (mostly tumor cells); these hormones are called *ectopic hormones* in contrast to eutopic (orthotopic) hormones secreted by normal endocrine cells. The term *ectopic hormone* was established by Liddle et al in 1969, refering to the products of tumor cells that cause remote metabolic effects resembling the known biologic action of hormones (41). The production of ectopic hormones, by comparison to that of eutopic hormones, is therefore a particular form of paraneoplasia, one of the most intriguing phenomena of endocrine physiology, which postulated that hormones are secreted only by specialized cells and organs, the endocrine glands (38).

The hormones secreted by neoplastic cells are biologically active polypeptides, similar structurally and antigenically to their normal hormones, and induce similar endocrine syndromes (Cushing's syndrome, hyperthyroidism, hyperparathyroidism, hypercalcitoninemia, inappropriate antidiuresis, and gynecomastia), called *paraneoplastic syndromes* or *ectopic hormone syndromes.* Hormone levels are always elevated and independent of the normal endocrine mechanisms or feedback control and decrease only after tumor removal, chemotherapy, or radiotherapy. They can also be synthesized in vitro by clonal tumor cells. Demonstration of these hormones in tumor tissue is also possible using biochemical and immunohistochemical methods. They are always secreted by nonendocrine tumors.

The active polypeptide or hormonelike substances occurring in a tumor should meet rigorous criteria to be genuine ectopic hormones. With the passage of time and increasing numbers of more sensitive methods (radioimmunoassays and biochemical, autoradiographic, and immunocytochemical methods) the number of recognized ectopic hormones continues to increase (33,42,44,57,58,78,79); however, in many instances, the ectopic hormone does not meet the strict criteria (described later) and consequently is not qualified for a real ectopic hormone syndrome. Until recently the production of ectopic hormones was considered a rare and bizarre manifestation of certain types of cancers, but in the last decade, biochemical evidence suggests that ectopic hormone production is much more common than suspected clinically and can be considered a general feature of neoplasia.

Until now, almost all polypeptides (but not steroid or thyroid hormones), including hypothalamic releasing factors (or hypothalamic hormones), have been described. Although most ectopic hormones are synthesized in neoplastic tissues, recent work suggests that some hormones previously considered as ectopic hormones can be also synthesized in small amounts outside of the endocrine glands (in adult nonendocrine tissues). An example is the chorionic gonadotropinlike substances (CG) occurring in nonpregnant women that suggest that fetal genes for CG are incompletely repressed (by defective or lack of operon repressors) in the adult tissue.

It is also possible that tumors consistently producing ectopic hormones are tumors containing neuroendocrine cells. Electron microscopic evidence from different laboratories, (including ours) reveals the presence of characteristic dense granules similar to those in neuroendocrine tumors.

Although it may be artificial to classify any tumor hormone as ectopic or eutopic, it is still convenient to define the hormones secreted by tumors as ectopic hormones.

Most of ectopic hormones are quite specific for different types of cancers and can be used as tumor markers. Their determination is valuable for detecting tumors, monitoring therapy, and following tumor evolution in several cases. Sometimes the presence of tumor markers in patient serum is detected even before the tumor is located (79). Because tumor ectopic hormones cause metabolic and systemic effects similar to those of specific endocrine gland, even though the respective gland is generally suppressed, the ectopic hormones are of great importance for the study of cancer.

This study outlines some criteria required for identifying ectopic hormones, commonly occurring ectopic hormones and their origin tumor tissue, the mechanism of ectopic hormone secretion, ectopic hormone or paraneoplastic syndromes, and comments on their biological and clinical significance.

CRITERIA FOR IDENTIFYING ECTOPIC HORMONES

Before we define criteria for more accurate characterization of genuine ectopic hormones, it is important to mention that hormones philogenetically evolved before plants and animals diverged; consequently, plants and animals should produce similar hormones. Only when animals evolved toward extreme cell differentiation and organization did specialized tissues or endocrine glands produce these hormones for body homeostasis and survival in a hostile environment. Animal cells contain a certain number of genes for each hormone, and only one gene is ordinarily expressed in a particular cell for synthesis of a particular or specific hormone. Which gene is expressed by a given cell type is still arbitrary.

It is important to mention that under normal conditions, most genes are in a repressed state, and only one gene is derepressed, becoming the active gene. The gene repression and derepression are mostly related to the degree of cell differentiation. What happens during neoplastic transformation is a progressive loss of cell differentiation and consequent derepression of many genes that later synthesize abnormal proteins or ectopic hormones.

This process probably happens frequently to cancer cells, which can secrete hormones that can cause severe metabolic disorders; therefore, ectopic hormone synthesis provides an interesting model for the study of gene expression in cancer cells and factors that can modulate this synthesis. Despite conflicting reports, some criteria can help identify a true ectopic hormone:

1. Conclusive evidence that the hormone is produced by the tumor must be established
2. Ectopic hormone production is usually independent of normal regulatory endocrine mechanisms (eg feedback mechanisms)
3. Lack of decreasing plasma hormone levels or regression of the clinical syndrome following extirpation of the normal gland of origin

4. Fall in plasma hormone levels and regression of the clinical syndrome after removal or treatment of the tumor
5. Demonstration of an arteriovenous difference of plasma hormone levels across the tumor vascular bed
6. Demonstration of hormone synthesis and secretion in the tumor tissue using biochemical and immunocytochemical methods
7. Incorporation of radioactive amino acids into tumor tissue and in vitro demonstration of ectopic hormone secretion by the tumor tissue (clonal tissue culture isolated from the tumor tissue)
8. Precise cytologic classification of the tumor and the presence of cytoplasmic secretory granules detected by electron microscopy
9. Although the primary amino acid sequences of ectopic hormones closely resemble those of their normal or eutopic hormones, the structure of ectopic hormones is more heterogeneous than eutopic hormones, containing a greater proportion of high molecular weight subunits (precursors) as in "big" and "little" adrenocorticotropin (ACTH), parathyroid hormone (PTH), and calcitonin, which also contain high molecular weight (HMW) subunits and low molecular weight forms and are also heterogeneous (54,55).

The structure of ectopic hormones still remains a problem of great biological and clinical importance; therefore, ectopic hormones contain more precursor subunits and fragment forms than do eutopic or authentic hormones secreted by normal endocrine glands. These differences probably reflect changes in posttranslational tumor hormone metabolism and storage rather than abnormalities in coding for the primary genes (54).

From all ectopic hormones, the structure of ectopic ACTH is better known. Evidence from analysis of cultural tumor cells, pituitary extracts, and recombination DNA work demonstrates that the prohormone molecule (stem hormone) of ACTH contains several sequences: authentic ACTH (position 1–39) or "classic" ACTH secreted by the corticotropic cells of the anterior pituitary, which contains α-melanocyte-stimulating hormone (MSH; position 1–13) and corticotropinlike intermediate lobe peptides (CLIP; position 18–39). Both α-MSH and CLIP are peptides normally found in species with a distinct intermediate lobe in the pituitary gland.

Although the 39 amino-acid form or "classic" ACTH predominates in normal pituitaries, larger and more acidic forms with minimal steroidogenic activity and more immunologic activity ("big" ACTH or high molecular weight ACTH) occur in greater relative amounts in tumors and plasma from patients with ectopic ACTH syndrome. "Big" ACTH accounts for more than 20% of total ectopic ACTH immunoactivity compared to less than 10% of eutopic ACTH. "Big" ACTH is generally the major constituent of bronchogenic carcinoma extracts and constitutes only a minor fraction of pituitary extracts.

Thirty percent of patients with chronic obstructive lung disease (COLD) reportedly had elevated "big" ACTH values (20,58). The presence of both "big" and "little" ACTH has been described in plasma and tumor tissue of patients with ectopic ACTH-producing tumors (78,79). "Big" ACTH is considered the precursor of "little" ACTH and also the biosynthetic precursor of authentic or eutopic ACTH. "Big" or HMW-ACTH, due to its high immunologic activity, should be considered a good tumor marker. In addition, Gamma-MSH (γ-MSH; position 53–48) was also isolated; Beta-lipoprotein (β-LPH; position 42–134) which contains gamma-lipoprotein (γ-LPH; position 42–101) and beta-MSH (β-MSH; position 84–101); Met-enkephalin (position 104–108) and beta-endorphin (β-endorphin; position 104–134) (7,46) were recently isolated from this common precursor (7,46). "Big" ACTH is the prohormone molecule, also called proopiocortin, which can be split into many biologically active fragments, including adrenal gland stimulation, to synthesize corticosteroids and androgens (by ACTH); melanocyte stimulation or hyperpigmentation (by MSH-containing pep-tides); and opiatelike activity (β-LPH, β-endorphin, met-enkephalin). Recent studies examined the biologic activity of these opioid peptides (β-LPH, β-endorphin, met-enkephalin) which mimic the action of morphine (24,32).

Cleavage of the promolecule in neoplastic syndromes is important because cleavage patterns change during development and may be different in tumors than in adult pituitary tissue. "Big" ACTH or proopiocortin is a glycosylated protein, and glycosylation may play an important role in its proteolysis.

Although ectopic ACTH production is thought to be unresponsive or unregulated, some in vitro studies revealed that some tumor tissues still exert control over ACTH secretion through cyclic AMP (cAMP)-dependent mechanisms (29). Recently peptides with corticotropin-releasing factor (CRF) activity have been identified in tumor extracts, a finding that may explain clinical observations that patients with ectopic ACTH syndrome sometimes respond to the adrenal inhibitor, *metyrapone*. It has been postulated that tumor tissue stimulates both the adrenal cortex and the pituitary gland through CRF mechanisms (1), but further studies are needed to estimate the pathologic significance of CRF in some bronchogenic carcinomas. The structure of other ectopic hormones is less well established.

Material resembling arginine-vasotocin (AVP) has been identified in patients with lung tumors who developed the syndrome of inappropriate antidiuretic hormone secretion (SIADH), which causes water retention to the extent that patients can suffer convulsions or go into coma. It is interesting that other posterior peptides (oxytocin and neurophysin) are also commonly found in these tumors, and they can make arginine vasotocin, the water retention hormone in birds, fish, and lower animals. An ectopic PTH (parathormone) has also been isolated. This PTH is heterogeneous and contains HMW forms and fragments, in addition to sequences found in normal or authentic PTH (1–84 sequences). It is possible that nonmetastatic hypercalcemia is due to the production of either PTH-like peptides or osteolysins. A role of ectopic prostaglandins, especially that of E series (prostaglandin E) is also suspected.

Ectopic calcitonin (CT) has also been found in excessive amounts in C-cell type tumors (medullayer carcinomas of the thyroid). Calcitonin (eutopic CT) is normally secreted by the C cells of the thyroid gland, which are of neuroectodermal origin (17). Ectopic calcitonin is also heterogenous with HMW, monomeric, and low molecular weight forms.

Ectopic gonadotropin, appears to resemble chorionic gonadotropin more than luteinizing or follicle-stimulating hormone (FSH). Both α- and β-chorionic gonadotropins were secreted by some tumors. Beta-human chorionic gonadotropin (β-hCG) is commonly used as a marker for detecting, monitoring, and therapy of placental and testicular tumors.

An ectopic insulin (insulinlike activity) has been also identified. Insulin can be made by the tumor of the pancreatic islets, but a number of other cancers, including liver and adrenal gland cancers, make insulinlike substances that may act like insulin but are not detected by the radioimmunoassays for insulin. Tumor hypoglycemia appears to be due to peptides with nonsuppressible insulin activity (probably somatomedins) rather than insulin itself.

The definition and criteria for identification of ectopic hormones should not be too rigidly judged because, recent studies using modern hormone detection techniques revealed that certain ectopic hormones are found in a variety of tissues as well as their major site of production. For instance, ectopic ACTH was found not only in lung tumors (oat cell carcinomas, bronchogenic carcinoma) but also in pancreatic islets and gastrointestinal cells (33,36); therefore, in these cases, ACTH is not an ectopic hormone.

In the case of ectopic hCG production, the problem is more complex. Ectopic production of hCG has been reported in patients with carcinomas of the lung, liver, stomach, kidney, and adrenals, but recent studies using specific radioimmunoassays for hCG reveal that immunoreactive hCG is widely distributed in a variety of normal nontrophoblastic tissues, such as testis, sperm, liver, and colon of adults and the kidney, ovary, and thymus of fetuses. The hCG producing tumors arising from the liver and colon are no longer ectopic.

The rigid differentiation of ectopic from eutopic hormone production has also become difficult; however, the detection of a hormone in some tissues by radioimmunoassays or immunohistochemical techniques does not necessarily imply the synthesis of the hormone by that tissue. This immunoreaction can be due to the existence of cross-reacting substances. For instance, serine proteases share common amino acids with glycoprotein hormones and thus show cross-reactivity with antisera against these hormones.

Although a strict differentiation between ectopic and eutopic hormones is sometimes difficult, we have to hold tentatively the definition of ectopic hormones as hormones produced by a neoplasm arising in an organ that is not unequivocally accepted as the site of production of that particular hormone.

Due to improvement in our technical procedures, the number of ectopic hormone syndromes has considerably increased in the recent years.

COMMONLY OCCURRING ECTOPIC HORMONES AND THEIR TUMOR ORIGIN

Several ectopic hormones are found in patients with nonendocrine tumors (see Table 9-1). From the data presented in this table, it appears that each ectopic hormone can be synthesized and secreted by different types of tumors, and one tumor can synthesize more than one (sometimes multiple) ectopic hormone.

It is also interesting that not only tumors but precancerous lesions or suspected lung cancers can synthesize ectopic hormones. Thirty percent of the patients with COPD (chronic obstructive pulmonary disease) reportedly have elevated serum "big" ACTH levels. This can be diagnostic of precancerous lesions and an objective test for tumor therapy (20). The presence of an ectopic hormone or even of multiple ectopic hormones is not always associated with typical clinical syndrome; some patients exhibit no typical paraneoplastic syndrome.

Recent cytological observations reveal that the cell population of a given tumor is functionally heterogeneous, thus some neoplastic cells can produce

Table 9-1 ECTOPIC HORMONES AND THEIR TUMOR ORIGIN

HORMONES	TUMOR ORIGIN
ACTH, MSH (α-and γ-MSH); β-endorphins, CLIP	Oat cell cancer, bronchogenic carcinoma (carcinoid) thymic cancer
PTH (parathyroid hormone)	Kidney tumors, hepatoma, pancreas, colon tumors, and squamous carcinoma of the lung
CT (calcitonin)	Medullary thyroid cancer, bronchus; breast cancer; pancreas tumors
hCG (human chorionic gonadotropin)	Liver tumors, large cell cancer (lung)
GH (growth hormone)	Lung cancer, uterine cancer
ADH (antidiuretic hormone)	Lung, pancreas cancer
Glucagon	Bronchus
Prolactin (PRL)	Bronchus, kidney, ovary, testis tumors
Erythropoietin (ESH)	Kidney tumor, hepatoma, cerebellar tumors
TSH (thyroid-stimulating hormone)	Gastrointestinal, bronchus
PGE (prostaglandins)	Bronchus, breast, kidney
Gastrin	Islets of Langerhans
Renin	Juxtaglomerular tumors, Wilms' tumor, kidney
Somatomedin (NSILA)	Retroperitoneal sarcoma, liver and stomach
Serotonin	Pancreas, bronchus

different active peptides that others do not. Some of these mixed cell populations of pancreatic tumors can produce several active peptides (37).

Ectopic ACTH was found to be almost indistinguishable from eutopic (pituitary) ACTH when subjected to a variety of physicochemical tests. Twenty-six tests are identical or common to pituitary ACTH (eutopic ACTH) and tumor ACTH (ectopic ACTH). Only one test, the response to dexamethasone, is different. Patients with ectopic ACTH exhibit a paradoxical response to dexamethasone, and the dexamethasone failed to inhibit or decrease the synthesis of 17-hydroxycorticosterone (17-OHCS). Although ectopic ACTH is identical to pituitary ACTH, its production is accompanied by abnormal ACTH analogues (38).

It is interesting that almost all eutopic (or authentic) hormones except steroid and thyroid hormones have their counterpart in ectopic hormones (ACTH, MSH, PTH, ADH, TSH, calcitonin, insulin, gonadotropin). No reports are available concerning the occurrence of ectopic steroid hormones or ectopic thyroid hormones. It is also important that the ectopic production of hormones may precede other signs of tumors, and ectopic hormones are good tumor markers for detecting and locating tumors and therefore may be important in prophylaxy and cancer therapy.

Carcinomas of the lung (oat cell carcinoma, bronchogenic carcinoma, and squamous cell carcinoma) are the most common underlying neoplasms that synthesize the greatest number of ectopic hormones. In several instances the ectopic hormone-producing tumors are malignant or carcinomas, and only in few instances, such as hypoglycemic syndromes, the tumor may be benign. In some instances, ectopic hormone production does not meet the criteria necessary for confirmation of an ectopic hormone syndrome.

Although the synthesis and secretion of ectopic hormones is not yet elucidated, ectopic hormones may act as a label for neoplastic cells and play an important role in localization of tumors, monitoring treatment, and in detecting the recurrence of tumors by serial measurements of serum ectopic hormone levels.

More data have recently become available regarding some of the new isolated ectopic hormones from various tumors. This is mainly due to a better purification and standardization of the prostaglandins: erythropoietin, gastrin, TSH, prolactin, and growth hormone.

Ectopic prostaglandins (PG) have been demonstrated in tumors, especially breast cancers, with a tendency to bone metastases. Cancers from patients with bone metastases synthesize more PG in vitro than do those with negative bone scans. More Pg-like material was found in breast cancers than in benign tumors or normal breast tissue (5). E series prostaglandins, namely PGE_2, are potent stimulators of bone resorption in vitro and also cause hypercalcemia in animal tumor models (73).

Indomethacin and aspirin, two inhibitors of enzyme prostaglandin synthetase, suppress osteolytic activity in some human cancers and the formation of bone metastases in rats and rabbits (18). It will be interesting to see if these prostaglandin inhibitors can reduce the incidence of bone metastases in cancer patients.

Ectopic erythropoietin production is associated with a number of different neoplasms. After renal carcinoma, which is the most productive because the kidney is the normal organ for erythropoietin synthesis, the second most responsible tumor is cerebellar hemangioblastoma, which accounts for approximately 20% of cases (42). Other tumors that exhibit an erythropoietinlike activity include hepatomas, uterine fibromyomas, ovarian tumors, and pheochromocytomas (52,59,74). Tumor removal promptly corrected the erythrocytosis.

Ectopic gastrin was originally found in nonbeta cell tumors of the pancreas (81) and has also been reported in tumors of the duodenum (30). Using radioimmunoassays, at least three ectopic gastrins were found in tumor extracts and in serum of patients with Zollinger–Ellison syndrome: in the resting period the principal component is a large molecule referred to us as "big, big" gastrin; the second is a larger, more basic molecule called "big" gastrin (heptadecapeptide amine); and "little" or "mini" gastrin (heptapeptide amine). The quantity and ratio of these ectopic gastrins varies. It has been reported that several patients with Zollinger–Ellison syndrome have up to 50% of immunoreactive gastrin as "little" gastrin and the remainder, often the major portion, as "big" gastrin. "Big, big" gastrin was found to comprise less than 2% (76).

Ectopic thyrotropin was isolated or extracted from a number of different tumors, mostly trophoblastic neoplasms, embryonal tumors of the testes, and bronchial epidermoid carcinoma (26,48). Four distinct substances have been isolated with TSH activity: thyrotropin (TSH), long acting thyroid stimulators (LATS), human chorionic thyrotropin (HCT), and molar thyroid-stimulating hormone (mTSH) (28). HCT is a polypeptide secreted by the normal placenta and has a biological activity similar to that of human pituitary TSH; its immunologic activity is more akin to that of bovine and porcine TSH (26,27). mTSH is secreted by trophoblastic tumors and it does not cross react immunologically with human or bovine pituitary TSH, LATS, or HCT. m-TSH does not appear to be closely related structurally to gonadotropins. Most of these patients exhibit symptoms of hyperthyroidism. Ectopic prolactin was isolated from different neoplasms such as renal cell carcinoma, oat cell carcinoma of the bronchus, and medullary carcinoma of the thyroid. Prolactin sometimes appears concomitant with other ectopic hormones, such as ACTH, β-MSH, and vasopressin.

Ectopic growth hormone was also found in tumors associated with acromegaly and hypertrophic pulmonary osteoarthropathy (64). Ectopically produced immunoreactive human growth hormone (IRhGH) appears to be immunologically and chemically similar to human pituitary growth hormone. In a patient with anaplastic large cell carcinoma of the bronchus and hypertrophic pulmonary osteoarthropathy, the level of IRhGH was elevated, and tumor cells in long term culture can incorporate ^{14}C-leucine and synthesize HGH-like material. Release of the ectopic hormone was stimulated by theophylline and cAMP but not by a sheep growth hormone releasing factor; therefore, the neoplastic cells behave similar to pituitary growth hormone secreting cells (22).

MECHANISMS OF SYNTHESIS AND SECRETION OF ECTOPIC HORMONES

The ectopic hormone production is one of the most intriguing phenomena of molecular biology and provides a good link between endocrinology and oncology.

Several hypotheses regarding the pathogenesis and pathophysiology of the ectopic hormone production and their inappropriate secretion were postulated during the last two decades, but the basic mechanisms of ectopic hormone secretion still remain to be elucidated. From the numerous hypotheses, five are the most important and will be discussed in detail: derepression hypothesis, abnormal regulation of gene expression, endocrine cell hypothesis, cell hybridization, and polyhormonal potential (33,61).

The Derepression Hypothesis

Until recently, the most common explanation for ectopic protein synthesis, and subsequently ectopic hormone production was the Derepression Hypothesis. According to this theory, all differentiated somatic cells contain the genetic information necessary for synthesis of all body proteins, including polypeptide hormones. The fact that only specific cells or endocrine cells can manufacture hormones is presumably due to repression (or suppression) or deletion of the genes in all other somatic cells. The genes necessary for hormone synthesis are repressed (or maintained in an inactive state) in all somatic cells, except endocrine cells in which in normal conditions can synthesize specific hormones. During the process of neoplastic transformation, a random derepression of these latent or suppressed genes can occur, and consequently a "chaotic protein metabolism" takes place in many transformed or neoplastic cells, which explains the ectopic production of one or more hormones.

This chaotic protein metabolism is also expressed in a high incidence of other abnormal proteins (α-fetoproteins, CEA, or oncofetal antigens) that frequently occur in several neoplasms.

The fact that ectopic hormones are all polypeptides and no reports involving ectopic steroid or thyroid hormones have been made can be explained by the fact that derepression takes place mostly in one gene and it happens in peptide synthesis, which is genetically coded as a single step.

In steroid hormone synthesis, which is more complicated and involves sequential steps, each step is catalyzed by a specific enzyme so the chances for ectopic steroid hormone synthesis are infinitesimally small. This hypothesis does not explain the association of a particular neoplasm with a particular hormone. For instance, ectopic ACTH production is common in lung cancer but uncommon in stomach cancer. This cannot be explained by simple and random derepression, which by chance includes genes involved only in polypeptide hormone production, so Williams proposed that genes are classified into four groups: a group of DNA is inaccessible by the normal effector but derepressed in neoplastic condition (76). Ectopic hormone production according to the derepression theory, is therefore a consequence of derepression of normally inactive genes. While this is a possible explanation in some instances, several observations are inconsistent with gene derepression as a general mechanism of ectopic hormone synthesis: direct measurements using nucleic acid hybridization have failed to detect significant gene derepression in neoplastic cells (77), and improved immunological techniques revealed the presence of ectopic proteins in normal tissue.

Abnormal Regulation of Gene Expression

It seems the most likely explanation for ectopic hormone secretion is deregulation of the regulatory mechanisms of gene expression with increase in the abundance of mRNA coding for ectopic protein synthesis rather than new synthesis from previously inactive genes.

Despite the recent progress of molecular biology, little is known about the regulatory mechanisms of gene expression. There may be several groups of phenotype-specific genes: A, genes of which transcription is irreversibly restricted during development; B, genes of which transcription is terminated during development, but irreversible transcription takes place at some time after the genes have ceased being actively transcribed; C, genes of which transcription has been restricted, but the restriction is reversible, being activated by hormones, regeneration, or wounds; and D, genes that are never repressed and are actively transcribed (13). The predominance of one group of genes or another is different in each tissue because of different developmental stages. Neoplastic transformation may cause a switch in gene transcription by activating the transcription of genes from group C, thus inducing the ectopic hormone production.

A close relationship between regulation of gene expression, cell growth, and cell differentiation and the synthesis of ectopic proteins has been suggested, but these relationships between cell growth, cell differentiation, and protein synthesis are not confined to ectopic proteins, but to other various proteins. The production of ACTH in regenerating bronchial epithelium (20) and production of hCG and α-fetoprotein (α-FP) in the regenerating liver and hepatomas can therefore be explained by an increased transcription of genes from group C.

Some close relationships between DNA synthesis and ectopic hormone production are observed in various tumors and sodium butyrate-induced hormone synthesis; therefore, ectopic synthesis of hCG in HeLa cells, mediated by sodium butyrate, is associated with cell cycle phase in late G_1 or early S phase where decondensation of chromatin is maximal. Inhibitors of culture that block HeLa cells in earlier stages of G_1 do not increase hormone production. The time course of butyrate-mediated hCG synthesis correlates directly with the degree of chromatin decondensation in synchronized HeLa cells. Using synchronized cultures, both late G_1 and butyrate-treated G_2 cells synthesized large amounts of hormone, but the chromatin of butyrate-treated G_2 HeLa cells resembles late G_1 chromatin in its maximal decondensation. These findings suggest that ectopic hormone production in neoplastic cells is related to decondensation of chromatin, irrespective of the position of cells in the cycle (16).

The relation between cell cycle stage and subsequent alterations in gene expression are not known. By using two potent inhibitors of DNA synthesis at late G_1 or early S phase, respectively, sodium butyrate and hydroxyurea were found to arrest HeLa cell multiplication at this stage. It was also found that a maximum chromosome decondensation is present at this stage which suggests that chromatin decondensation and the chromatin cycle may play a major role in the induction of ectopic hCG synthesis.

A human bronchogenic carcinoma cell line, ChaGo, also exhibits ectopic hCG synthesis that is markedly stimulated by sodium butyrate. Ultrastructural studies have shown a striking increase in decondensed chromatin in ChaGo cells grown with sodium butyrate (67). The ectopic synthesis of polypeptidic hormones by malignant tumors derived from nonendocrine tissues therefore provides a good system for studying gene expression and factors that modulate the ectopic hormone production.

Further studies should clarify the regulation of hormone biosynthesis in normal developmental cells. It is known that there are similarities between ectopic hormones and hormones produced in the fetus. Also, cell fusion between orthotopic and ectopic cells that results in the ectopic hormone production is another pathogenetic mechanism but remains to be proved (75). The morphologic and biologic similarity between ectopic hormones and some fetal hormone is postulated to be due to cell differentiation because cancer represents some sort of dedifferentiation to a more embryonic form.

The Endocrine Cell Hypothesis

The most favorably received and the most quoted hypothesis of ectopic hormone secretion at the present time is based on the concept that hormone synthesis can occur not only in endocrine glands but also in many other tissues (57). It has been suggested that all tumor producing ectopic hormones are linked by a single progenitor cell type, which is pluripotential and migratory in nature, normally associated with peptide synthesis (3).

These cells are characterized cytochemically by their amine precursor uptake and decarboxylation (APUD) of certain amino acids. The APUD cell system in the original concept proposed by Pearse (53) originates from the neural crest, from which these cells migrate to the primitive layer of ectoderm. The migration of APUD cells throughout the primitive gut has been demonstrated with a high concentration occurring in foregut; they appear in different organs derived from the primitive endoderm, such as thyroid and parathyroid glands and the pancreatic islets and endow these organs with their specific endocrine function. Further, as the gastrointestinal tract is formed from the primitive endodermal canal, the APUD cells retain their secretory capacity and become the primary source of hormones originating from the stomach, duodenum, and intestine. Many of the polypeptide secreting cells, including the pituitary corticotropins, have the same APUD characteristics as those found in chromaffin and argyrophil cells of the stomach and intestine and the Kulchitsky cells of the bronchial mucosa (which are not known to synthesize polypeptides).

Others argued that the neural crest origin does not apply to the gastrointestinal APUD cells and have postulated two distinct APUD cell systems: the neuroectoderm, which is the source of thyroid C cells and pheochromocytes; and the endoderm, which is the source of enterochromaffin and argyrophil cells of the gastrointestinal tract and pancreas (2). Under normal conditions, these cells are restricted to synthesize only a few hormones appropriate to their anatomic site (catecholamines and 5-hydroxytrypta-mine). When neoplastic transformation takes place, presumably a shift in gene function occurs and the genes for the polypeptide synthesis are subsequently readily derepressed, initiating ectopic hormone production.

The APUD cell hypothesis provides an endocrine explanation for ACTH production by oat cell carcinomas of the bronchus and by pancreatic islet cell tumors; the oat cells are deriving from Kulchitsky cells.

The separation of APUD cells into endodermal and neuroectodermal groups is in accordance with the separation of the familial multiple endocrine adenomatosis (MEA) into two types. The first MEA type, type I, includes tumors arising from enterochromaffin or argyrophil cells, such as carcinoid syndrome and Zollinger–Ellison syndrome, which arise in pancreatic islets. This MEA$_1$ syndrome includes the pituitary secreting ACTH and parathyroid tumors.

The second group, MEA type II, includes pheochromocytomas, medullary carcinoma of the thyroid and parathyroid adenomas; however, this hypothesis fails to explain why other tumor cells that do not belong to the APUD system may secrete ectopic hormones or why these cells can secrete gonadotropins and parathyroid hormone, neither of which is normally secreted by cells belonging to APUD system. It is therefore possible that tumor cells differ not only at the transcriptional level but also at RNA of posttranslational level (63).

A recent study using a large number of ectopic hormone producing tumors found that calcitonin (CT) was the major hormone (almost 97%) detected in APUD cell tumors, and it was quite often associated with production of ACTH and β-MSH. The source of ectopic hormone production should be the small, dense granules (80 to 60 μm) with a crystaloid core. Ultrastructural studies indicate that these so-called neurosecretory granules are the sites of synthesis and storage of ectopic hormones. These granules are transported towards the cell surface close to a blood capillary and discharged into capillary lumen. Their number varies greatly according to the cell function. These granules are characteristic and can be good markers for identifying an ectopic hormone producing cell (34). A quite frequent production of CT was found also in non-APUD tumor series (37%), which can be due to a polyclonal differentiation that can take place during neoplastic transformation. Transplantation of oat cell carcinoma (which is an APUDoma) in athymic nude mice showed the ability of tumor cells to differentiate towards both exocrine (endodermal) and endocrine (ectodermal) lines; therefore, the APUD concept can not explain the occurrence of ectopic hormones in a large series of non-APUD tumors. The APUD concept does have the advantage of explaining the relationship between hormone production and tumor histogenesis. In addition to CT and ACTH, APUDomas contain also lipotropin (LPH) and vasopressin (AVP).

Cell Hybridization Hypothesis

The ectopic hormone production in other tumors (nonapudomas) can be due to formation of hybrid cells arising from fusion of neoplastic nonendocrine cells (or ectopic cells) with endocrine cells (or orthotopic cells), such that a mixed hormone secreting phenotype is produced (75).

Polyhormonal Potential

During neoplastic transformation, some cell lines undergo dedifferentiation and subsequently acquire a polyhormonal potential of producing several hormones at the same time. An endocrine tumor therefore produces the hormone appropriate to its site together with the ectopic production of another hormone (eg medullary thyroid carcinoma producing CT and ACTH). Rarely, a tumor may produce the hormone of its origin and several other ectopic hormones; therefore, a certain tumor may produce a variety of ectopic hormones (eg ACTH, calcitonin, MSH, AVP, and LPH), and an ectopic hormone syndrome can be caused by different tumor types (eg ectopic Cushing syndrome can be caused by oat cell carcinoma, medullary thyroid carcinoma, thymic carcinoid, pancreatic islet tumor, gastric tumor and carcinoid of the mediastinum) (25).

At the moment, no unifying concept explains all phenomena in ectopic hormone production. No evidence of gross abnormalities in structural genes has so far been obtained because most ectopic and native or eutopic hormones are identical. The regulatory mechanism(s) of ectopic hormone production are not yet fully understood (33,55,61).

ECTOPIC HORMONE SYNDROMES (OR PARANEOPLASTIC SYNDROMES)

At present, several clinicopathologic entities produced by ectopic hormones are similar or almost identical to that occurring in original endocrine syndromes (see Table 9–2).

Ectopic Cushing's Syndrome

From these syndromes, ectopic Cushing's syndrome resulting from ectopic ACTH production is the best known.

The first case of ectopic Cushing's syndrome was reported by Brown in 1928 (11) in a woman with adrenal hyperplasia, oat cell carcinoma of the bronchus, and typical symptoms of Cushing's syndrome: obesity, hirsutism, hypertension, and diabetes mellitus. He made no comment on the possible relationship between the lung neoplasm and the endocrine disorders. It was later found that these patients exhibit elevated plasma ACTH levels, and corticotropic activity in both primary and metastatic tumor tissue was demonstrated. The term *ectopic ACTH* was coined (40).

Both "big" and "little" ACTH were detected in plasma and tumor tissue of patients with ectopic ACTH-producing tumors. The "big" ACTH is

Table 9-2   **THE MOST COMMON ECTOPIC HORMONE SYNDROMES AND THEIR RESPONSIBLE HORMONES**

ECTOPIC HORMONE	CLINICAL SYNDROME
ACTH (and CRF) and MSH, MSH alone, PTH, PGE$_2$, OAF	Cushing's syndrome, hyperpigmentation, hypercalcemia
CT (calcitonin)	unknown
Gonadotropins	Gynecomastia, precocious puberty
Insulin (NSILA-somatomedin)	Hypoglycemia
TSH	Hyperthyroidism
Erythropoietin	Erythrocytosis
Vasopressin (ADH)	Hyponatremia, convulsions, coma, SIADH (syndrome of inappropriate secretion of ADH)
Prolactin (PRL)	Galactorrhea
Gastrin	Zollinger–Ellison syndrome
Glucagon	Malabsorption
GH (growth hormone)	Hypertrophic osteoarthropathy
Renin	Hypokalemic alkalosis
Serotonin and 5-OH tryptophan	Carcinoid syndrome

considered to be the precursor of the "little" ACTH. Ectopic Cushing's syndrome is most frequently associated with carcinoma of the bronchus, which is predominantly an oat cell carcinoma (approximately 50% of all cases) (41). The second most commonly associated are thymic and pancreatic tumors and very rarely, medullary carcinoma of the thyroid. "Big" ACTH is an immunoreactive form of the hormone with a large molecule but without any significant steroidogenic activity. Like "big" insulin, it is considered a prohormone because trypsinization in vitro converts "big" ACTH into normal ACTH with 39 amino acid polypeptides that exhibit steroidogenic activity. In a study including 28 bronchial carcinomas without clinical evidence of Cushing's syndrome, most patients contained only "big" ACTH in their plasma and tumor tissues (20); therefore, when ectopic ACTH production results in Cushing's syndrome, the tumors are nearly always the oat cell type. This suggests that only oat cell carcinomas have an enzymatic mechanism for the conversion of "big ACTH to "little" ACTH or steroidogenic hormone.

Recently, peptides with corticotropin releasing factor (CRF) activity were identified in tumor extracts of patients with ectopic ACTH syndrome (two oat cell carcinomas and two pancreatic cancers) (1). A similar case of CRF production was reported in a patient with medullary carcinoma of the thyroid. Some authors speculated that the ectopic secretion of CRF by the tumor may be not autonomous but subject to a feedback regulation. Tumor extracts contained both ACTH and CRF. It was suggested that the tumor CRF stimulates tumor secretion of ACTH and consequently of plasma cortisol and that a regulatory feed back mechanism exists between tumor CRF and plasma cortisol. These patients with ectopic ACTH syndrome respond to metyrapone (65) (Fig. 9-1), which inhibits the 11β-hydroxylase activity in the adrenal cortex.

It should be mentioned that not all patients with ectopic ACTH syndrome exhibit the typical Cushing's syndrome. For instance, some patients do not exhibit typical trunkal obesity and cutaneous striae. Hypokalemia, asthma, and edema are more common among patients with ectopic Cushing's syndrome than among patients with other forms of Cushing's syndrome. The edema is often misdiagnosed as being caused by heart failure or venous obstruction.

Ectopic ACTH and lipoprotein hormone, pro-ACTH/LPH can be used for early cancer detection. A significant pro-ACTH/LPH blood elevation was found in 92% of pancreatic cancers, 72% of lung cancers, 54% of gastric cancers, 41% of breast cancers, and 27% of colon cancers (51). Some of the ectopic ACTH producing tumors can secrete opiate peptides, such as β-endorphins, which may relieve some cancer symptoms (pain).

Unfortunately the prognosis of ectopic Cushing's syndrome, due to its frequent association with bronchogenic carcinoma, is very poor. The management of these patients depends on the extent of the disease, the clinical state, and the severity of hypercortisolism. Only in rare cases the surgical

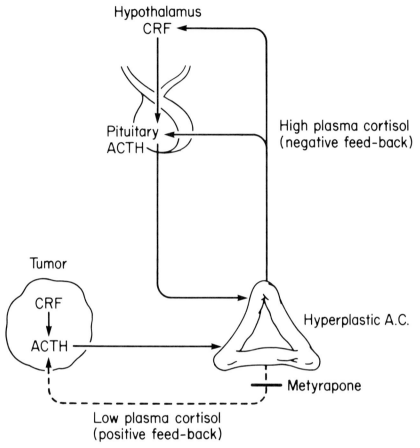

Figure 9-1 Feedback mechanism of corticotropin-releasing factor (CRF) and adrenocorticotropic hormone (ACTH) in ectopic tumors as compared to pituitary ACTH.

removal of the tumor is possible, producing immediate reversal of Cushing's syndrome. When the tumor is unresectable and the course of the disease is rapid, bilateral adrenalectomy is an alternative, but in only few cases was successful.

Medical adrenalectomy uses inhibitors of cortisol synthesis such as metyrapone, which blocks the activity of 11β-hydroxylase, and aminoglutethimide, which blocks the conversion of cholesterol to pregnenolone (see Fig. 10–3). Although both drugs may ameliorate symptoms, the doses should be very large (14).

Ectopic MSH (Melanin-Stimulating Hormone) Syndrome

Ectopic MSH syndrome appears always to occur with ACTH syndrome and its presence and symptoms are overshadowed by those of ACTH. Most patients exhibit hyperpigmentation, and radioimmunoassay detects β-MSH in their plasma or tumor extracts. In addition, β-, α-, and γ-LPH (lipoprotein hormone) were found. Electron microscopy studies in one patient with oat cell carcinoma, hyperpigmentation, and ectopic Cushing's syndrome (both ACTH and β-MSH) revealed large populations of neurosecretory granules (Fig. 9-2). Also both immuno-reactive ACTH and β-LPH were found by using immunocytochemistry in the same cells of a patient with malignant pancreatic endocrine tumor and Cushing's syndrome (Fig. 9-3a, 3b).

Ectopic PTH (Parathyroid Hormone) Syndrome

A variety of tumors can be associated with the occurrence of hypercalcemia attributable to ectopic PTH production, but the most common are squamous cell bronchial carcinomas, hypernephroma, hepatoma, carcinoma of the

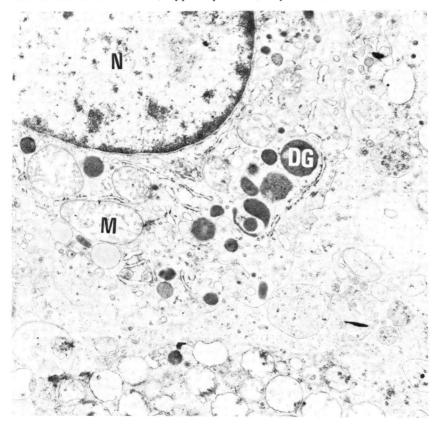

Figure 9-2 Electron micrograph of lung tissue from a patient with oat cell carcinoma. Several small characteristic neurosecretory granules (arrow) and also "big" granules (DG) are scattered throughout the cytoplasm. Mitochondria (M) and nucleus (N). Patient has Cushing's syndrome and hyperpigmentation due to ectopic ACTH and β-MSH. Epon, uranyl acetate, and lead citrate, ×15,000.

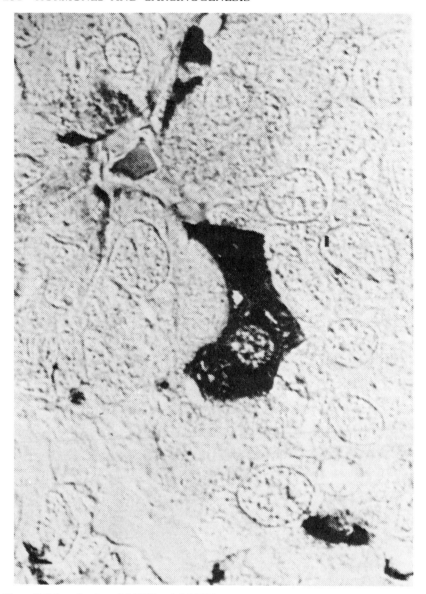

Figure 9-3 Localization of ACTH-and β-LPH-immunoreactivity in the same cells of a patient with malignant pancreatic endocrine tumor and Cushing's syndrome: (a) ACTH-immunoreactivity, (b) -LPH-immunoreactivity. Serial semithin sections, unlabeled antibody enzyme method, differential interference contrast optics, ×1000. [from Heitz et al (25), reproduced with permission of the author.]

pancreas and colon, and breast cancer. It is interesting that most lung tumors that secrete ectopic PTH were squamous cell carcinomas, and only very few oat cell carcinomas, in contrast with lung tumors that produce ectopic ACTH syndrome, which are predominantly oat cell carcinomas (57,58).

Clinical and laboratory evidence suggests that there are differences

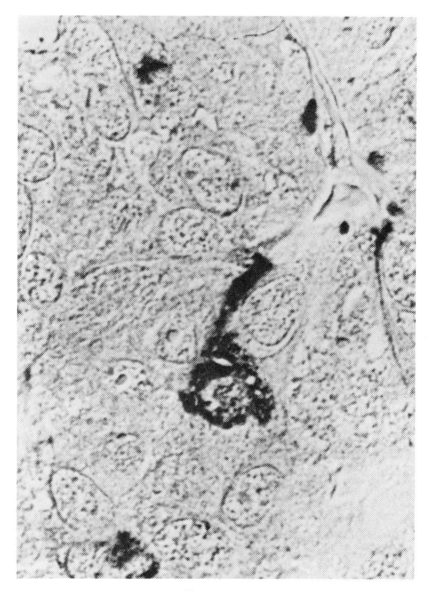

Figure 9–3b.

between parathyroid gland secreted PTH (eutopic PTH) and ectopic PTH produced by tumors. There are immunoreactive differences that result in a varied ratio of immunologic-to-biologic activity. It is therefore possible to distinguish between immunoreactive PTH found in serum of patients with primary hyperparathyroidism and ectopic hyperparathyroidism (pseudohyperparathyroidism).

Using a specific antiserum directed against the C terminal and fragments (—COOH) of the PTH molecule, it was found that most eutopic PTH is active by increasing the serum calcium level (hypercalcemia), but despite hypercalcemia in ectopic PTH-producing tumors, it was impossible to detect PTH at all with serum (56). This can be due to the fact that tumor cells may synthesize a PTH precursor, but are unable to convert it into the active PTH (which is normally secreted by the parathyroid gland) due to the absence of an enzyme that splits the molecule and separates the biologically inactive C-terminal fragments from the biologically active N-terminal fragment. The concentration of the active fragment of the hormone from the NH terminal is similarly increasing in both ectopic and primary hyperparathyroidism, explaining the hypercalcemia is present in both syndromes.

Immunologic studies showed that in some patients with the ectopic PTH syndrome, there is a striking increase of a higher molecular weight component that occurs in advance of both pro-PTH and eutopic PTH. It has been suggested that this is the *prepro-PTH* described previously by Kemper, et al. (35,55). Clinically, the features of ectopic PTH syndrome are that of hypercalcemia, hypophosphatemia, and hypercalciuria with anorexia, weight loss, polydipsia, polyuria, vomiting, dehydration, azotemia, mental confusion, and coma. In contrast with primary hyperparathyroidism, renal calculi and bone resorption are never seen in ectopic PTH syndrome, and patients with ectopic hyperparathyroidism always have low serum phosphorus levels (hypopyosphatemia) as do those with primary hyperparathyroidism.

Treatment consists primarily in the tumor removal, which induces a prompt decrease of hypercalcemia and relief of symptoms. When surgery is not possible, hypercalcemia may be controlled by medical means, such as sodium sulfate infusions and administration of calcitonin or mithramycin (39).

Ectopic Calcitonin (CT) Production

Calcitonin is a polypeptide hormone normally produced by the parafollicular (or C) cells of the thyroid gland, which are of neuroectodermal origin. Calcitonin is found in excess in medullary thyroid carcinoma, which is a C cell tumor, but does not represent ectopic hormone production. Radioimmunoassay of calcitonin is an accurate test to monitor patients with medullary thyroid carcinomas.

With the development of the radioimmunoassays for calcitonin in biological fluids, calcitonin was found in other neoplasms such as oat cell carcinoma, pheochromocytomas, breast cancers, intestinal and ovarian carcinoids, and malignant melanomas (62). Calcitonin is indeed the most constant hormone found in APUD tumors.

In a few cases, breast cancer is accompanied by elevated calcitonin secretion and hypocalcemia; it has been postulated that this is due to the ectopic production of calcitonin. Also, a circulating immunoreactive calcitonin has been found in some patients with carcinoid tumors associated with hyperparathyroidism. Although ectopic calcitonin and ACTH were found in the same lung tumors (oat cell carcinoma, squamous cell carcinoma), malignant carcinoids, medullary thyroid carcinomas, breast cancer, melanoma, colon, gastric, pancreatic and ovarian cancers, most of the studies failed to show that calcitonin and ACTH have a common precursor molecule, but they did show a high molecular weight of calcitonin (44). Hypercalcitoninemia is not usually associated with specific clinical manifestations, and an ectopic CT syndrome is still unknown.

Ectopic Gonadotropin Syndrome

The fact that gonadotropins are normally produced by both pituitary and trophoblastic tissue implies a nonpituitary, nontrophoblastic source for ectopic production of gonadotropins. The most common tumors associated with excessive gonadotropin secretion are carcinoma of the lung, germ cell tumors of testis and ovary, and less commonly, tumors such as hepatoma, or hepatoblastoma, and melanoma. This excessive ectopic gonadotropin secretion by tumors is frequently associated with precocious puberty in children, gynecomastia in men, and oligomenorrhea in premenopausal women. Hyperthyroidism may result from the excessive gonadotropin production.

Immunologic and biochemical studies reveal that both pituitary gonadotropins, follicle-stimulating hormone (FSH) and luteinizing hormone (LH), share biochemical properties with each other and with the hCG produced by a human trophoblast. They share an identical α-subunit, which is not hormone specific, and a discrete β-subunit, which has specific biologic and immunologic properties (71). Recently, specific radioimmunoassays for the β-subunit of hCG (β-hCG) were developed, and ectopic β-hCG secretion can now be accurately estimated. High serum levels of β-hCG have been found in a variety of tumors such as lung, breast, liver, and ovarian tumors. A high β-hCG level associated with high prolactin (PRL) and estradiol (E_2) levels were also reported in patients with testicular and ovarian tumors. Although the α-subunit is not hormone specific, several tumors make the biologically inactive α-chain of gonadotropins, and its demonstration in serum may be indicative of tumor. Both α- and β-subunits are therefore good tumor markers. Five to ten percent of patients with nonmalignant chronic diseases also have elevated hormone levels, which shed some doubt on their specificity. Both α- and β-subunits have been shown to be produced by human tumor cells in vitro (66). The incidence of the ectopic gonadotropin syndrome is rare, and many of these tumors respond to chemotherapy.

Ectopic Insulin (and Insulinlike Substances) Syndrome

Hypoglycemia associated with nonislet cell tumors is interesting because hormone production has not been definitely demonstrated. This syndrome is not a well-characterized paraneoplastic syndrome. Hypoglycemia can be produced by a variety of extrapancreatic tumors, but the most common (approximately 2 out of 3) are those of mesenchymal origin (fibrosarcoma, neurofibromas, mesotheliomas, rhabdomyosarcomas, spindle cell carcinomas, and lymphosarcomas) followed by hepatomas (21%), adrenal carcinomas (6%), and miscellaneous (5%).

The symptoms are those of hypoglycemia with neurologic findings (coma and occasionally focal findings). The mechanism of hypoglycemia associated with nonpancreatic tumors has not yet been elucidated, and there are potentially many ways by which tumors can cause hypoglycemia, including ectopic insulin production, production of insulinlike activity or nonsuppressible insulinlike activity (NSILA), over consumption of glucose by the tumor, tumor production of leucine and tryptophan, which can stimulate the eutopic insulin secretion, and massive infiltration of the liver by the tumor, inhibiting glucose output. At present, the most likely mechanism, although not well documented, is the tumor production of nonsuppressible insulinlike activity (NSILA), which is an atypical insulin, also called *sulfation factor of somatomedin* (72).

Somatomedins are a family of peptide hormones produced by the liver and normally under the control of growth hormone; therefore, patients with cancer hypoglycemia appear to have NSILA-producing tumors. NSILA has a molecular weight of 7400; it behaves biologically like insulin in vitro and in vivo, but immunologically is not reactive (does not react with anti-insulin antibodies).

Although it has been shown that NSILA is increased only in some patient sera, not all patients with secondary hypoglycemia due to extrapancreatic tumors have elevated NSILA (43). Further purification using receptor assays and tissue culture studies of tumor cells from these patients are required to establish whether the tumor cells produce the NSILA. Clinically, the paraneoplastic hypoglycemia should be considered in any patient with an extrapancreatic tumor who meets the criteria for organic hypoglycemia (induced by insulinomas): symptoms of hypoglycemia in fasting state, serum glucose less than 50 mg/ 100 ml during an attack, and relief of these symptoms by glucose infusion. The principal symptoms are of neurological origin (due to neuroglycopenia): headache, impaired vision, and mental confusion. The glucose tolerance test (GTT) is similar to that occurring in organic hypoglycemia (due to insulinomas); however, the characteristic marked hypoglycemia that occurs in patients with organic hypoglycemia after intravenous tolbutamide, does not occur. When possible, treatment includes the surgical removal of the tumor, which normally corrects the symptoms. If surgical intervention is not possible (inoperable cases), the paraneoplastic hypoglycemia should be controlled by glucose infusion (for acute symptoms): long-acting glucagon (or zinc-glucagon) and streptozotocin may also be effective. Glucocorticoids are less effective. Diet is also recommended, but there are little data regarding longterm effectiveness of any surgical, chemotherapeutic, radiotherapeutic, or medical approach in controlling cancer hypoglycemia.

Ectopic Thyrotropin (TSH) Syndrome

Several patients with hyperthyroidism associated with trophoblastic tumors have been reported (48). The material extracted was active biologically, but not immunologically similar to human TSH. There are four isolated substances with thyrotropic activity: pituitary TSH, LATS (long-acting thyroid stimulator), hCT (human chorionic thyrotropin) and mTSH (molar thyroid stimulating hormone). The ectopic TSH syndrome has been also described in patients with epidermoid carcinoma of the lung and mesotheliomas; all patients had tachycardia and laboratory findings similar to hyperthyroidism (^{131}I-thyroidal uptake, BMR, and serum thyroxine are elevated), but TSH was immunologically unreactive. The measurements of the β-subunit of TSH will be of particular interest for identifying this syndrome.

Ectopic Erythropoietin (ESH) Syndrome

Erythropoietin (ESH) is elaborated by cells in the kidney, which have not yet been identified. It acts on erythropoietin cells from the bone marrow in response to anemia, hypoxemia, or other conditions of impaired circulation. It produces an increased number of erythrocytes; therefore, patients have an abnormal increase of the erythrocytes, hematocrit, and hemoglobin (Hb). Ectopic erythrocytosis by tumors should be differentiated from polycythemia vera by the absence of pancytosis and splenomegaly. The ectopic ESH shares most of the physical properties of normal erythropoietin.

The most common tumors associated with ectopic ESH syndrome are renal cell carcinomas (but these can not be considered ectopic if the kidney is the normal site for erythropoietin secretion) and most important if renal carcinomas are excluded, cerebellar hemangioblastomas, which account for nearly 20% of associated tumors. Other tumors in which erythropoietinlike material can be found include fibromyomas of the uterus, hepatomas, pheochromocytomas, and Wilms' tumors. Ectopic erythropoietin syndrome can be corrected by surgical removal of the tumors.

Ectopic ADH Syndrome

Although the first description of this syndrome dated from 1938 in a patient with carcinoma of the lung, hyponatremia, and elevated urinary sodium levels with normal renal and adrenal function, the syndrome of inappropriate secretion of antidiuretic hormone (SIADH) was fully described 20 years later

(4). It was convincingly shown that the neoplastic cell produces an aberrant peptide, probably identical to ADH. It was also demonstrated that ADH could be synthesized in vitro by bronchogenic carcinoma. Tumor stimulation of posterior pituitary was the mechanism proposed at that time. Tumor tissue from patients with SIADH can incorporate in vitro ^{3}H-labeled arginine into a peptide chemically similar to arginine vasopressin (19).

The most common tumors producing ectopic ADH are oat cell carcinoma of the lung, pancreas, duodenum, thymus, breast, and esophagus, but oat cell carcinoma of the lung is the major cause of SIADH (almost one-third of all cases). This ectopic ADH appears to be biologically, chemically, and immunologically indistinguishable from original or eutopic ADH.

Laboratory findings are predominantly hyponatremia with hypotonicity of the plasma, excretion of sodium in the urine, hypokalemia, hypocalcemia, decrease of renin secretion and normal kidney function. Clinically, most patients with SIADH syndrome develop symptoms of water intoxication with headache, anorexia, nausea, and vomiting. With low sodium levels (less than 115 mEq/liter) neurologic symptoms are common (mental confusion, areflexia, pseudobulbar palsy, and convulsions); when serum sodium levels are very low (less than 100 mEq/liter), death occurs frequently (8,44). The clinical and laboratory features are widely dependent on the tumor evolution; thus, a mild SIADH can frequently be seen in the early stages or severe form in advanced tumor stages and metastases.

Treatment should be directed to hyponatremia and water intoxication by restricting fluids and giving hypertonic saline solution, especially in cases with very low serum sodium levels, where hyponatremia is life threatening. This will correct the hyponatremia within a few days and reverse the symptoms of water intoxication. Lithium and demeclocycline can interfere with the action of ADH on the renal tubule and are effective in some cases, but the mechanism of lithium action is not clear, is associated with serious complications (central nervous system dysfunction, thyroid dysfunction, and myocardial irritability), and is therefore not a safe drug.

Demeclocycline is less toxic and has been used with success in treating this syndrome. It is possible that it interferes with cAMP synthesis, which is the intracellular mediator of ADH. Surgical resection of tumor (namely oat cell carcinoma) can produce prompt remission of symptoms.

Ectopic Prolactin (PRL) Syndrome

Only few cases of the ectopic prolactin syndrome have been reported to date, but high immunoreactive serum prolactin (hyperprolactinemia) has been reported in patients with renal cell carcinoma, bronchogenic carcinoma, ovarian and testicular tumors, and medullary carcinoma of the thyroid (9,69). Most of these cases are associated with galactorrhea (gynecomastia, in some cases). The ectopic production of prolactin was demonstrated by its synthesis in tissue culture and in some cases is associated with other ectopic hormones, such as ACTH, β-MSH, ADH, and TSH (55).

Surgical resection of the tumor produces a prompt reduction of serum prolactin and relief of clinical symptoms.

Ectopic Gastrin and Enterogastrin Syndrome

Ectopic gastrin syndrome was described in 1955 by Zollinger and Ellison and is known as Zollinger-Ellison syndrome (81). They reported on patients with severe gastrin hypersecretion associated with peptic ulcer and non–insulin-secreting adenomas of Langerhans islets. The clinical syndrome is dominated by peptic ulcerations and diarrhea. The original hypothesis was that gastrin was produced by pancreatic adenomas, and two heptadecapeptides of identical amino acid sequence (gastrin I and II) were recently isolated from these tumors (23).

Using radioimmunoassays, it was found that ectopic gastrin occurs in blood in several forms: *such as* "big, big" gastrin, "big" gastrin, and "little" or "mini" gastrin. It was recently found that sera from patients with Zollinger-Ellison syndrome contain up to 50% "little" gastrin and the remainder, often the major portion, as "big" gastrin. Only less than 2% is "big, big" gastrin (78).

Gastrin is normally secreted by the antral part of the stomach, but it was recently shown that gastrin also normally occurs in D cells of the islets of Langerhans, and most of the pancreatic tumors of the patients with Zollinger–Ellison syndrome are composed of this type of cell, D cells (23). In this case, the ectopic production of gastrin is not more ectopic. Treatment of choice is total gastrectomy, but recently cimetidine (Tagamet) has been shown to markedly inhibit gastrin secretion, allowing ulcers to heal. Cimetidine is probably the drug of choice in Zollinger–Ellison syndrome.

In addition to gastrin, other ectopic enterogastrins, such as a vasoactive intestinal polypeptide (VIP) with a stimulating effect on intestinal muscle and a relaxant effect on gastric and gallbladder muscle, was found in carcinomas of the pancreas, ganglioblastomas, and pheochromocytomas. A gastric inhibitory peptide (GIP) also inhibits gastric secretion and shares some amino acid sequences with glucagon. By using histoimmunofluorescent methods, both VIP and GIP were detected in non-β cell pancreatic tumors (57).

Interesting, a recent study of 81 patients with primary ovarian carcinoids and intraovarian metastases from six midgut carcinoids showed large amounts of immunoreactive gastroenteropancreatic peptides (GEP). The incidence of GEP was higher (53%) in the trabecular carcinoids, 42% in the strumal carcinoids, and low (only 7%) in the insular carcinoids. Less commonly found were substances P, VIP, calcitonin, neurotensin, β-endorphin, and ACTH (62). Some of these strumal ovarian carcinoids also contain calcitonin, triiodothyronine (T_3), and thyroxine (T_4) (21).

The close relationship between histologic patterns and the production of these neurohormonal peptides indicates that these tumors are heterogenous cell tumors, each cell type producing its own peptide or cell types that can synthesize several immunoreactive peptides.

Ectopic Glucagon Syndrome

Ectopic glucagon production was recently demonstrated in renal tumors that contain some APUD cells and histologically resemble a carcinoid or a pancreatic islet α-cell tumor. It was also found in bronchogenic carcinoid and ovarian carcinoids (62). Immunohistochemical studies demonstrated large amounts of glucagonlike immunoreactive material in these bronchial, renal, and ovarian tumors, which appeared to be identical with enteroglucagon.

Clincal pattern is characterized by severe constipation, malabsorption and villous hypertrophy of intestinal mucosa.

Ectopic Growth Hormone (GH) Syndrome

Ectopic production of immunoreactive human growth hormone (IRhGH) or of growth hormone releasing hormone by tumors is sometimes associated with acromegaly and hypertrophic pulmonary osteoarthropathy (64).

High plasma IRhGH levels were found in some patients with carcinoma of the bronchus and gastric cancer associated with hypertrophic pulmonary osteoarthropathy. Although the surgical removal of the lung tumor may be followed by improvement in the course of hypertrophic pulmonary osteo- arthropathy, there are doubts that GH is responsible for this disease. These patients also exhibit an abnormal glucose tolerance and unsuppressed IRhGH level after glucose loading.

Ectopically produced IRhGH appears to be immunologically and chemically similar to human pituitary GH. In a patient with anaplastic large cell carcinoma of the bronchus and hypertrophic pulmonary osteoarthro- pathy, the circulating plasma IRhGH concentration was elevated and the tumor extract contained high levels of this polypeptide. It is interesting that tumor cells in tissue culture are able to incorporate ^{14}C-leucine and synthesize hGH-like material. The release of hGH from tumor cells was stimulated by theophylline and dibutyril cAMP, but not by a sheep growth hormone releasing factor; thus, these neoplastic cells behave similarly to somatotrophic pituitary cells (22).

High levels of IRhGH were also found in other tumors, such as cancer of the breast and endometrial carcinoma; however, it is not certain whether the ectopic growth hormone secretion is responsible for these clinical abnor- malities.

Ectopic Renin Syndrome

Ectopic renin production was found in juxtaglomerular cell tumors and Wilms' tumor and is frequently associated with hypokalemic alkalosis.

Ectopic Serotonin Syndrome

Ectopic serotonin production occurs in pancreas and bronchus carcinoids and is clinically characterized by symptoms similar to that of carcinoid syndrome, where serotonin is secreted as a eutopic or orthotopic hormone by argentaffine cells. These symptoms include facial flushing, edema of the head and neck, diarrhea, asthmatic symptoms, and telangiectasia. In addition to serotonin, these tumors secrete other vasoactive materials, such as histamine, prostaglandins, and VIP (vasoactive intestinal polypeptides) (45).

COMMENTS AND CONCLUSIONS

The ectopic hormone production by nonendocrine tumor cells is one of the most intriguing phenomena. Ectopic hormone production is controlled and regulated in the same way as it is in non-malignant cells. The neoplastic cells also seem to have hormone receptors on their surfaces. Cytogenetic studies of cultured cells revealed that oat cell cancer can derive from a pluripotent pulmonary endocrine cell. Both oat cells and the pulmonary endocrine cells secrete a variety of hormones including calcitonin, bombesin, arginine vasopressin and ACTH. Apart from their considerable theoretical value, they are also a source of interest to all clinicians because they produce clinical syndromes similar or almost identical to those produced by original or orthotopic (eutopic) hormones. They are also biologically, chemically, and immunologically similar to eutopic hormones. Their active molecules are bigger than those of natural hormones, and in some cases they should be considered as large precursor molecules, or "big" hormones ("big" ACTH, "big" gastrin, etc). Most of ectopic hormones contain these large precursor molecules and small fragment units, but despite that, they are biologically and chemically similar, and there are differences in their terminal amino acid sequences (–NH terminal), which are namely responsible for their immunological activity. This explains the immunologic differences between eutopic and ectopic hormones. Some ectopic hormones do not react with the natural hormone antisera, so their estimation in patient sera is still difficult even with radioimmunoassays.

   With improved radioimmunoassay methods, the number of ectopic hormones demonstrated in plasma serum and tumor extracts is markedly increased in the past few years; however, the real ectopic nature of these hormones remains more questionable. By using radioimmunoassays and immunohistochemical techniques it was also shown that the hormone-producing tumors are proliferating from cells that are ultrastructurally and histochemically identical to those that normally manufacture these hormones; thus, some of them are not ectopic hormones at all (most of APUD series).

   Almost all native or eutopic hormones have their counterparts or ectopic tumor hormones, except steroid hormones and thyroid hormones. This can be due to their complex biosynthetic mechanism. A tumor can secrete one or several ectopic hormones. It was originally assumed that tumor cells synthesize large precursor hormones from which (by enzyme splitting or cleavage) result different polypeptidic hormones. Due to a lack of enzymes, these precursors are sometimes not cleaved and remain biologically inactive, which further complicates the pathophysiology of ectopic or paraneoplastic syndromes. Although this may be true in some cases, it has also been demonstrated that these tumors contain a heterogeneous cell population. Ultrastructural and immunohistochemical studies reveal different cell lines or cell subpopulations, thus one cell line can elaborate its own hormone, which in turn produces a specific clinical syndrome.

The ectopic hormone syndromes may appear before any sign of malignancy, which allows an early detection of primary tumor. They can therefore be used as tumor markers in many cases, and their serum levels can be used as accurate criteria for management of cancer and its metastases. Several syndromes caused by inappropriate secretion of ectopic hormonelike substances, called paraneoplastic, paraendocrine or ectopic hormone syndromes, have been described, and it became apparent that ectopic hormone production is more common than has been appreciated in the past (25,34, 40,50,57,58).

Because the ectopic hormone production is of great importance for early recognition and detection of primary cancer and recurrence of metastases, for prognostic value, for monitoring the effects of various therapeutical methods by measuring the ectopic hormone levels, and for a better understanding of the mechanism of their synthesis and secretion, it is evident that the study of ectopic hormones became a major field in endocrinology and oncology.

Ectopic hormone production that quite often accompanies neoplastic disease and induces metabolic disorders that are sometimes more grave than neoplastic disease itself exerts an aggravating and unfavorable effect on the patient well being; however, ectopic hormone production may act as a label for the neoplastic cells, becoming a valuable marker of tumor location and monitoring response to treatment. Because the production of most ectopic hormones is not governed by the same mechanisms (eg feedback mechanism) as that of original or authentic hormones, their clinical manifestations run parallel to that of neoplastic disease, their therapy and prognosis is markedly influenced by that directed to primary tumor, and in most cases the surgical resection of tumor is the only effective treatment.

Although great progress has been made in the past decades regarding the accurate detection and estimation of ectopic hormone production, a number of questions remain concerning their basic mechanisms of synthesis and secretion:

Why the ectopic hormone synthesis occurs during carcinogenesis; is it beneficial or detrimental to neoplasm evolution?
Why only certain tumors produce ectopic hormones and others do not.

Why specific ectopic hormone synthesis is often associated with a limited range of tumors (e.g. ectopic ACTH occurs mainly in lung cancers but not in gastric cancers).

Which are the governing factors and regulating mechanisms of the ectopic hormone production?

Despite numerous proposed explanations or hypotheses, it seems that their mechanism is more complex and not yet elucidated. Perhaps it is better understood than occurrence and synthesis of ectopic or abnormal proteins, such as α-fetoprotein (α-FP) or all oncofetal proteins, which are easier to explain by a loss of cell differentiation or gene expression due to a derepression mechanism. It is more difficult to explain the production of ectopic hormones that involve more complex biosynthetic mechanisms and are specifically related to endocrine glands.

Each cell contains in its genome all genes necessary for protein and hormone synthesis and cell function. This is expressed mainly by the derepressed or active gene at a specific time during its evolution; during neoplastic transformation, repressed genes can be derepressed and start to express their biological potential. Consequently, the cell function is shifted toward more abnormal or ectopic protein production (eg ectopic hormones). Gene derepression is therefore an important feature of neoplasia, but the question why not all tumors synthesize ectopic hormones—ectopic hormone production is not universal phenomenon of neoplasia—remains unclear.

Production of multiple ectopic hormones in tumors and expression of ectopic hormone receptors may indicate that activation of either repressed (or normally inactive genes) or rarely transcribed unrepressed genes takes place in a relatively wide range of genomes. Further studies on the ontogeny of gene expression should be done in order to determine whether ectopic hormone production is mainly due to undifferentiated or loss of cell differentiation, such as in embryonic tissues or tumors.

It is possible that the hormones synthesized by tumors are required for the tumor to "autostimulate" its growth (eg the tumor may produce its own growth factors). This will justify the ectopic hormone production in different neoplasms (15,50). The demonstration of a hormone in tumor tissue is sometimes firm evidene that it is synthesized by tumor cells. It was suggested that neoplastic cells can absorb hormones from circulation like a sponge ("sponge" hypothesis); in this way, polypeptide hormones are taken up by receptors on the tumor cell surface (70). Such receptors for growth hormone, prolactin, and insulin have been demonstrated in some breast cancers (31).

To clarify the origin of ectopic hormones, further studies on the synthesis of these hormones in tissue culture of tumor cells is required. These studies are hampered by the difficulty of obtaining longterm tissue culture of cancer cell lines. Recently, the neurophysin biosynthesis in a transplantable human oat cell carcinoma of the lung with ectopic vasopressin production was studied in vitro. Tumor cells incubated in vitro incorporate ^{35}S-cysteine and form two neurophysins with different molecular mass, 10K and 20K respectively. Kinetic studies revealed that 20K neurophysin appears after a short time (approximately 1 hour), whereas 10K neurophysin required a longer time period. These results suggest that neurophysin is synthesized in ectopic vaso-pressin-producing tumors by posttranslocational process from a glyco-sylated proneurophysin with an apparent molecular mass of 20,000 daltons and a pH of 5.7 (80).The synthesis of neurophysin in cell-free systems is therefore directed by mRNA. The synthesis of ectopic hormones by tumor cells in tissue culture is more convincing evidence that these are really ectopic hormones. Studies in vitro can isolate the hormone precursors (or prohor-mones) as well as their different active forms.

Immunocytochemical and electron microscopic studies have also demonstrated that the ectopic hormone-producing tumors are mixed cell tumors, composed of heterogenous cell populations, each cell producing one hormone. Sometimes a tumor of bizzare cell origin, such as pelvic tumor of nerve origin, can synthesize insulin and peptides with insulinlike activity and consequently hypoglycemia. Analysis of tumor extracts revealed that this nerve origin tumor (neurofibrosarcoma) contained insulin, proinsulin, and secretory type of granules (60).

Ectopic hormone production is often associated with occurrence of abnormal antigens, such as carcinoembryonic antigen (CEA). For instance, thyroid tumor cells from a poorly differentiated follicular carcinoma can synthesize and secrete both antigen and hormone. The association of CT (calcitonin) and CEA is a good marker for differentiation of certain histologic types of poorly differentiated follicular carcinoma; thus, CT and CEA occur only in type II (trabecular structure), whereas no CT or CEA can be found in type I (follicular structure). CT secreting trabecular carcinoma can be con-sidered a different type of neoplasm, possibly an ectopic CT-producing tumor (12).

Recent work also demonstrated that oat cell carcinoma, which is one of the most frequent neoplasms associated with production of polypeptide hormones (over 50% of these tumors secrete ectopic ACTH and CT), may also synthesize growth factors. These tumor cells in tissue culture can synthesize a fibroblast growth factor (FGF), a mitogenic agent that stimulates cell division in normal fibroblasts and interacts with the membrane receptors for epidermal growth factor (EGF). It is a peptide with a molecular weight of approximately 13,400 that initiates DNA synthesis and proliferation of fibroblast and produces a marked fibrosis (oat cell carcinoma with fibrosis) (47).

Despite the similarities of these two growth factors, their role in "auto-crine," stimulation of neoplastic growth must still be defined. Even so, the most attractive hypothesis for ectopic protein synthesis that can explain the pluripotential of these cells is that of gene derepression (derepression of normally inactive or dormant genes) with an increase of messenger RNA (mRNA) coding for ectopic proteins rather than new synthesis from previously inactive genes (61).

Another important role of ectopic hormones and ectopic proteins is their use as tumor markers, for early cancer detection as a mass screening program. For instance, plasma and tumor ACTH evaluation in carcinoma of the lung revealed the presence of ectopic ACTH in 47 of 49 specimens of epidermoid carcinoma, in 15 of 17 specimens of adenocarcinomas, and in 7 of 8 specimens of large cell carcinoma.

In addition to oat cell carcinoma, which is the main source of ectopic ACTH production, immunoreactive ACTH is found in almost all extracts of lung carcinoma irrespective of their cellular type, but the levels in adenocarcinoma are generally smaller than in oat cell carcinoma and epidermoid carcinoma. Most of ectopic ACTH appears as "big" ACTH (precursor form), which is biologically inactive (79).

Ectopic ACTH can be found in preneoplastic lesions or carcinoma in situ. Extracts of lung tissue from a "smoking" dog without invasive carcinoma but showing atypical histologic changes (basal cell hyperplasia and atypical proliferation of alveolar cells) contained ACTH, mainly in the "big" or precursor form, whereas no ACTH was detected in the lung tissue from other "smoking" dogs without significant histologic changes (79).

High ACTH values were also found in patients with chronic obstructive pulmonary disease (COPD). Although these results suggest that preneoplastic cells can also elaborate ectopic hormones there are no convincing data to indicate in which stage of neoplastic transformation the ectopic hormone production occurs.

REFERENCES

1. Amatruda, T., and Upton, G.: Hyperadrenocorticism and ACTH releasing factor. *Ann. NY Acad. Sci. 230*:168–180 (1974).
2. Andrews, A.: A study of the developmental relationship between enterochromaffin cells and the neural crest. *J. Embryol. Exp. Morphol. 11*:307–324 (1963).
3. Azzopardi, J., and Williams, E.: Pathology of "nonendocrine" tumors associated with Cushing's syndrome. *Cancer 22*:274–286 (1968).
4. Bartter, F., and Schwartz, W.: The syndrome of inappropriate secretion of antidiuretic hormone. *Am. J. Med. 42*:790–806 (1967).
5. Bennett, A., Charlier, E., McDonald, A., Simpson, J., Stamford, I., and Zebro, T.: Prostaglandins and breast cancer. *Lancet 2*:624–626 (1977).
6. Berson, S., and Yalow, R.: Nature of immunoreactive gastrin extracted from tissues of gastrointestinal tract. *Gastroenterology 60*:215–222 (1971).
7. Bertagna, X., Nicholson, W., Pettengill, W., Sorenson, G., Mount, C., and Orth, D.: Corticotropin, lipotropin, and β-endorphin production by a human non-pituitary tumor in culture: Evidence for a common precursor. *Proc. Natl. Acad. Sci USA 75*:5160–5164 (1978).

8. Bewsher, P.: Ectopic hormone production by tumors: Clinical aspects. *Scott. Med. J. 25*:142–145 (1980).
9. Birkenhäger, J., Upton, G., Seldenrath, H., Krieger, D., and Tahsjian, A.: Medullary thyroid carcinoma: Ectopic production of peptides with ACTH-like, corticotropin-releasing factor like and prolactin production stimulating activities. *Acta Endocrinol. (Copenh) 83*:280–292 (1976).
10. Bloom, S.: An enteroglucagon tumour. *Gut 13*:520–523 (1972).
11. Brown, W.: A case of pluriglandular syndrome: "Diabetes of bearded women." *Lancet 2*:1022–1023 (1928).
12. Calmettes, C., Cailou, B., Moukhtar, M., Milhaud, G., and Gerard–Merchant, R.: Calcitonin and carcinoembryonic antigen in poorly differentiated follicular carcinoma. *Cancer 49*:2342–2348 (1982).
13. Caplan, A., and Ordahl, C.: Irreversible gene expression model for control of development. *Science 201*:120–130 (1978).
14. Coll, R., Horner, I., Kraiem, Z. and Gafni, J.: Successful metyrapone therapy of the ectopic ACTH syndrome. *Arch. Intern. Med. 121*:549–553 (1968).
15. DeLarco, J., and Todaro, G.: Growth factors from murine sarcoma virus transformed cells. *Proc. Natl. Acad. Sci USA 75*:4001–4005 (1978).
16. Falton, R., and Cox, R.: Relation of cell cycle position and chromatin decondensation to ectopic hormone synthesis in HeLa cells. *Somat. Cell Genet. 7*:193–204 (1981).
17. Foster, G., Baghdiantz, A. Kumar, M., Slack, E., Soliman, A., and MacIntyre, I.: Thyroid origin of calcitonin. *Nature 202*:1303–1305 (1964).
18. Galasko, C., and Bennett, A.: Relationship of bone destruction in skeletal metastases to osteoclast activation and prostaglandins. *Nature 263*:508–509 (1976).
19. George, J., Capen, C., and Phillips, A.: Biosynthesis of vasopressin in vitro and ultrastructure of a bronchogenic carcinoma. *J. Clin. Invest. 51*:141–148 (1972).
20. Gewirtz, G., and Yalow, R.: Ectopic ACTH production in carcinoma of the lung. *J. Clin. Invest. 53*:1022–1032 (1974).
21. Greco, M., Livolsi, V., Pertschuk, L., and Bigelow, B: Strumal carcinoid of the ovary. An analysis of its components. *Cancer 43*:1380–1388 (1979).
22. Greenberg, P., Beck, C., Martin, T., and Burger, H.: Synthesis and release of human growth hormone from lung carcinoma in cell culture. *Lancet 1*:350–352 (1972).
23. Gregory, R., Grossman, M., Tracy, H., and Bentley, P.: Nature of the gastric secretagogue in Zollinger–Ellison tumors. *Lancet 2*:543–544 (1967).
24. Guillemin, R: Endorphins, brain peptides that act like opiates. *N. Engl. J. Med. 296*:226–228 (1977).
25. Heitz, P., Kloppel, G., Polak, J., and Staub, J.: Ectopic hormone production by endocrine tumors: Localization of hormones at the cellular level by immunocytochemistry. *Cancer 48*: 2029–2037 (1981).
26. Hennen, G.: Characterization of a thyroid stimulating factor in a human cancer tissue. *J. Clin. Endocrinol. Metab. 27*:610–614 (1967).
27. Hennen, G., Pierce, J., and Freychet, P.: Human chorionic thyrotropin: Further characterization and study of its secretion during pregnancy. *J. Clin. Endocrinol. Metab. 29*:581–594 (1969).
28. Hershman, J., Higgins, H., and Starnes, W.: Differences between thyroid stimulator in hydatidiform mole and human chorionic thyrotropin. *Metabolism 19*:735–744 (1970).
29. Hirata, Y., Yamamoto, H., Matsukura, S., and Imura, H.: In vitro release

and biosynthesis of tumor ACTH in ectopic ACTH producing tumors. *J. Clin. Endocrinol. Metab. 41*:106–114 (1975).

30. Hoffmann, J., Fox, P., and Wilson, S.: Duodenal wall tumors and the Zollinger–Ellison Syndrome: Surgical management. *Arch. Surg. 107*:334–339 (1973).
31. Holdaway, U., and Friesen, H.: Hormone binding by human mammary carcinoma. *Cancer Res. 37*:1946–1952 (1977).
32. Hughes, J.: Opioid peptides and their relatives. *Nature 278*:394–395 (1979).
33. Imura, H.: Ectopic hormone production viewed as an abnormality in regulation of gene expression. *Adv. Cancer Res. 33*:39–75 (1980).
34. Kameya, T., Shimosato, Y., Abe, K., and Takenchi, T.: Morphologic and functional aspects of hormone producing tumors. *Pathol. Annu. 15*:351–386 (1980).
35. Kemper, B., Habener, J., Mulligan, R., Potts, J., and Rich, A.: Pre-proparathyroid hormone. A direct translation product of parathyroid messenger RNA. *Proc. Natl. Acad. Sci USA 71*:3731–3735 (1974).
36. Larsson, L.: Corticotropin like peptides in central nerves and in endocrine cells of gut and pancreas. *Lancet 2*:1321–1323 (1977).
37. Larsson, L., Grimelius, L., Hakanson, R., Rehfeld, G., Stadil, F., Holst, J., Angervall, L., and Sundler, F.: Mixed endocrine pancreatic tumors producing several peptide hormones. *Am. J. Pathol. 79*:271–284 (1975).
38. Liddle, G.: The adrenals. In *Textbook of Endocrinology*. (Philadelphia, W. B. Saunders, 1981), pp. 273–276.
39. Liddle, G., and Ball, J.: Manifestations of cancer mediated by ectopic hormones. In Holland, J., and Frei, E. (eds.): *Cancer Medicine*. (Philadelphia, Lea & Febiger, 1973), pp. 1046–1057.
40. Liddle, G., Island, D., and Meador, C.: Normal and abnormal regulation of corticotropin secretion in man. *Rec. Prog. Horm. Res. 18*:125–166 (1962).
41. Liddle, G., Nicholson, W., Island, D., Orth, D., Abe, K., and Lowder, S.: Clinical and laboratory studies of ectopic humoral syndromes. *Rec. Prog. Horm. Res. 25*:283–305 (1969).
42. Lipsett, M., Odell, W., Rosenberg, L., and Waldmann, T.: Humoral syndromes associated with non-endocrine tumors. *Ann. Intern. Med. 61*:733–756 (1964).
43. Megyesi, K., Kahn, C., Roth, J., and Gorden, P.: Hypoglycemia in association with extra-pancreatic tumors: Demonstration of elevated plasma NSILA's by a new radioreceptor assay. *J. Clin. Endocrinol. Metab. 38*:931–934 (1974).
44. Minna, J., and Bunn, P.: Paraneoplastic syndromes. In DeVita, T., Hellman, S., and Rosenberg, S. (eds.): *Principles and Practice of Oncology*. (Philadelphia, J. B. Lippincott, 1982), pp. 1476–1517.
45. Mullins, J., and Hillard, G.: Cervical carcinoid ("argyrophil-cell" carcinoma) associated with an endocervical adenocarcinoma: A light and ultrastructural study. *Cancer 47*:785–796 (1981).
46. Nakanishi, S., Inoue, A., Kita, T., Nakmura, M., Chang, A., Cohen, S., and Numa, S.: Nucleotide sequence of cloned DNA for bovine corticotropin-B-lipotropin precursor. *Nature 278*:423–427 (1979).
47. Newcom, S., and O'Rourke, L.: Oat cell carcinoma with fibrosis: Evidence for release of a growth substance. *Cancer 49*:2358–2364 (1982).
48. Odell, W., Hertz, R., Lipsett, M., Ross, G., and Hammond, C.: Endocrine aspects of trophoblastic neoplasms. *Clin. Obstet. Gynecol. 10*:290–302 (1967).
49. Odell, W., and Wolfsen, A.: Humoral syndromes associated with cancer.

Annu. Rev. Med. 29:379-406 (1978).

50. Odell, W., and Wolfsen, A.: Hormones from tumors: Are they ubiquitous? *Am. J. Med. 68*:317-318 (1980).

51. Odell, W., Wolfsen, A., Bachelot, I., and Hirose, F.: Ectopic production of lipotropin by cancer. *Am. J. Med. 66*:631-638 (1979).

52. Ossias, A., Zanjani, E., Zaluski, R., Estren, S., and Wasserman, L.: Case report: Studies on the mechanism of erythrocytosis associated with a uterine fibromyoma. *Br. J. Haematol. 25*:179-185 (1973).

53. Pearse, A.: The cytochemistry and ultrastructure of polypeptide hormone producing cells of the APUD series and the embryologic, physiologic and pathologic implications of the concept. *J. Histochem. Cytochem. 17*:303-313 (1969).

54. Ratcliffe, J.: Ectopic hormones—biochemical aspects. *Scott. Med. J. 25*:146-150 (1980).

55. Rees, L.: The biosynthesis of hormones by non-endocrine tumors: A review. *J. Endocrinol. 67*:143-175 (1975).

56. Riggs, B., Arnaud, C., Reynolds, J., and Smith, L: Immunologic differentiation of primary hyperparathyroidism from hyperparathyroidism due to non-parathyroid cancer. *J. Clin. Invest. 50*:2079-2083 (1971).

57. Rose, D.: The ectopic production of hormones by tumors. In Rose, D. (ed.): *Endocrinology of Cancer*, vol. II. Boca Raton, Fl., CRC Press, 1979), pp. 95-123.

58. Samaan, N.: Ectopic hormone producing tumors. In Kellen, J., and Hilf, R. (eds.): *Influences of Hormones in Tumor Development*. (Boca Raton, Fl., CRC Press, 1979), pp. 95-113.

59. Schonfeld, A., Babbott, D., and Gundersen, K.: Hypoglycemia and polycythemia associated with primary hepatoma. *N. Engl. J. Med. 265*:231-233 (1961).

60. Shetty, M., Boghossian, H., Duffell, D., Freel, R., and Gonzales, J.: Tumor-induced hypoglycemia. A result of ectopic insulin production. *Cancer 49*:1920-1923 (1982).

61. Shields, R.: Ectopic hormone production by tumours. *Nature 272*:494 (1978).

62. Sporrong, B., Falkner, S., Robboy, S., Alumets, J., Hakanson, R., Ljungberg, O., and Sundler, F.: Neurohormonal peptides in ovarian carcinoids: An immunohistochemical study of 81 primary carcinoids and of intra-ovarian metastases from six mid-gut carcinoids. *Cancer 49*:68-74 (1982).

63. Steiner, D.: Processing of protein precursors. *Nature 279*:674-675 (1979).

64. Steiner, H., Dahlback, O., and Waldenstrom, J.: Ectopic growth hormone production and osteoarthropathy in carcinoma of the bronchus. *Lancet 1*:783-785 (1968).

65. Suda, T., Demura, H., Wakabayashi, I., Namura, K., Odagiri, E., and Shizuma, K.: Corticotropin-releasing factor like activity in ACTH producing tumors. *J. Clin. Endocrinol. Metab. 44*:440-446 (1977).

66. Tashjian, A., Weintraub, B., Barowsky, N., Rabson, A., and Rosen, S.: Subunits of human chorionic gonadotropin: Unbalanced synthesis and secretion by clonal cell strains derived from a bronchogenic carcinoma. *Proc. Natl. Acad Sci USA 70*:1419-1427 (1973).

67. Traika, T., Rosen, S., Weintraub, B., Lieblich, J., Engel, L., Wetzel, B., Kingsbury, E., and Rabson, A.: Ultrastructural concomitants of sodium butyrate enhanced ectopic production of chorionic gonadotropin and its alpha subunit in human bronchogenic carcinoma (Cha Go) cells. *J. Natl. Cancer Inst. 62*:45-61 (1979).

68. Trump, D., and Baylin, S.: Ectopic hormone syndromes. In Abeloff, M. (ed.): *Complications of Cancer: Diagnosis and Management.* Baltimore, John Hopkins University Press, 1979), pp. 211–241.

69. Turkington, R.: Ectopic production of prolactin. *N. Engl. J. Med. 285*:1455–1458 (1971).

70. Unger, R., Lochner, J., and Eisentraut, A.: Identification of insulin and glucagon in a bronchogenic metastasis. *J. Clin. Endocrinol. Metab. 24*:823–831 (1964).

71. Vaitukaitis, J., Braunstein, G., and Ross, G.: A radioimmunoassay which specifically measures human chorionic gonadotropin in the presence of human luteinizing hormone. *Am. J. Obstet. Gynecol. 113*:751–758 (1972).

72. VanWyk, J., Underwood, L., Hintz, R., Clemmons, D., Voina, S., and Weaver, R.: The somatomedin: A family of insulin like hormones under growth hormone control. *Rec. Prog. Horm. Res. 30*:259–318 (1974).

73. Voelkel, E., Tashjian, A., Franklin, R., Wasserman, E., and Levine, L.: Hypercalcemia and tumor-prostaglandins: The VX_2 carcinoma model in the rabbit. *Metabolism 24*:973–986 (1975).

74. Waldmann, T., and Bradley, J.: Polycythemia secondary to a pheochromocytoma with production of an erythropoiesis stimulating factor by the tumor. *Proc. Soc. Exp. Biol. Med. 108*:425–427 (1961).

75. Warner, T.: Cell hybridization in the genesis of ectopic hormone secreting tumours. *Lancet 1*:1259–1260 (1974).

76. Williams, E.: Tumours, hormones and cellular differentiation. *Lancet 2*:1108–1110 (1969).

77. Williams, J., Hoffman, R., and Penman, S.: The extensive homology between mRNA sequences of normal and SV40 transformed human fibroblasts. *Cell 11*:901–907 (1977).

78. Yalow, R., and Berson, S.: Characteristic of "big ACTH" in human plasma and pituitary extracts. *J. Clin. Endocrinol. Metab. 36*:415–423 (1973).

79. Yalow, R., Eastridge, C., Higgins, G., and Wolf, J.: Plasma and tumor ACTH in carcinoma of the lung. *Cancer 44*:1789–1792 (1979).

80. Yamaji, T., Ishibashi, M., Katayama, S., Itabashi, A., Ohsawa, N., Kondo, Y., Mizumoto, Y., and Kosaka, K.: Neurophysin biosynthesis in vitro in oat cell carcinoma of the lung with ectopic vasopressin production. *J. Clin. Invest. 68*:1441–1449 (1981).

81. Zollinger, R., and Ellison, E.: Primary peptic ulceration of the jejunum associated with islet cell tumors of the pancreas. *Ann. Surg. 142*:709–728 (1955).

Chapter 10

HORMONES AS THERAPEUTIC AGENTS: A SELECTIVE HORMONOTHERAPY FOR CANCERS

BASIC PRINCIPLES OF HORMONE THERAPY FOR CANCERS

A few years after the role of hormones in the induction and development of tumors was demonstrated, it was also proved that hormones are important in the regression and extinction of cancers (27,28). This was the cornerstone for hormone therapy of cancers. Some mammary and prostate cancers can be regressed in their evolution or even extinguished by concomitant administration of hormones of opposite sex (androgens in mammary cancer, estrogens in prostate cancer). Because cancer has a plurifactorial etiology, the treatment of malignant disease by combined methods is recommended. In the last three to four decades, experimental and clinical investigations demonstrated that hormones are potential therapeutic agents in treating and managing cancers.

For many years the practice of hormone therapy in cancer management was mostly empirically based. At present, due to our improved knowledge regarding the role of hormones, hormonelike substances (or hormonomimetic agents), and hormone antagonists in pathogenetic and invasive (metastatic) mechanisms of cancers, the endocrine therapy and hormone therapy are gaining an important place in the treatment of a variety of cancers (mammary tumors, prostatic cancer, thyroid, uterus, ovary, kidney, and melanocarcinoma).

Experimental investigations using more accurate procedures revealed that neoplastic transformation is not an irreversible process leading to death; the precancerous cells and some cancerous cells are still sensitive and responsive to homeostatic regulatory mechanisms; thus the carcinogenic process can be slowed or regressed in its evolution. Among the controlling factors, hormones and hormonomimetic agents can play an important role in the regression or extinction of tumors. The benign tumors can be stopped in their evolution toward malignancy and maintained in a stage of latency or dormancy for many years.

A long time ago, before the endocrine concept was established, it was shown by empirical observation that removal of the ovaries (ovariectomy) and thyroid extract exerts a beneficial therapeutic effect in women with advanced breast cancer; also, ovariectomy prevents the occurrence of mammary cancer in mice (37). Thus, ablative endocrine therapy plays an important role in cancer treatment, namely those hormone-dependent cancers.

Administration of large amounts of opposite hormones, such as androgens (testosterone) in mammary cancers or synthetic estrogens (stilbestrol) induces a remarkable shrinkage and regression of breast cancers or malignant prostatic tumors.

Another principle of hormone therapy for cancers has been established: cancerous cells can be stopped or regressed in their neoplastic transformation by hormone excess. When the hormone level is either too little or too much, cancer evolution can be markedly delayed; therefore, administration of large doses (pharmacological doses) is another important principle of hormone therapy.

In hormone therapy, then, cancers are effectively treated with *antagonistic hormones* (androgens vs. estrogens, progesterone), *deficient hormones* (ablative endocrine therapy, ovariectomy, hypophysectomy, adrenalectomy, thyroidectomy), *cytotoxic effects* of large hormone doses (cortisone, ACTH) in lymphomas and leukemias, and *additive hormone effects* to cytostatics, radiation therapy, and so-called hormone manipulations.

It is important to distinguish between the therapeutic role of hormones in hormone-dependent cancers, where the role of hormones for cell growth and maintenance is critical; without hormones the cells cannot grow, will shrink, and will finally die, whereas in nonhormone-dependent cancers cell growth and proliferation only can be delayed for months or several years and thus hormones exert some beneficial therapeutic effects.

Large amounts of hormones may exert specific cytotoxic effects of hormones causing death only for cancer cells and leaving the normal cells undamaged (28). Another explanation cites the property of some steroid hormones to counteract the toxic action of carcinogens (catatoxic steroids) (54). A long time ago, investigators tried to stop the tumor growth by treatment with organic extracts (opotherapy) (49); this procedure produced many failures, primarily because only one extract was used. Later it was assumed that neoplastic transformation is usually multifactorial in origin, and the general belief was that many inhibitory factors should be used as a combined therapeutic method. The era of *multivalent hormonotherapy* had begun.

Substances that cannot act alone act harmonically when combined and induce a marked inhibition of tumor growth in rat cancers or in transplanted tumors. From this came the hope that it will be possible to cure the human cancers. Following administration of these hormonoids (hormonelike substances), marked histological changes, especially in the nerves and blood vessels, were described in animal and human cancers. In these nerve and blood cells the impulses originate and are stimulated by the reticuloendothelial system (RES), which in its turn exerts a favorable influence on cancer treatment (14).

In one study, a number of 114 cases with various cancers (stomach, colon, intestine, mammary, lung, skin, uterine, and ovarian) were treated by this multivalent hormone therapy. Metastases always react faster than primary tumors. All the above tumors with the exception of skin cancer were not recommendable for surgery or radiotherapy. The degenerative cellular changes in nerves and blood vessels were specific to hormonotherapy because they do not occur following radiation. An accurate description of the hormone combinations used was not provided but it is likely that adrenalin was one of the hormones (9).

Several experimental investigations and clinical observations demonstrated that a limited number of cancers, namely hormone-dependent cancers, which occur in target tissue, are dramatically influenced in their evolution by hormones and hormonelike substances; however, a larger number of tumors are hormone responsive at least during their initial stages.

The favorable effect of endocrine therapy or hormonotherapy depends largely on the degree of their hormone dependence, namely how far the cells have advanced along the carcinogenic process; the effect of hormones on tumor growth is greater during benign stages compared to malignant or autonomous stages. In the last stages, only few cancers remain hormone responsive; for this reason, an accurate estimation of cellular or nuclear abnormalities by histological or ultrastructural studies is important in the patient's choice of either hormone or ablative therapy. The evaluation of hormone cellular receptors provides a good indication for responsiveness. Low amounts of receptors indicate poor responsiveness.

Recent cytologic, autoradiographic, and endocrinologic studies have also revealed that tumors are composed of heterogeneous cell sublines; they are a "mosaic" or mixture of various cell populations. Some of these sublines are hormone-responsive or hormone-dependent, contain hormone receptors, and are well differentiated; whereas others are hormone-independent or hormone-insensitive, contain no hormone receptors, and are poorly differentiated. This new concept explains why tumor response to the same hormone, drug, or endocrine ablation is variable or unpredictable and mainly depends on the ratio of hormone-sensitive cells to insensitive or independent cells. Treatment by removal of the hormone source does "kill" dependent tumors; dependent tumor cells will succumb while the independent cells will take over.

Autoradiography using ^{3}H-thymidine can be useful for the study of DNA synthesis in tumor cells from drug-treated and control specimens and thus become a useful in-vitro assay for predicting the cancer drug effectiveness.

Combined hormonal therapy with radiation or chemotherapy should be advised because cells that escape hormonal action will be killed by radiation or chemotherapeutic drugs.

Resistance to a single hormone administration does not rule out response to another hormone or combination of this hormone with radiation therapy or cytostatic agents. Optimal timing of chemotherapy is after endocrine therapy.

It is important that hormones or hormone antagonists act continuously and their action be sustained in order to exert favorable effects. Otherwise, tumor development or regression can not be maintained.

All these principles provide a rational basis for hormone therapy. At present we know most of the mechanisms that activate neoplastic growth, but we do not know the mechanisms that deactivate it.

HORMONES AS POTENTIAL THERAPEUTIC AGENTS

Most of experimental investigations demonstrated the role of hormones in the induction and control of the rates of tumor growth and differentiation. Despite the fact that there is no firm conclusion regarding the role of hormones in initiating the carcinogenic process, valid data documents their role in tumor growth or regression.

Lacassagne (1932) first demonstrated the role of estrogens in the induction of mammary adenocarcinomas of male mice, a strain that never developed spontaneous mammary cancer. Only few years later (1939) it was shown that androgens (testosterone propionate), when given at an early age, can prevent the occurrence of mammary cancer in C_3H female mice. No effect was observed if the testosterone was given later, even in large doses (see ref. 78, ch. 4). Extinction of mammary cancers was later successful using combined administration of estradiol-17β and progesterone in chemically induced mammary carcinoma of rats. Large amounts of estradiol-17β and progesterone induced almost complete regression and extinction of cancers; 52% of rats were cancer free even 6 months later after treatment was discontinued (30). The same hormone combination injected intramuscularly over a long period of time produced significant clinical improvement in patients with advanced breast cancer (females and males) (36). Similarly, it was shown that androgens play an important role in tumor growth (40).

The era of hormonotherapy for cancers began by 1942 to 1944, when Huggins found in his studies on spontaneous dog prostate tumors that testosterone administration accelerated tumor growth; whereas castration or injection of estradiol benzoate or stilbestrol caused a dramatic and long-lasting regression in dogs as well as human prostatic cancers (29). Stilbestrol (a synthetic estrogen discovered by Dodds et al., 1939) was the first anticancer drug, and the era of cancer chemotherapy had begun (Fig. 10–1).

Hormonotherapy is a modern approach to the management and cure of cancer. Whereas surgery and radiotherapy are methods used mostly for local removal or treatment of tumors, hormonal therapy is mostly a part of systemic therapy when cancer is well spread or metastazing. It should be used with other methods: chemotherapy (cytostatics), radiation, and surgery. Hormones or hormonelike substances can act as antitumor agents, somewhat similar to cytotoxic substances, killing mainly the cancerous cells and leaving the normal cells almost intact. This is especially evident in hormone-dependent cancers, in which the cells from target tissue are in critical need of hormones, which maintain their growth and differentiation. Without hormones these cells soon die. In non–hormone-dependent cancers, hormones exert mostly an anti-inflammatory or palliative role, which is also important for cancer therapy. Hormonotherapy is not intended to cure cancer, but to control and stop or delay cancer development and metastasis. Hormones are

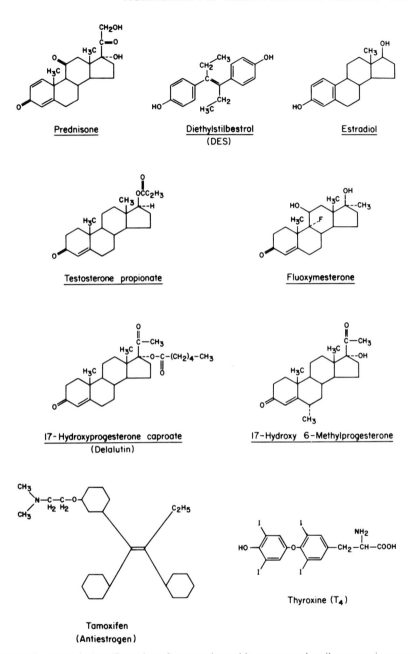

Figure 10-1 Chemical configuration of commonly used hormones and antihormones in cancer treatment.

potent therapeutic agents in cancer therapy because they direct cell division and differentiation, which are the cornerstone of neoplastic transformation. Hormones are less toxic than most cytostatic agents and work better in advanced or metastatic cancers.

At present, we do not know with certainty whether hormones act directly in initiating cancers, being carcinogenic per se; however, a tremendous amount of data demonstrate the role of hormones as important modifiers or modulators of cancers and justify their wide use in the treatment and management of cancers.

Basically, three different approaches apply to the use of hormones in cancer therapy. First, is use of *opposite hormones* (such as estrogens in the treatment of prostate cancers, androgens and progesterone in breast cancer, and thyroxine and triiodothyroxine in thyroid cancers), which can regress or even extinguish the hormone-dependent cancers. The second approach is to *deprive or remove the main source*, the endocrine gland—*ablative endocrine therapy* (ovariectomy, orchiectomy, adrenalectomy, or hypophysectomy). The third is use of *hormones in large doses* (pharmocologic doses), such as corticosteroids (cortisone, prednisone) and ACTH to treat lymphomas, leukemias, and Hodgkin's disease, where they exert a cytotoxic effect by killing the neoplastic cells.

The last effect was based on the cornerstone observations of Heilman and Kendall (26), who induced a dramatic and apparently complete regression of transplanted lymphosarcomas in mice (mostly female mice), following large amounts of cortisone. The hormone failed to regress the same tumors in male mice. The lymphosarcomas of male mice are rapidly reabsorbed only after combined treatment with cortisone plus estradiol-17β. A few years later, similar results were obtained by using cortisone and ACTH, which produced temporary regression of human leukemias and lymphosarcomas (51).

ABLATIVE ENDOCRINE THERAPY

Castration—Ovariectomy or Oophorectomy and Orchiectomy

Removal of gonads (ovary, testis), the main source of sex hormones (estrogens, progesterone, androgens), usually induces a marked regression of hormone-dependent breast cancer and prostate tumors in some laboratory animals and in humans. Spontaneous mammary cancer is common in dogs, mice, and humans.

Ovariectomy produces no tumor regression in dogs or mice, but induces significant cancer regression in human and rat mammary cancers, which are hormone-dependent. A similar shrinkage and regression of cancer was observed in spontaneous prostate cancers of humans and dogs following orchiectomy. Ovariectomy was used as a therapeutical method almost a century ago by British surgeon Beatson (4), who observed important beneficial effects and tumor regression in two out of three women with advanced metastatic breast cancer, following ovariectomy and administration of thyroid extract. In some experimental series, chemically induced (by 3-methylcholanthrene) mammary cancer regressed or was inhibited in 72% of cases by ovariectomy compared to 87% induced by hypophysectomy (34). Approximately one-third (30% to 40%) of premenopausal women with breast cancer respond to surgical castration (ovariectomy) with tumor regression; no changes were observed in postmenopausal women. Hormone determinations showed a sharp fall in estrogen levels within 2 to 3 days after surgical castration; it takes 3 to 5 months to reach a comparable level after radiation castration, which can be achieved in 4 days by administration of relatively high doses (1200 to 1600 rad) to the ovaries.

Castration acts mainly on the evolution of the primary tumor and less on distant metastases (bones, lungs, brain, or liver); however, some regression of visceral and bone metastases has been reported (57). Tumor histology reveals distinctive cytologic changes, such as destruction of cancer cells, flattening of acinar epithelium, and increase in acinar lumina, in all tumors that diminish after ovariectomy.

The marked effect of castration only in premenopausal women compared to postmenopausal women in which no effects can be seen, is similar to observations made by Loeb (41). He found that ovariectomy performed by the sixth week reduced to zero the incidence of mammary cancer in mice compared to ovariectomy performed after 6 months, when no changes were observed.

Recommendation for castration should be made according to several criteria, such as cytological methods, x-rays, ultrasonic scans, hormone estimation using radioimmunoassay (RIA), and estrogen receptors (ER). It was found by using these more sensitive methods that approximately 60% of tumors containing ER respond to castration; 30% of women with metastatic cancer respond to castration, whereas only a few (5%) tumor lacking these receptors are responsive. Studies for other hormone receptors (progesterone, insulin, androgens) should be conducted to explain the failure or lack of success in nonresponsive cases.

Orchiectomy

Castration in males with breast cancer produces significant relief. Here the castration is considered essential to therapy regardless of age. Approximately 68% of male breast cancer patients show objective signs of tumor regression and clinical improvement following castration. The average duration of such remission is approximately 30 months. Beneficial effects on skeletal metastases have also been reported (19,20). Subcapsular orchiectomy is the method of choice, but the removal of testicular tissue should be complete. Rationale of orchiectomy in male breast cancer is the fact that these tumors

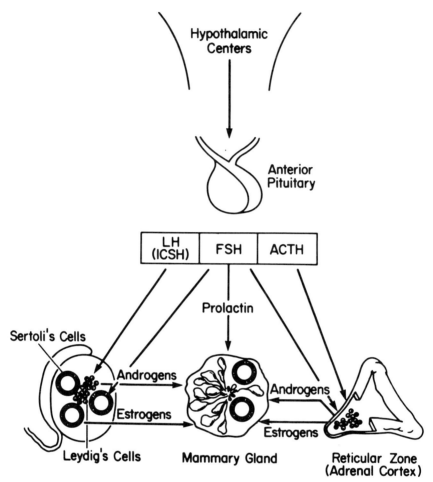

Figure 10-2 Hormonal control of male breast. ICSH, Interstitial cell stimulating hormone; FSH, follicle-stimulating hormone; LH, luteinizing hormone; ACTH, adrenocorticotropic hormone.

are androgen-dependent (see Fig. 10–2), they quickly lose their hormone dependence, and become more malignant than female breast cancer.

Orchiectomy for Prostate Cancers

Castration (orchiectomy) and estrogen therapy are well-established methods for treatment of prostate cancer. Although both are beneficial for relief of pain, dysuria, and spread of metastases, there is no general consensus that castration is superior to estrogen therapy, and many surgeons still hesitate to recommend it first, because many cancer symptoms can be relieved by estrogen therapy. Total orchiectomy has the advantage of removing the whole source of androgens, but it is difficult for patients to accept because of emptiness of the scrotum, andropause symptoms, and psychological disturbances. Subcapsular orchiectomy is therefore recommended most often, even though there are still disadvantages because many Leydig cells remain that can multiply and provide an adequate androgen secretion that still responds to interstitial cell-stimulating hormone (ICSH).

The greatest prolongation of life was achieved when orchiectomy and estrogen therapy are used simultaneously, and then estrogens are used indefinitely. Debate continues between advocates of surgery as a first therapeutic trial and endocrinologists recommending estrogen therapy. Due to cardiovascular complications of estrogen therapy (increased deaths due to cardiovascular accidents, including thromboembolism) shown by some cooperative studies, some prefer surgical castration (32,39).

It has been demonstrated that in spontaneous canine prostate cancers the cells are totally androgen-dependent in their growth and proliferation. If treatment is androgen deprival (castration), the cells will die, the tumor will regress, bone pain will be alleviated, acid phosphatase will sharply decrease, and urinary obstruction will be relieved (27). A good histologic or cytologic evaluation of the prostate tumor should be first done using electron microscopy and androgen receptor studies of prostatic cells. In this way, the stage of hormone dependence is more accurately assessed. If the tumor is in the first stages of its growth, the most beneficial therapeutic effects will certainly follow endocrine manipulation. This is also true when the tumor is well spread with bone metastases, which are unresponsive to cytotoxic agents, but mostly for palliative effects. If the tumor is well localized and encapsulated, surgery (prostatectomy and castration) or radiation therapy are first recommended.

Adrenalectomy

Adrenalectomy is performed by surgical or chemical methods (chemical or medical adrenalectomy). The rational basis for this procedure is removal of the adrenal source of estrogens and androgens. It is mostly recommended supplementary to castration. Experimental evidence suggesting its use is still controversial because adrenalectomy alone was found to increase the number and size of DMBA-induced rat mammary carcinomas by increasing prolactin secretion (15), and also dog mammary cancers are not regressed following adrenalectomy. Patients for adrenalectomy should be carefully selected because randomly performed adrenalectomy will not be beneficial in two-thirds of patients.

Patients who respond well to castration or other hormone therapy are good candidates for adrenalectomy. Estimation of estrogen receptors showed that about 59% of women with positive estrogen receptors are responsive to adrenalectomy or other ablative surgery, whereas only 8% with negative estrogen receptors respond to endocrine ablation. Estrogen receptors are good indicators for ablative surgery in both primary and metastatic tumors.

Adrenalectomy is still preferable to hypophysectomy because it is easier for surgeons to perform and its postoperative management is not so difficult. Replacement therapy is always recommended and includes hydrocortisone or some other synthetic steroid (prednisone, fluorohydrocortisone). The mortality rate is approximately 5%, so adrenalectomy should not be recommended for very ill patients and is of no value in patients who do not respond to castration. Adrenalectomy is mostly recommended in postmenopausal women with breast cancer in whom beneficial effect can rise to 30% to 50%. The reason is to eliminate the adrenal source of estrogens, which remain an important stimulus of tumor growth in many menopausal and postmenopausal women (see Fig. 10–2).

It is advisable to treat menopausal and postmenopausal women by simultaneous ovariectomy and adrenalectomy. In premenopausal women, ovariectomy is the first choice; only if tumor growth resumes should adrenalectomy be performed. Adrenalectomy should always be bilateral. The favorable response to bilateral adrenalectomy largely depends on the stage of tumor and its hormone responsiveness, age, and the general health of the patient.

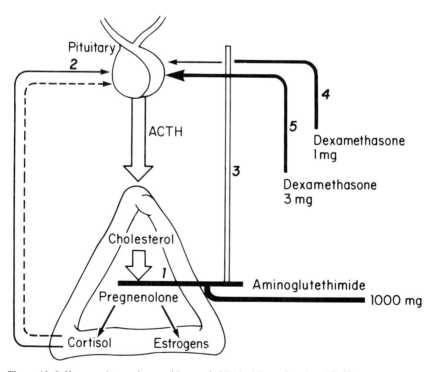

Figure 10–3 Hormonal steps in steroidogenesis blocked by aminoglutethimide.

If the patient responds well to castration or hormone therapy, 30% to 50% can also respond well to adrenalectomy. Transient relief of pain is described in most cases. Regression of primary tumor has an average duration between 18 and 26 months, and the influence of adrenalectomy on the evolution of metastases is still uncertain. The poorest palliative effects occur in the postmenopausal women following 5 to 6 years of menopause.

Chemical or medical adrenalectomy is also recommended, using aminoglutethimide, a potent adrenal steroid inhibitor. Association of this drug with cortisol was found to be nontoxic and capable of producing tumor regression and palliation of clinical symptoms (the same as surgical adrenalectomy). A 1-mg dosage aminoglutethimide combined with 40 mg cortisol was found effective in inducing medical adrenalectomy, by blocking pregnenolone synthesis (Fig. 10-3). Controlled randomized trials showed that the effectiveness of the medical adrenalectomy is about the same as surgical adrenalectomy (61).

Hypophysectomy

Hypophysectomy is more difficult to perform and is still less recommended than adrenalectomy; it is also supplimentary to castration. If patients respond well to castration, a 30% to 50% beneficial therapeutic effect following hypophysectomy can be expected. The rational basis for hypophysectomy is removal of all pituitary tropic hormones (ACTH, TSH, prolactin, growth hormone, and FSH) that control the growth and tumor progression in target tissues.

In spite of the fact that in most experimental carcinomas (mammary carcinomas, thyroid carcinomas) the inhibitory rate induced by hypophysectomy is high, attaining 87% in some cases (34); its effectiveness in human hormone-dependent cancers is still less effective. Effectiveness depends largely on the presence or absence of estrogen or androgen receptors on the cancerous cells, Hypophysectomy has no effect in about two-thirds of randomly selected patients and is effective in only 30% of patients responsive to castration or hormone therapy. The duration of tumor regression is 1 to 1½ years and depends on the anatomical completeness of pituitary removal.

Transfrontal hypophysectomy provides better results than transphenoidal hypophysectomy or radiotherapeutic hypophysectomy by implantation of [90]yttrium. More recent cryohypophysectomy or ultrasonic ablation have been used; their effectiveness is not higher than that of previous methods. In addition to some palliative effects (relief of pain), some advocates claim an objective tumor remission, especially in soft tissue (lung, pleural) and bone metastases which can reach 30% to 40%. This remission also depends on the size of the tumors; it is more efficient when tumors are smaller (43). At present, hypophysectomy (a more complicated surgical procedure with a more difficult postoperative management) is less recommended than previously discussed ablative endocrine therapies.

In summary, ablative endocrine therapy is appropriate and important in managing and controlling advanced and metastatic cancers. It is always less toxic than other procedures (e.g., chemotherapy and radiotherapy). Selection of patients should be carefully made, weighing advantages and disadvantages compared to use of hormones (additive hormone therapy) or hormone antagonists. It is important to be mindful that in most cases ablation of an endocrine gland produces a dramatic effect on tumor regression, prolongation of life, and relief of pain. Tumor responsiveness largely depends on the presence or absence of hormone receptors, the anatomical and histological stage of tumor evolution, and the general health status of the patient. In some cases the ablative methods produce psychological and emotional problems and are less safe compared to hormone administration, which is less dramatic but safer. Hypophysectomy should not be recommended for terminally ill patients or in patients whose tumors are deficient in hormone receptors.

HORMONE ADMINISTRATION—ADDITIVE HORMONE THERAPY

The use of hormones in large (pharmacologic) doses was for a long time tried alone or in combination with other methods (ablative therapy, chemotherapy, or radiation therapy) for treatment of cancers. Hormone therapy is therefore an important part of endocrine manipulation or endocrine control of malignant disease. Steroid therapy (estrogens, androgens, progestins, corticosteroids) is commonly used in the treatment of cancers, especially when ablative therapy (ovariectomy, hypophysectomy) failed to control tumor growth and progression. Administration of steroid hormones alone or in combination in large or pharmacologic doses interferes with hormonal equilibrium or homeostasis (principle of hormone interference) and inhibits the original source; the tumor therefore shrinks and regresses. Both endocrine deprival (ablative therapy) and hormone administration (hormonal interference), especially in human hormone-dependent cancers, are sometimes recommended. Selection of one of these procedures depends on the developmental stage of the tumor, its hormone responsiveness, general health status of the patient, and the judgement of the physician (29).

Estrogens

Estrogens have been used for a long time in the treatment of cancers, mostly in breast cancers and prostate cancers. Their use is more cautious and limited in postmenopausal women because uterine adenocarcinoma, or rarely other tumors, have been reported.

Experimental investigations demonstrated extinction of DMBA-induced mammary cancer in rats, following combined administration of estradiol-17β with progesterone; 52% of the rats treated with this hormonal combination were cancer free after 6 months (30). Similar beneficial therapeutic effects were reported in human breast cancers following the same combined hormone therapy (50 mg progesterone and 5 mg estradiol benzoate injected IM daily) mostly in patients in whom castration or adrenalectomy failed to control the growth and progression of malignant disease. In human prostate cancer, administration of estradiol benzoate or a synthetic estrogen (stilbestrol) caused a long-lasting remission of cancer. Estrogens inhibit the effect of androgens on androgen-dependent tumors of the prostatic gland. In breast cancer, the effects of estrogens are dose dependent; small doses stimulate tumor growth and large doses inhibit, probably by accumulating within the cells and exerting a toxic effect by killing the cells. Intracellular estrogen receptors were found in target cells, and it is possible that estrogens bind to the intracellular receptor sites and become toxic, causing cells to die.

Stilbestrol was the first anticancer drug. Of many estrogen analogues, diethylstilbestrol (DES) is the most commonly used in oncology because it is less toxic, less expensive, and longer lasting compared to natural estrogens (Fig. 10–1). In breast cancers, which are estrogen-dependent tumors, DES is used mostly in postmenopausal women in doses ranging from 1.5 mg to 150 mg daily. Standard dose is approximately 15 mg daily. In premenopausal women, DES should be cautiously tried only if ovariectomy failed. DES should be given three times daily, in a dosage of 5 mg. In carcinoma of prostate, 1 mg daily is sufficient to control the progression of disease. Higher doses are recommended only in advanced cancers with metastases.

This potent and nonsteroidal estrogen is rapidly absorbed after oral administration and metabolized in the liver. Major side-effects include nausea, vomiting, water retention, changes in libido, trombophlebitis, and embolism. Toxic effects are dose-dependent and appear mostly following large doses. In male breast cancer, estrogen therapy is preferred to cortico-steroid therapy if the castration failed. Several hormones can influence the growth of mammary gland in males (see Fig. 10–2).

Progestins

Progesterone alone accelerates the incidence and development of mammary carcinoma in female rats; a concomitant administration of progesterone and estradiol-17β extinguishes cancer in almost 52% of DMBA-treated rats. The same combination has produced long-lasting beneficial effects in human cancers. Progestins should be tried only in cases in which castration, adrenalectomy, or estrogen therapy have failed. Progesterone has also been used with some success in male breast cancer or in prostate carcinoma, especially as cyproterone acetate (which exhibits antiandrogenic properties).

Progestins are usually administered IM and orally. Commonly used progestins are 17-hydroxyprogesterone caproate (Delalutin), 1 mg twice weekly, and megestrol acetate (Megace), orally, 160 mg daily. In endometrial carcinoma, progestin induced a 30% to 35% favorable response lasting 27 months (58). Because progestin therapy is simple, nontoxic, and moderately effective, it is also used with controversial effects in the treatment of hypernephromas and in prostatic carcinoma.

Androgens

Androgens are mostly used in cases of advanced breast cancer with bone metastases in postmenopausal women. Favorable responses appear, namely in cases with estrogen receptors. Pharmacologic doses of androgens have produced a regression in 50% to 80% of DMBA-induced mammary carcinomas in rats (65) and in 15% to 30% of breast carcinomas in human subjects. This correlated with the presence of ER in tumors. A dramatic decline of ER was observed in all regressed tumors following androgen treatment. These studies suggest that androgen can induce tumor regression by depletion of estrogen receptors (65). Experimentally, they are also used in cases with hypernephroma, to improve secondary anemia, and in debilitated patients as anabolic steroid therapy, especially after chemotherapy or ionizing radiation. Most often used is testosterone propionate, 100 mg IM, three times weekly. For oral administration, fluoxymesterone may be chosen in dosages of 20 mg daily with same effect as 100 mg testosterone propionate. Higher doses (20 mg to 40 mg daily) produced an even greater decrease in tumor growth, but with increased virilization. This is the most common complication especially in women; other side-effects include hirsutism, acne, deepening of the voice, amenorrhea and occasionally jaundice, nausea, fluid retention, hypercalcemia, and prostatic obstruction.

Corticosteroids

Corticosteroids produce a variety of changes in cancer cells because of their catabolic, anti-inflammatory, and cytotoxic actions. Corticosteroids bind to their intracellular receptors and translocate to the nucleus. Commonly used are hydrocortisone, prednisone, and dexamethasone; they are mostly used to treat leukemias, Hodgkin's disease, lymphomas, or multiple myelomas, producing dramatic effects alone or in combination with ACTH. In treating breast cancer or prostatic carcinoma, they are used mostly for their beneficial effects on tumor complication (relief of pain, dyspnea). Tumor regression occurred only in 10% to 15% of treated cases. Most often used is prednisone, 4 mg, qid. Other tumor complications (such as hypercalcemia from bone metastases, coma from brain tumors, and dyspnea of lung tumors) can also be improved following corticosteroid therapy. In experimental pulmonary tumors corticosteroids induced a significant regression of tumor growth (see ref. 56 Chapter 4). Also in human lung cancers, cortisone produces tumor regression and reduces the peritumoral inflammatory reaction. Association of testosterone increases the effects of cortisone in the management of lung cancers (3).

Thyroid Hormones

Thyroid hormones (thyroxine, T_4) have been used with beneficial effects in the treatment of thyroid carcinomas. Most experimentally induced thyroid carcinomas in mice, rats, or hamsters are TSH-dependent (hormone dependent); almost 70% to 75% of human carcinomas (papillary thyroid carcinoma) and 40% of undifferentiated carcinomas are responsive to thyroid hormones (namely thyroxine) as demonstrated by tumor regression and survival for 10 years or more. The effects of thyroid hormones are less beneficial in advanced thyroid cancers (autonomous tumors) with bone, lung, or brain metastases. Use of thyroid hormones in breast carcinoma is based on the fact that hyperthyroid patients develop less mammary carcinoma than euthyroid subjects.

Experimental and clinical investigations show that hypothalamic-pituitary–thyroid–ovarian axis may play an important role in the causation and development of breast cancer (see Chapter 4). Thus, in a study of 14 patients, after mastectomy and use of thyroid hormones, 13 patients remained cancer free at a 4-year follow-up (13). Some toxic effects can occur: hyperthyroidism, arrhythmia, and angina pectoris.

NEW HORMONE ANTAGONISTS—THEIR ROLE IN CANCER TREATMENT

Hormone antagonists are synthetic, nonsteroidal compounds that exert antagonist effects for estrogens, androgens, and prostaglandins.

Antiestrogens

Antiestrogens (estrogen antagonists) recently synthesized include clomiphene (Clomid), nafoxiden, and tamoxifen (TAM) (Nolvadex); they are weakly estrogenic substances that can bind to cytoplasmic estrogenic receptors and thereby deplete the cell from estrogen receptor sites. They are less effective in premenopausal patients with breast cancer. Doses vary for each compound: 100 mg to 300 mg daily for clomiphene; nafoxiden, 100 mg to 200 mg daily; and tamoxifen, 10 mg to 80 mg daily. All three antiestrogens are nontoxic. Tamoxifen (Nolvadex) in doses of 20 mg daily is the drug of choice for postmenopausal women with metastatic breast cancer (47). This drug has also been tried in other hormone-dependent cancers, such as prostatic carcinoma, endometrial carcinoma, and kidney cancer (38).

Recent studies in human oncology indicate that the nonsteroidal antiestrogen, tamoxifen, is an effective antitumor agent. Its efficacy and safety as a single agent in the treatment of advanced breast cancer are well established. The overall objective response rate to therapy (greater than 50% of tumor regression) is about 32%, and side-effects are generally mild.

Because an estrogen binding activity has been reported in several tumors (including those of prostate, endometrium, hypernephroma, malignant melanoma, ovary, rat pancreas, and gastrointestinal tract), it was assumed that some of these tumors may be hormone-sensitive, and tamoxifen was tried. Some objective regression was observed only in prostate and endometrial cancers, but tamoxifen seems to offer little effect against renal cell carcinoma. It does not seem to block the effects of ectopic hormones released from some lung tumors, and more data are required regarding the efficacy of this drug in other tumors (50). There are no clear cut differences between these three compounds. All induce responses in about 28% to 35% of patients with breast cancer and a survival of 9 months or more.

Antiandrogens

Despite the fact that these drugs significantly depress plasma levels of testosterone, androstendione, and dehydroepiandrosterone in experimental animals and humans, they have no significant benefits over orchiectomy or in estrogen refractory prostate carcinomas. Cyproterone, a testosterone-blocking agent, was tried experimentally, in doses of 200 mg to 300 mg daily in the treatment of prostate cancer with some beneficial results, namely in patients who do not respond to estrogens.

Prostaglandin Inhibitors

Prostaglandins are implicated in the development and metastases of some cancers (mammary cancers, skin cancers); thus, indomethacin, a prostaglandin synthetase inhibitor, reduces the growth of tumors induced in mice by Moloney sarcoma virus. A new prostaglandin synthesis inhibitor, called *flurbiprofen*, induces significant inhibition of tumor growth and increases survival rates of mice with tumors. Similar effects were reported, especially a tendency to increase survival time and an enhancement of tumor response to chemotherapy and radiotherapy (6).

MULTIVALENT HORMONE THERAPY

Hormones are now used alone or combined with other systemic methods in order to inhibit or delay tumor progression or to relieve symptoms of incurable malignant disease. In many cases of advanced metastatic cancer, hormones can enhance the response of tumor growth to chemotherapy or radiotherapy. When more than one type of hormonal therapy is recommended, sequential therapies are defined as a pattern to attain a prolonged control of cancer disease. In patients who do not respond to one hormonal therapy, the addition of a second or third hormonal procedure should be tried in order to achieve improvement. Multiple hormone therapy can be recommended by using two- to three-hormone preparations concomitantly or alternately. These combined hormone therapies, as well as the introduction of new synthetic hormone antagonists (tamoxifen, aminoglutethimide, cyproterone), may replace the major endocrine ablation or fit them as a second or third additive procedure.

In some cases surgical ablation may be necessary. In principle, one hormone is tried, if patients do not respond or exhibit a low response, then it is better to recommend an additional, second or third, hormonal preparation, cytostatic agents, or radiation therapy as adjuvant in order to enhance the responsiveness of a primary tumor or its metastases.

Advanced Cancer of the Breast

Hormone therapy for breast cancer largely depends on the menopausal status of patients, presence of estrogen receptors (ER), and the histological stages of lesions (42,44,45). In premenopausal women, the ideal treatment of advanced cancer is bilateral ovariectomy. At least one-third (15% to 56%) of the patients with advanced cancer will respond to endocrine therapy, namely ovariectomy. In patients who fail to respond to ovariectomy, a second endocrine manipulation should be tried. The most commonly used steroid hormones are androgens, progestogens, and corticosteroids. Use of estrogens in premenopausal women is still controversial, and there is insufficient information regarding the use of antiestrogens or newer compounds. Treatment of choice is still ovariectomy or combined ovariectomy and adrenalectomy. The response is favorable in 30% to 35% and can be increased to approximately 60% if the treatment is confined only to patients with estrogen receptors.

There is a direct relationship between the content of steroid receptors and response to endocrine therapy and cytotoxic chemotherapy in metastatic breast cancer. Most patients with advanced breast cancer respond favorably to hormonotherapy (estrogens, progestins), especially tumors that contain both estrogen and progesterone receptors (ER, PR). In selecting cases for hormonotherapy, both receptors should be assayed. In patients treated with cytotoxic drugs, the presence of ER and PR in the tumors seems to favor an objective response to chemotherapy (64). In premenopausal women older than 35 years, ovariectomy has no therapeutic value, and synthetic estrogens (DES) in large doses improves only 10% to 12% of cases. Most clinicians use tamoxifen alone or combined with androgens, progestogens, and corticosteroids, which induce the same rate of improvement.

In patients who relapsed after castration, a second endocrine manipulation, particularly adrenalectomy, should be performed (surgical or medical adrenalectomy [aminoglutethimide]). In postmenopausal women, the treatment of choice is DES or tamoxifen. DES is a nonsteroidal estrogen, inexpensive and effective in oral administration. Preferable doses of 15 mg daily (3 × 5 mg) give beneficial results. Higher doses are more toxic and should be tried only in patients who failed to respond or respond slowly to standard doses. Toxic reactions include nausea, vomiting, aggravation of chronic cystic mastitis, endometriosis, uterine bleeding, thrombophlebitis, and embolism; liver dysfunction can occur in advanced stages with bone metastases. Hypercalcemia can also occur and in these cases, DES therapy should be stopped. In male breast cancer, DES may produce decreased libido, impotence, and gynecomastia. Histologically the mammary cancer of the male is similar to that of the female. Since 1941 when Farrow and Adair (and Treves in 1944) obtained good results with bilateral orchiectomy, this method has been used as treatment of choice in male breast cancer (20). Estrogens and progestin receptors were found in mammary tumors of males and these patients respond more favorably to endocrine therapy. Hormone administration, especially DES and tamoxifen, should be tried as an alternative to orchiectomy.

Tamoxifen (Nolvadex) is a synthetic antiestrogen that is preferable to many clinicians because it is a less toxic drug and easier to handle in cancer management. Standard doses of 20 mg (2 x 10 mg) are used, and favorable responses occur in 15% of cases. Current trials in advanced breast cancer are seeking to improve the response rates to treatment and duration of response by combining tamoxifen with other agents (cytotoxics) (62).

Prostate Cancer

It has been demonstrated that prostate tumors are hormone-dependent or mostly androgen-dependent cancers (see Chapter 4); consequently, castration (bilateral orchiectomy) was recommended as treatment of choice. In dogs as well as in humans, castration induces marked remission with shrinkage of tumors due to the removal of androgens. In breast cancer and prostate carcinoma, endocrine manipulation and hormone therapy are firmly established, and their therapeutic effects are remarkable, mostly during the first stages (stages I and II) of tumor development and much less during advanced stages (stages III and IV) (59,60).

There are four stages in the development of prostate cancers. The first three stages are related to local development of tumor (intraprostatic or confined to pelvis); acid phosphatase and alkaline phosphatase are not elevated. In these stages, there is hope for a cure using endocrine therapy. About 80% of cases are responsive to castration during these stages. During the fourth stage with distant metastases when acid phosphatase is elevated, these patients are no longer cured by endocrine therapy.

If because of emotional problems the castration is not accepted by the patient, estrogen therapy should first be tried. Among different estrogen preparations (DES, ethinylestradiol, or premarin), DES is the most commonly used drug. Dosages of 1 mg, three times daily, are recommended. Higher dosages provide no substantial advantage over standard dosages, besides increasing the toxic effects. Estrogen therapy provides the same therapeutic effects as bilateral orchiectomy.

The schedule of DES is almost the same as in postmenopausal women with breast cancer. In only a few cases, higher doses of 15 mg (5 mg, tid) should be tried for a short period of time. The most common complications of DES treatment are cardiovascular, including cardiac failure and edema. Groups including the U.S. Veterans Administration Cooperative Urological Research Group (VACURG) reported an increase of 75% in death rate due to cardiovascular accidents in estrogen-treated patients compared to untreated patients (32).

Cyproterone, a testosterone-blocking agent, has also been tried experimentally with some promising results. Dosages of 200 mg to 300 mg daily can provide some symptomatic relief and are used when effects of castration or estrogen therapy wear off. A critical appraisal of castration and estrogen therapy reveals that both produce the same symptomatic relief and that the preference for one over the other depends on the physician's experience with each; individualization of therapy is also important. In addition to cardiovascular complications, a decreased libido, impotence, and gynecomastia occur quite often following DES treatment; when urethral obstruction is important, orchiectomy or transurethral resection of prostate should be immediately recommended.

It is interesting that various proteic hormones (prolactin, GH, FSH) that normally act through membrane receptors may exert important regulatory effects on prostatic cell growth and intracellular biochemistry. Epidemiological studies suggest a relationship between the onset of sexuality and the occurrence of prostate cancer; thus the patient with prostate carcinoma can be hormonally different from the normal male.

Ovarian Cancer

Cancer of the ovary accounts for 5% of malignant tumors in women, fewer than endometrial carcinoma. Classification of ovarian tumors is based mostly on their histogenesis (53). There are benign or hormone-secreting tumors and malignant or non–hormone-secreting (nonfunctional) tumors.

Treatment of ovarian tumors should be individualized. Commonly used methods are surgery, radiotherapy, chemotherapy, hormonotherapy, and immunotherapy. Selection of methods and patients should be according to the stage of disease and the presence of hormone receptors. An integration therapy is sometimes advised. The presence of estrogen and progesterone receptors was recently reported in some ovarian tumors (22). The existence of receptors in ovarian cancer cells was correlated with the nuclear grade and its response to surgery, radiotherapy, and hormonotherapy (progestins, DES).

Endometrial Carcinoma

Endometrial carcinoma is the second most frequent malignant tumor of the female genital tract and the third most frequent malignancy among American women. This hormone-sensitive tumor is especially sensitive to progestins and estrogens. Progestogens produce regression of experimentally induced carcinoma (40). Exogenous estrogens used in the last decades to relieve climacteric symptoms showed a dramatic increase (fourfold to eightfold) in the risk to endometrial cancer compared to control studies. Administration of estrogens can therefore induce endometrial cancer in animal studies, and ovariectomy can inhibit the methylcholanthrene-induced endometrial cancer in rabbits (39). Massive doses of progesterone (500 mg of hydroxyprogesterone caproate, 3 times weekly, IM) have induced objective remission in 25% of women with endometrial cancer (33). Palliation of advanced or metastatic endometrial adenocarcinoma may be achieved with large doses of medroxyprogesterone (400 mg IM weekly or 100–200 mg orally daily). The treatment of choice is still surgery combined with radiation.

Recent studies in monkeys showed that estrogens are necessary for persistance of endometriosis but not for its initiation. The role of exogenous and endogenous estrogens was widely investigated in recent years. There is evidence from several sources that endometrial carcinoma is estrogen sensitive (24). A higher risk of endometrial cancer was reported among women at menopause and following estrogen administration (66). In the United States an increased incidence of endometrial cancer was also observed in the past 5 years; this is coincidental with the increased use of estrogens in postmenopausal women. There is a dose relationship; the higher the use of estrogens the greater the incidence of endometrial carcinoma.

More interesting is the role of endogenous estrogens. In postmenopausal women, estrone is derived largely from the adrenal cortex due to the conversion of androstendione, synthesized by the adrenal cortex, and converted to estrone in the liver, adipose tissue, and skin. Experimental and epidemiologic data reveal that prolonged stimulation of uterus by exogenous or endogenous estrogens increases the occurrence of endometrial carcinoma. Logically, progestins protect against endometrial cancer.

The review of these data is not intended to rule out the use of estrogens in postmenopausal women. Certainly they exert beneficial effects on the menopause symptoms and osteoporosis, and the physician should balance the advantages against the increasing incidence of endometrial cancer. The use of drugs that suppress ovarian function and retrograde menstruation offer the best chance of clinical remission. These drugs are synthetic androgens, for example, danazol (Danocrine), 800 mg in two dosages for at least 3 to 6 months and should begin during menstruation. Remission induced by progestens can be due to a stromal reaction against tumor, whereas synthetic androgens suppress ovarian function. Oral contraceptives (which contain estrogen and progestins) are not as effective in treating endometriosis.

Renal Cell Carcinoma

Although the renal cell carcinoma can be induced by chronic administration of synthetic estrogens (diethylstilbestrol) in male golden syrian hamsters and progesterone, testosterone, and deoxycorticosterone can inhibit their onset and development, no conclusive evidence supports the beneficial effects of hormone therapy in human renal cell carcinoma (RCC). Androgen receptors have been found in both normal and malignant renal tissue. It is important in resected tumors to estimate androgen receptors by autoradiographic studies using radioactive hormones.

Bloom was the first investigator to try to inhibit the estrogen-induced renal adenocarcinoma in golden hamsters by hormone manipulation using progestational agents. He later tried the same technique in human renal carcinoma. During the early 1960s, he treated patients with advanced renal carcinoma with androgens and progestogens. By 1973 he reported significant improvement in 11 of 80 patients (8). Others at UCLA, using the same hormone combination (androgens and progesterone) were unable to report a single objective remission (10,32).

Thyroid Cancer

Most of the experimental and clinical investigations demonstrated that thyroid tumors are TSH-dependent. Administration of thyroid-stimulating hormone (TSH) or thyrotropin stimulates growth and development of these tumors, whereas its suppression induces regression of thyroid carcinoma. Thyroid suppressive therapy was used for a long time in the treatment of cancers. Dessicated thyroid, thyroxine, or triiodothyronine were mostly used to treat papillary and follicular carcinoma.

The response rate to thyroid suppressive therapy largely depends on early detection using biopsy and consequently studies with electron microscopy and autoradiography of resected thyroid tumors. Estimation of thyrotropin receptors in the thyroid cells in benign and some differentiated malignant thyroid carcinomas is also an important factor in response to hormone therapy and prognosis. Recent investigation revealed that the so-called cold nodules, which are less effective in incorporating the radioiodine than the surrounding tissue, still respond to TSH administration and consequently to thyroid suppressive therapy.

Doses a little larger than those of standard therapy should be used, and the response rate is favorable in almost 75% of patients with papillary adenocarcinoma and 40% of undifferentiated carcinomas. Response rate is even higher in benign thyroid tumors or hot nodules such as papillary or follicular adenomas. There is no conclusive evidence supporting the use of thyroid therapy as primary therapy, but it has been used as an adjuvant therapy with surgery or radiation. Some investigators do believe, however, that suppressive therapy can be used as a primary therapy and that its effectiveness depends on the early detection and staging of thyroid tumors using EM studies, TSH receptors on thyroid cancerous cells, and radioiodine incorporation using autoradiographic studies. Thyroid suppressive therapy is widely used after subtotal or total thyroidectomy to prevent recurrent disease or spread of metastases to bone, lung, and brain. Thyroid suppression provides favorable results in almost 70% of papillary and follicular adenomas or carcinomas. Adverse effects of thyroid hormone administration occur with hyperthyroidism, arrhythmia, or angina pectoris.

Leukemias and Lymphoid Tumors

Adrenocorticosteroids were long used in the treatment of chronic lymphatic leukemia and Hodgkin's disease due to their cytolytic effects, especially when used in large or pharmacologic doses. This use was based on experimental investigations that showed dramatic remission of transplanted lymphosarcomas in mice following cortisone administration (26,51). Temporary remission of human lymphatic leukemia and Hodgkin's disease were reported early in 1950 following administration of cortisone and ACTH (51). The beneficial therapeutic effects can be explained by antilymphocytic effects of adrenocorticosteroids and the presence of glucocorticoid receptors.

These glucocorticoid receptors are intracellular receptors located in the cytoplasm of target cells. The steroid hormones are known to interact with the receptor of the soluble cytoplasm and form a complex that is later translocated to a nuclear site, thereby eliciting cellular response. Some human cell lines contain glucocorticoid receptors and consequently are hormone sensitive and responsive to corticosteroid therapy and rapidly killed by hormones; others lack these receptors and are hormone resistant. A quite fair correlation therefore exists between the presence or lack of glucocorticoid receptors and response to hormone therapy.

Most hormones used are prednisone and dexamethasone in dosages of 40 mg daily or 5 mg to 10 mg daily, respectively. Corticosteroids can be used alone or in combination with cytostatics (chlorambucil [Leukeran]) in chronic lymphatic leukemias (CLL), acute lymphocytic leukemia (ALL), malignant lymphoma, Hodgkin's disease, and multiple myelomas; the response rate varies between 60% and 70% as does improved survival rate in other types of cancers, (lung cancer) mostly due to their anti-inflammatory and supportive effects. Glucocorticoids can also increase responsiveness to chemotherapy or radiotherapy, and their association to other therapeutic agents as adjuvant therapy is justifiable (23).

POSSIBLE MECHANISMS BY WHICH HORMONES EXERT THEIR THERAPEUTIC EFFECTS

Present status of our knowledge indicates that the exact mechanism of hormones on normal, precancerous, and cancerous cells is still unclear. It is possible that hormones interfere in cell metabolism and exert their effects in several ways. Important achievement in this field was made during the last decade due to the use of autoradiographic studies and cell markers, electron microscopic studies, and tissue culture, which expanded our knowledge regarding the cytokinetic cell-line sensitivity and the effects of hormones on cancer cell populations. For example, light and electron microscopic autoradiography revealed that in most tumors there are two different cell compartments: one smaller, proliferative compartment represented by cells that proliferate at any time (so-called growth fraction) and a large compartment of dormant or silent cells, which can remain for years in this stage. Most hormones, namely steroid hormones, act on this rapidly proliferating pool.

It has also been demonstrated that most cancer cells undergo the same cell cycle as do normal cells. Cell cycle is divided into at least four distinct phases: G_1 (presynthetic phase) is quite long in normal cells (18 to 22 hours); a synthetic phase (S phase) in which DNA synthesis takes place (approximately 6 to 8 hours); G_2 (postsynthetic or premitotic phase), which is short (2 to 3 hours); and M (or mitotic) phase, which is approximately 1 hour long and divided into four phases (prophase, metaphase, anaphase, and telophase; see Chapter 2).

Compared to normal or control cells in which the G_1 phase is very long, in cancer cells this G_1 is short, only a few hours, indicating that cancer cells divide rapidly. Due to a short G_1 period, they enter the cell cycle very fast and thus rapidly divide. This is one of the most important characteristic of cell cycle in cancer cells. At present we do not understand the controlling factors of this shorter G_1 phase in the cell cycle of cancer cells; this will be an important clue for the cell biology of cancer cells as well as for developing new therapeutic or cytostatic agents. We do know that most hormones that are widely used in treating cancers interfere in the cell cycle, namely during the S phase or DNA synthesis, and they are called *cell cycle specific (CCS)* agents.

Hormones, mainly steroid hormones, are antimitotic agents that exert a specific toxicity on the rapidly dividing cancer cells only in one phase, the S phase of their cell cycle. Thus, hormones are useful therapeutic agents for all tumors with a high proliferating or growth fraction, especially leukemias and lymphomas and some genital tract tumors. Most of the other cytostatic agents act nonspecifically, regardless of whether the cells are proliferating, by making complexes with DNA. These are *cell cycle nonspecific (CCNS)* agents (most of cytostatic or alkylating agents), and they are mainly used in the treatment of solid tumors with a low growth fraction or slowly dividing cancer cells.

Another possible mechanism of hormonal intervention can be due to the interaction of hormones with the intracellular receptor sites located in the cytoplasm of cells. This complex between steroid hormone and the receptor or soluble cytosol fraction is later translocated to the nuclear acceptor site where it combines with DNA and initiates mRNA synthesis (transcription) and is then transferred to polysomes where the synthesis of new proteins takes place (translation).

The presence of hormone receptors is very important in eliciting cellular responses and consequently, to the effectiveness of hormone therapy (see Chapter 5). Lack of hormone receptors indicates a failure of therapy. Hormone antagonists (antihormones) such as tamoxifen compete with estradiol for the same cytoplasmic receptor, which it translocates to the cell nucleus, failing to stimulate a full estrogenic response. Tamoxifen is effective against most estrogen receptor-positive, dimethylbenzanthracene (DMBA)-induced mammary rat tumors, and the response is similar to that seen in human mammary tumors. Experimental data suggest that tamoxifen given continuously is more effective than ovariectomy and is a most effective clinical treatment.

These exciting achievements, which are still incompletely understood, can predict the prognosis and effectiveness of endocrine therapy. Thus, hormones and hormone antagonists may exert their therapeutic effects by using one of the following mechanisms: blocking the diffusion of hormone from plasma into the cell; blocking the binding of the hormone to its receptor and formation of hormone receptor complexes, which are translocated to the nucleus; blocking the growth response, resulting from the cell; blocking the recycling of spent receptors or synthesis de novo; and blocking the hypothalamic–hypophyseal axis (Fig. 10–4).

Hormones may also act by inhibiting or delaying the rate of transformation of preneoplastic cells towards neoplastic cells and thus delaying the tumor growth and preventing the spread of micrometastases. Previous investigations demonstrated that hormones are important controlling factors of preneoplastic cells and their transformation into cancer cells (see Chapter 3).

Hormones may act differently in cancer cells than in normal cells. Besides their cytolytic, cytotoxic, and modulating effects on cancer cells, hormones also exert anti-inflammatory and anti-edematous effects on stroma surrounding the tumor. Despite the substantial progress made in the last two decades regarding the role of hormones on normal cells, investigations into the role of hormones on cell metabolism and growth of precancerous and cancerous cells is just beginning to approach the root of the matter. A better understanding of the basic controlling mechanisms of hormones on precancerous and cancerous cells will enlighten the role of hormones in cancer treatment.

COMMENTS AND CONCLUSIONS

Hormone therapy is an important therapeutic method for cancer treatment and management. It is difficult to judge its effects in all cases due to recurrence

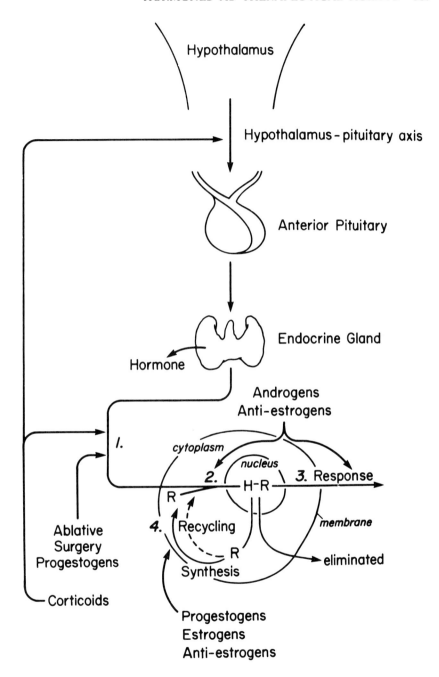

Figure 10-4 Different mechanisms by which hormones exert their therapeutic effects. I, blocking hormone in plasma before entering the cell; 2, blocking the formation of the hormone–receptor complex; 3, blocking the elicited response; 4, blocking the recycling receptors; 5, blocking the hypothalamic–pituitary axis.

of tumor. Compared to other methods such as surgery, radiotherapy, and chemotherapy, it produces equal effects, is less toxic, and can also act on metastases. Hormone therapy is a systemic therapy; others are mostly local. We should keep in mind, however, that hormones are not inoffensive agents, especially in large amounts. We do not know how hormones act on cancerous and precancerous cells, and their mechanisms can be different from those involved in normal cells.

In almost all hormone-dependent cancers, the endocrine manipulations, ablative methods, and hormones (additive methods) are the ideal therapeutic methods and should be tried before other therapies. They provide in all hormone-sensitive cancers prolongation of life and remission of tumor growth and can be tried again after recurrence. Because there are no specific ultrastructural or autoradiographic differences between cancer cells and normal cells (cancer cells are almost identical to normal cells), most therapeutic agents (cytostatics, radiation, or immunotherapy) act similarly by destroying both cell lines. The principal difficulty of cancer therapy is that we have no selective therapeutic agents for cancer cells only. Consequently, most of the side-effects and toxic systemic effects limit use and effectiveness.

From the multivalent agents tried, hormones act mainly on the cancer cells, interfering in cancer cell metabolism and producing tumor regression and extinction (in hormone-dependent cancers). Hormones are also enhancer, potentiator, or adjuvant factors when combined with cytostatics, radiation, or immunotherapy; hence, they are used mostly in combination with chemotherapy, radiotherapy, or immunotherapy. It is amazing that hormonal control of cancer can be achieved by two diametrically opposed methods: removal of the endocrine glands (ablative endocrine therapy) or administration of their hormone (additive hormone therapy), for example, castration and adrenalectomy or the administration of progestins, estrogens, or corticosteroids.

Although the endocrine therapy was used a long time ago, mostly as an empirical method, several beneficial therapeutic effects on tumor regression were reported only in recent years. At present, hormone therapy is recommended largely not to cure the cancer, but to control the cancer disease, achieving tumor remission and prolongation of life in many cancer patients (23,33,44). Even more than 50 years ago when hormone therapy was in its empirical stage, this method was judged to be superior to surgery or radiation therapy (16,17). During that time, cancer was assumed to be a systemic disease caused by dysfunction of endocrine glands, especially thyroid and adrenal secretions.

Before the modern era of hormones, several glandular extracts (opotherapy) were used to treat cancers. Naame (1921) successfully treated uterine cancer by mammohypophyseal and thyromammary extracts; breast cancer by thyro-ovarian extracts, and different types of epithelioma with thyroid and pancreatic extracts in combination (49). Cummings (16,17) also found that endocrine therapy removed most cancer symptoms and is distinctly superior to other therapeutic procedures.

Engel (1922) in detailed experimental studies showed that tumor growth in mice is under strong hormonal control. Using several glandular extracts (or optonen), such as hypophysisopton, thymusopton, ovarialopton, and thyroidopton, he found that pituitary extract slightly stimulates tumor growth, whereas thymus and thyroid extracts inhibit tumor development. Only the thymus extract exerts a constant tumor inhibitory effect. Interestingly, he assumed that the cancer treatment and cancer prevention would be possible, controlled by hormones or their components. Thus, cancer is a systemic disease, mainly due to a hormonal disequilibrium (or imbalance), and its treatment should be a systemic therapy.

Engel also stated that systemic hormone therapy is superior to local therapy (surgery, radiation) in several kinds of carcinoma (18). Thymus extract exerts the strongest inhibitory effect, whereas ovarian and testicular extracts have no effect. Ovariectomy may exert its beneficial therapeutic effects by reviviscence of thymus.

This was the era of glandular therapy or opotherapy. Because the cell growth and proliferation required several factors, among them hormones, the use of hormones to suppress or kill the cancer cells was justifiable and provided significant relief for the cancer patient. Both the lack of hormones in deprival or ablative endocrine therapy and the administration of large doses in additive hormone therapy can produce significant improvement, remission, and prolongation of life, mainly in hormone-dependent cancer, as well as palliation as an adjuvant therapy in most hormone-sensitive tumors.

Hormonotherapy is sometimes used alone in hormone-dependent cancers, in which hormones play a critical role in maintenance and cell growth or as an adjuvant therapy with chemotherapy and radiation therapy by increasing the responsiveness to cytostatics or radiation.

A critical appraisal showed that endocrine therapy produced equally beneficial therapeutic effects as surgery, chemotherapy, radiotherapy, or immunotherapy; because it is less toxic it can be recommended in recurrent cases. Hormone therapy is a systemic therapy compared with surgery and radiation therapy, which are mostly local therapies. It is also more accepted by patients because it is less desfigurating and without psychological complications. The idea of hormonotherapy emerged from studies and progress made in the last three to four decades that revealed that cancer is not always autonomous, self-perpetuating, and resulting in death; it is still a controllable disease.

Among several factors that can control the cell growth and proliferation, hormones are important because they interfere in the cell environment by changing the so called "milieu interieur" or "milieu de la vie" and thus changing the rate of cell growth and proliferation and inducing tumor remission or extinction. With advancement in cytokinetics and pharmacokinetics, most endocrine ablative therapy will be less and less used and replaced by the use of synthetic hormone antagonists (or antihormones) that can provide equal therapeutic effects.

Hormone therapy is now routinely used after surgery (mastectomy, prostatectomy, thyroidectomy, in breast, uterine, prostate, or thyroid cancers) to prevent recurrent disease and metastases (21,23,27,33,52,56,59) There are not yet conclusive studies on controlled, randomized patients in which hormone therapy alone can significantly reduce or regress the cancer growth (1,5,46,63). However, due to its lesser toxicity and aggressiveness, hormone therapy should be considered an ideal therapeutic method and used more frequently in the management and treatment of malignant diseases, especially during early stages.

REFERENCES

1. Ackland, T.: An evaluation of endocrine ablation therapy. In Stoll, B. (ed.): *Endocrine Therapy in Malignant Disease.* (Philadelphia, W. B. Saunders, 1972), pp. 401–419.
2. Armilage, J., Corder, M., Leimert, J., Dick, I., and Elliott, T.: Advanced diffuse histiocytic lymphoma treated with cyclophosphamide, doxorubicin, vincristine and prednisone (CHOP) without maintenance therapy. *Cancer Treat. Rep. 64*:649–654 (1980).
3. Ballestero, L.: El tratamiento del cancer de pulmon con esteroides. *Prensa Med. Argent. 41*:2974–2979 (1954).
4. Beatson, G.: On the treatment of inoperable cases of carcinoma of the mamma: Suggestions for a new method of treatment with illustrative cases. *Lancet 2*: 104–162 (1896).
5. Beck, J.: In search of hormonal factors as an aid in predicting the outcome of breast carcinoma. *Can. Cancer Conf. 6*:3–35 (1966).
6. Bennett, A., Houghton, J., Leaper, D., and Stamfor, I.: Tumor growth and response to treatment. Beneficial effect of the prostaglandin synthesis inhibitor flurbiprofen. *Proc. Br. Pharm. Soc.* 1978.
7. Bischoff, I., and Maxwell, G.: Hormones and cancer: Effect of glandular extirpation. *J. Biol. Chem. 92*:30 (1937).
8. Bloom, H.: Adjuvant therapy for adenocarcinoma of the kidney: Present position and prospects. *Br. J. Urol. 45*:237–257 (1973).
9. Blumenthal, F., Jacobs, E., and Rosenberg, H.: Zur behandlung der Krebs krankheit. Eine multivalente hormone therapie. *Schweiz. Med. Wchschr. 66*:6405 (1936).
10. Bondy, P.: Medical treatment of hormone dependent cancers. In Beeson, P., McDermott, W., and Wyngaarden, J. (eds.): *Cecil's Textbook of Medicine* (Philadelphia, W. B. Saunders, 1979), pp. 1918–1922.
11. Briele, H.: Endocrine treatment of advanced cancer of the breast. *Curr. Surg. 37*: 149–151 (1980).
12. Brodie, A.: Inhibition of estrogen biosynthesis: An approach to treatment of estrogen dependent cancer. In Iacobelli, S., et al. (eds.): *Hormones and Cancer* (New York, Raven Press, 1980), pp. 507–514.
13. Burrow, G.: Thyroid hormone therapy in nonthyroid disorders. In Werner, S., and Ingbar, S. (eds.): *The Thyroid.* (Hagerstown, MD., Harper & Row, 1978), pp. 974–980.

14. Caillian, R.: Histologic studies of effect of hormone therapy on animal and human subjects. *Schweiz. Med. Wchschr. 66*:642–645 (1936).
15. Chen, H., Bradley, C., and Meites, J.: Stimulation of carcinogen induced mammary tumor growth in rats by adrenalectomy. *Cancer Res. 36*:1414–1417 (1976).
16. Cummings, W.: The endocrine vs. surgery in the treatment of cancer. *Clin. Med. (Chicago) 31*:693–696 (1924).
17. Cummings, W.: The endocrine evolution and therapy of cancer. *Cancer 2*:143–147 (1925).
18. Engel, D.: Experimentelle studien uber die beeinflussung des tumor wachstum mit abbauprodukten (Abderhaldenschen Optonen) von endokrinen drüsen bei maüsen. *Z. Krebsforsch. 19*:339–380 (1922).
19. Farrow, J.: The management of metastatic breast cancer by hormone manipulation. *Bull. NY Acad. Med. 38*:151–162 (1962).
20. Farrow, J., and Adair, F.: Effect of orchidectomy on skeletal metastases from cancer of the male breast. *Science 95*:654 (1942).
21. Foulds, L.: Hormones and cancer. *Practitioner 192*:370–375 (1964).
22. Gonzalez, E.: Estrogen, progesterone receptors in ovarian cancer. *JAMA 245*:1626 (1981).
23. Greenblatt, R.: Role of hormones in the management of cancer. *NY State J. Med. 64*:383–387 (1964).
24. Gusberg, S.: Hormone dependence of endometrial carcinoma. *Obstet. Gynecol. 30*:287–293 (1967).
25. Hardy, J.: Hormones in cancer growth and treatment. *Bull. Soc. Int. Chir. 34*:210–211 (1975).
26. Heilman, F., and Kendall, E.: The influence of 11-dehydro-17-hydroxycorticosterone (compound E) on the growth of a malignant tumor in the mouse. *Endocrinology 34*:416–420 (1944).
27. Hubay, C., Pearson, O., and Marshall, J.: Adjuvant chemotherapy, antiestrogen therapy and immunotherapy for stage II, III breast cancer. *Eur. J. Cancer* (in press).
28. Huggins, C.: Two principles in endocrine therapy of cancers: Hormone deprival and hormone interference. In Sharma, R., and Criss, W. (eds.): *Endocrine Control of Neoplasia.* (New York, Raven Press, 1978), pp. 1–9.
29. Huggins, C., and Hodges, C.: Studies on prostatic cancer: I. The effect of castration, of estrogen and of androgen injections on serum phosphates in metastatic carcinoma of the prostate. *Cancer Res. 1*:293–297 (1941).
30. Huggins, C., Moon, R., and Morii, S.: Extinction of experimental mammary cancer. I. Estradiol-17β and progesterone. *Proc. Natl. Acad. Sci USA 48*:379–386 (1962).
31. Jacobs, E.: Klinische erfolge mit der multivalenten hormon therapie an 114 Kranken. *Schweiz. Med. Wchrshr. 66*:640–642 (1936).
32. de Kermion, J.: Cancer of the prostate: Hormone therapy. In Haskell, C. (ed.): *Cancer Treatment.* (Philadelphia, W. B. Saunders, 1980), pp. 363–367.
33. Kennedy, B.: Hormone therapy in cancer. *Geriatrics 25*:106–112 (1970).
34. Kim, N., and Furth, J.: Relation of mammary tumors to mammotropes. II. Hormone responsiveness of 3-methylcholanthrene induced mammary carcinomas. *Proc. Soc. Exp. Biol. Med. 103*:643–645 (1960).
35. Koeffler, H., and Golde, D.: Humoral modulation of human acute myelogenous leukemia cell growth in vitro. *Cancer Res. 40*:1858–1862 (1980).
36. Landau, R., Ehrlich, E., and Huggins, C.: Estradiol benzoate and progesterone in advanced human breast cancer. *JAMA 182*:632–636 (1962).

37. Lathrop, A., and Loeb, L.: Further investigations on the origin of tumors in mice. III. On the part played by internal secretion in the spontaneous development of tumors. *J. Cancer Res. 1*:1–19 (1916).

38. Legha, S., and Muggia, F.: Antiestrogens in the treatment of cancer. *Ann. Intern. Med. 84*:759 (1976).

39. Lipsett, M.: Estrogen use and cancer risk. *JAMA 237*:1112–1115 (1977).

40. Lipschütz, A., and Vargas, L.: Prevention of experimental uterine and extrauterine fibroids by testosterone and progesterone. *Endocrinology 28*:669–675 (1941).

41. Loeb, L.: Further observations of the endemic occurrence of carcinoma, innoculability of tumors. *Univ. Penn. M. Bull. 20*:2 (1907).

42. Matsumato, K., and Sugano, H.: Human breast cancer and hormone receptors. In Sharma, R., and Criss, W. (eds.): *Endocrine Control of Neoplasia.* (New York, Raven Press, 1978), pp. 191–208.

43. McCallister, A., Welbourn, R., Edelystyn, G., Taylor, A., Gordon, D., and Cole, J.: Factors influencing response to hypophysectomy for advanced cancer of the breast. *Br. Med. J. 1*:613 (1961).

44. Meyer, J., Rao, B., and Stevens, S.: Low incidence of estrogen receptor in breast carcinomas with rapid rates of cellular replication. *Cancer 40*:2290–2298 (1977).

45. McGuire, W.: Hormone receptors: their role in predicting prognosis and response to endocrine therapy. *Semin. Oncol. 5*:428–433 (1978).

46. Moreno, J.: Hormones do not cure cancer. *Prensa Med. Argent. 31*:973 (1944).

47. Mouridsen, H., Palshof, T., Patteron, J., and Battersby, L.: Tamoxifen in advanced breast cancer. *Cancer Treat. Rev. 5*:131–141 (1978).

48. Murlin, J., Kockakian, C., Spur, C., and Harvey, R.: Androgens and tumor growth. *Science 90*:275 (1939).

49. Naame, O.: Cancer et opotherapie (Cancer and glandular therapy). *Gaz. d. Hôp. (Paris) 1*:667–672 (1921).

50. Patterson, J. and Battersby, L.: Tamoxifen: An overview of recent studies in the field of oncology. *Cancer Treatm. Rev. 64*:775–778 (1980).

51. Pearson, O., Eliel, L., Rawson, R., Dobriner, K., and Rhoads, C.: ACTH and cortisone induced regression of lymphoid tumors in man. *Cancer 2*:943–945 (1949).

52. Reymond, C.: Hormonotherapie des tumeurs. *Rev. Med. Suisse Rom. 82*:303–316 (1962).

53. Scully, R.: Ovarian tumors. A review. *Am. J. Pathol. 87*:685–720 (1977).

54. Selye, H.: Catotoxic steroids. *Can. Med. Assoc. J. 101*:51 (1969).

55. Segaloff, A.: Hormonal therapy in cancer of breast: Effect of methylandrostendiol on clinical course and hormonal excretion. *Cancer 5*:271–274 (1952).

56. Segaloff, A.: Alterations in hormone balance as cancer therapy. *Proc. Natl. Cancer Conf. 4*:195–198 (1960).

57. Stoll, B.: The basis of endocrine therapy. In Stoll, B. (ed.): *Endocrine Therapy in Malignant Disease.* (Philadelphia, W. B. Saunders, 1972), pp. 111–137.

58. Underwood, P., Miller, C., Kreutner, A., Joyner, C., and Lutz, M.: Endometrial carcinoma: The effect of estrogens. *Gynecol. Oncol. 8*:60–73 (1979).

59. Voigt, W., and Castro, A.: Androgen and androgen receptors in prostatic cancer. In Sharma, R., and Criss, W. (eds.): *Endocrine Control of Neoplasia.* (New York, Raven Press, 1978), pp. 291–301.

60. Wagner, R., Schulze, K., and Jungblut, P.: Estrogen and androgen receptor in human prostate and prostatic tumor tissue. *Acta Endocrinol (suppl.) 193*:52 (1975).

61. Wells, S., Santen, R., Lipton, A., Haagensen, D., Ruby, E., Harvey, H., and Dilley, W.: Medical adrenalectomy and aminoglutethimide: Clincial studies in postmenopause patients with metastatic breast carcinomas. *Ann. Surg. 187*:475–484 (1978).
62. Westerberg, H.: Tamoxifen and fluoxymesterone in advanced breast cancer: A controlled clinical trial. *Cancer Treatm. Rep. 64*:117–121 (1980).
63. Wynder, E., and Schneiderman, M.: Exogenous hormones: Boon or culprit? *J. Natl. Cancer Inst. 53*:729–731 (1973).
64. Young, P., Ehrlich, C., and Einhorn, L.: Relationship between steroid receptors and response to endocrine therapy and cytotoxic chemotherapy in metastatic breast cancer. *Cancer 46*:2961–2963 (1980).
65. Zava, D., and McGuire, W.: Estrogens receptors in androgen induced breast tumor regression. *Cancer Res. 37*:1608–1610 (1977).
66. Ziel, H., and Finkle, W.: Increased risk of endometrial carcinoma among users of conjugated estrogens. *N. Engl. J. Med. 293*:1167–1170 (1975).

INDEX

Note: Italicized numbers indicate figures; page numbers followed by *t* indicate tables.

ABOUT THE AUTHOR

Aurel Lupulescu, *MD* (Federal License in Medicine & Surgery), *MS* (Endocrinology), *PhD* (Biology), is an Associate Professor at Wayne State University School of Medicine, Detroit, Michigan. He has published over 200 scientific papers, 4 textbook chapters, and 5 monographs in the United States and elsewhere. He is also an active member in 12 scientific and medical societies.

He has worked for almost 30 years in Endocrinology and Tumor Cell Biology, studying the effects of various hormones on cancer development and regression. He has studied the mechanism of action of hormones at cellular and macromolecular levels (DNA, RNA and protein synthesis), extending our knowledge of hormones and cancer cell biology.